Crossroads in Psychiatry: A History of The McLean Hospital

Crossroads in Psychiatry: A History of The McLean Hospital

By

S. B. Sutton

American Psychiatric Press, Inc.
1400 K Street, N.W.
Washington, DC 20005

Manufactured in the United States

Library of Congress Cataloging-in-Publication Data

Sutton, S. B. (Silvia B.)
Crossroads in psychiatry.

Bibliography: p.
Includes index.
1. McLean Hospital—History. 2. Psychiatric hospital care—Massachusetts—History. 3. Psychiatry—History. I. Title. [DNLM: 1. McLean Hospital. 2. Hospitals, Psychiatric—history—Massachusetts. WM 28 AM4 S9c]
RC445.M4B447 1986 362.2′1′097444 86-14159
ISBN 0-88048-253-2

Contents

Foreword

This chronicle of McLean Hospital satisfies a need as well as a personal ambition.

Although the "Asylum" which became the McLean Hospital was founded as part of the Massachusetts General Hospital 175 years ago, no comprehensive history has been written. This book fills the gap. It documents the leading role which McLean played in certain periods of American psychiatry and in advancing scientific knowledge about mental illness. It does not, however, shy away from describing and explaining its less glorious days. As such, it fulfills a historical mission, not only with regard to McLean, but also in helping us understand the ups and downs of any institution over time and the factors—financial, professional, leadership, interpersonal, social, and political—which, in varying degrees, determine the destiny of organizations. It does so in the context of events that took place in the world at large as McLean evolved, and with an eye toward developments in medicine and psychiatry.

Many of us on the McLean staff enjoy a sense of shared adventure in its long history, as well as pride in our connection with the Massachusetts General Hospital and Harvard University, institutions whose own histories belong to the fabric of the country. My own association with the Massachusetts General Hospital and

McLean began in 1952 as a psychiatrist in training. For half of my life, and all of my professional life, I have been connected with these institutions. It has been a source of particular personal satisfaction to have been entrusted for a quarter of a century with responsibility for managing McLean. During these years while, with others, I was "making" McLean history, I was also promising myself that someday I would write it. There is a spirit about the place which I very much wanted to capture in writing—a spirit that has for generations attracted committed, talented staff and employees who have made possible some extraordinary contributions to the theory and practice of psychiatry. It is a difficult-to-define spirit. Central to it though is that McLean is a caring environment for both patients and staff. Its decentralized organization permits individuals to exercise their maximum potential.

McLean has traditionally operated with the belief that most people try their best, and therefore it gives them "room to perform" and is understanding of shortcomings and mistakes. McLean believes that the conditions of human existence can be improved, that what a person does makes a difference, and that individuals can have a powerful impact on each other and on the hospital's role. Though the very nature of psychiatry means we who work in institutions like McLean must be able to tolerate ambiguities and uncertainties, there is a deep commitment to doing the best we can with the knowledge we have today and a belief that tomorrow may bring McLean's and psychiatry's greatest glories.

Despite such personal affection for McLean, I have come to realize that I will probably never write the history of McLean, although I have not quite given up the dream of writing my personal memoirs of these important years.

The book ends in December of 1984 for several reasons. We wanted to have it ready for publishing in 1986, the hospital's 175th anniversary year. Also, after serving as McLean's psychiatrist in chief for 12 years, Dr. Shervert Frazier resigned in 1984 to become the director of the National Institute of Mental Health. That year, therefore, marked the natural end of an era and seemed a legitimate cutoff.

More importantly, as 1985 dawned, McLean was in the midst

of major events and decisions which would need more time to place into perspective. The sale of McLean to Hospital Corporation of America had been turned down, but discussions were continuing about the possibility of a leasing arrangement. Meanwhile, two other for-profit hospital companies were interested in exploring an affiliation with McLean: American Medical International and Psychiatric Institutes of America. McLean's purpose in these discussions was to find the capital needed to renovate McLean's antiquated physical plant and ensure the support of treatment and research in the years ahead. Other developments were in process. A McLean-Harvard Medical School search committee had been appointed to select a new psychiatrist in chief. Also, an expansion of McLean's Board of Trustees was planned to include individuals with a primary interest in McLean in addition to the trustees of the Massachusetts General Hospital.

By the spring of 1986, many decisions had been taken. The Board of Trustees had been broadened. The renovation and construction program was under way as a result of the $30 million worth of bonds sold through the Health and Education Facilities Authority (HEFA) in December of 1985. Last but not least, on February 27, 1986, McLean and American Medical International, Inc., the investor-owned hospital company, entered into an agreement to create a joint venture which would deliver various mental health services off the McLean campus. McLean's integrity as a nonprofit hospital, affiliated with Massachusetts General Hospital and Harvard Medical School, remains intact.

These events and decisions will clearly affect the history of McLean for years to come. They involve many stories and issues that only time can properly sort out. Their telling best rests with some future chronicler who will be able to place them into historical perspective.

Francis de Marneffe, M.D.
General Director,
The McLean Hospital

Acknowledgments

I am grateful to the following individuals for having taken time from their schedules to share their memories of McLean with me: Mr. Alexander Armour, Mr. Francis H. Burr, Mr. David C. Crockett, Ms. Golda Edinburg, Dr. Shervert H. Frazier, Dr. Paul M. Howard, Dr. Merton Kahne, Mr. John E. Lawrence, Ms. Mildred Makin, Dr. Francis de Marneffe, Mr. Frank Norton, Dr. Alfred Pope, Mr. George Putnam, Dr. Benson Snyder, Dr. Irene Pierce Stiver, Dr. Arlene Frank Vagi, Mr. George Zager, and a patient whose name must remain confidential. Their insights and observations supplemented the documentary evidence while aiding my understanding of several categories of technicalities, ranging from scientific matters to insurance coverage. I note with regret Mr. Armour's death in September 1985. He served as hospital steward for many years and, after his retirement, took great interest in McLean's history, wrote an informal account of its early years, and put together a talk illustrated by slides.

A number of people read and commented helpfully on all or parts of the manuscript: Dr. Thomas Bond, Mr. Terry Bragg, Dr. de Marneffe, Dr. Pope, and Mrs. Evelyn Stone. I especially appreciated Dr. Bond's assistance and Mrs. Stone's warm encouragement and practiced editorial instincts.

The administrative and secretarial staff in the general director's office and in the offices for Research Administration and Resources at McLean helped make it possible for this manuscript to be written and revised in a relatively short time. However, I could never have managed without the moral and practical support of Terry Bragg, registrar and archivist, and his colleagues, Lynne Wighton and Bernice Bindman. Mr. Bragg answered my endless requests with unfailing good humor and imagination, while volunteering sources I might never have found by myself. His familiarity with the resources at Clark University proved particularly helpful. I should like to acknowledge as well the cooperation of the Clark University Archives (G. Stanley Hall collection), the Houghton Library of Harvard University, and The Johns Hopkins Medical Institutions (Alan Mason Chesney Medical Archives).

Martin Bander and Doris Schreckengaust of the Massachusetts General Hospital kindly arranged access to nineteenth-century records of the Massachusetts General Hospital-McLean trustees. I am also grateful to Dr. John A. Popplestone, director of the Archives of the History of American Psychology, University of Akron, for his assistance in identifying the equipment pictured in the photograph of the McLean psychology laboratory.

Finally, I wish to thank Dr. de Marneffe for trusting me to fashion what was originally a vague assignment according to my own design and for his generous deployment of support services.

Readers will note that the last few chapters, which discuss McLean's modern history, name only a few individuals. Since 1955 the staff has grown so large that for every name I might have mentioned I would have slighted a dozen equally meritorious people by omission. Since the object of this book is to illuminate the concepts that guided McLean's evolution, and the specific shapes those concepts took, it seemed prudent to concentrate on programs rather than on individuals. Nevertheless, I recognize that an institution is not a collection of buildings, but the people who work in it and the traditions that govern it.

S. B. Sutton

PART I

The Asylum

CHAPTER

1

A Peculiar Claim

Item: "Mad is . . . not a complex idea, as has been supposed, but a complex term for all the forms and varieties of this disease. Our language has been enriched with other terms expressive of this affection, all of which have a precise meaning. Delirium, which we have borrowed from the Latin, merely means, *out of the track,* de lira, so that a delirious person, one who starts out of the track regularly pursued, becomes compared to the same deviation in the process of ploughing. *Crazy,* we have borrowed from the French *ecrasé,* crushed, broken; we still use the same meaning, and say that such a person is crack'd. Insane, deranged, or disarranged, melancholic, out of one's wits, lunatic, phrenetic, or as we have corrupted it, frantic, require no explanation. *Beside one's self* most probably originated from the belief of possession by a devil, or evil spirit."

(From *Observations on Madness and Melancholy,* 1809, by John Haslam, apothecary at Bethlehem Hospital in London.)

Item: "DR. ROBERTSON'S VEGETABLE NERVOUS CORDIAL *OR* NATURE'S GRAND RESTORATIVE is confidently recommended, as the most efficacious medicine, for the speedy relief and cure of all nervous complaints, impurities of the blood, seminal weakness, and various complaints, resulting from dissipated pleasures, residence in warm climates, the immoderate use of tea, the unskillful and excessive use of mercury, and diseases peculiar to females at a certain period of life.

"Under the denomination of nervous disorders in its full extent, are included several diseases of the most dangerous kind, and are so various that a volume would hardly suffice to complete a description of them. It pervades with its baleful influence the whole nervous system, writhing the heart with inexpressible anguish and exciting the most dreadful suggestions of horror and despair. To this demon have thousands fallen a sacrifice, in the direful transports of its rage.

"The most common symptoms at its commencement are weakness, flatulence, palpitations, watchfulness, drowsiness after eating, timidity, flashes of heat and cold, numbness, cramp, giddiness, pains in the head, back and loins, hiccup, difficulty of respiration, deglutition, anxiety, dry cough, etc.

"Since Dr. Robertson's first discovery of this invaluable medicine, upwards of two hundred thousand persons have experienced its happy and salutary effects, many of whom had been reduced to the last stage, and had given up all hopes of recovering.

Price: One dollar and fifty cents."

(Advertisement in the *Boston Patriot*, May 20, 1809.)

Item: "I was called in October last, to visit Mr. ________ , who had a large family; his wife had been recently and dangerously sick. He had long been known by his employers and neighbours, as a man of industry, punctuality, and the most regular habits. He had been able to support his family in a very decent and comfortable manner. When I saw him, he had been taken suddenly insane, and was raving violently. He made a determined resistance to all attempts at confining him, became outrageous, and repeatedly escaped, not without danger to his family and others. The situation of his wife rendered it impossible that he should be kept at home, and as there were no means of defraying his board in an expensive situation he was carried to the Boston Almshouse. There he was lodged in a small, dark and uncomfortable cell, without fresh air, and hardly long enough to allow him to lie down. In this situation he refused food, and was found every morning sitting naked on the straw of his crib, having divested himself of clothes during the night. He became rapidly emaciated and his strength sunk so far, that it was found necessary to remove him to the sick room, to save his life. By the humane attentions of the physician of the house, he recovered strength enough to be taken out and carried to the house of a relative, but his family having no means to support him or themselves their situation became very wretched."

(From a letter from a physician, unsigned, to the Board of Trustees of the hospital, March 21, 1816.)

There is no gentle introduction to the subject of mental illness and the treatment of the mentally ill in the early nineteenth century. It was an era of muddled notions and desperate therapies. The foregoing extracts appeared in the decade before the Asylum in Charlestown opened its doors; they reveal the language, the popular wisdom, and the experiences of the period. There had been no witches burned in Massachusetts since 1693. Explanations of mental afflictions had slowly shifted from the nether regions of superstition to the domain of medicine, and by the beginning of the nineteenth century educated people had learned to understand insanity as a condition of disease. No self-respecting, enlightened Bostonian would admit publicly to suspicions of satanic intervention. Yet such was the baffling and awful nature of the condition that discredited theories lurked in the recesses of individual imaginations: The asylum's first patient would be a young man whose father, believing him to be possessed by a devil, had subjected him to regular floggings.

However, the more usual practice when faced with an exhibition of strange and irrational behavior was to consult a physician. (For the moment I shall beg the issue of defining "strange" and "irrational" and ask the reader to share with me the understanding that "insanity," as used in the nineteenth century, applied to severe, usually psychotic manifestations of mental illness.) Unfortunately, doctors knew almost nothing about mental illness. Insofar as they paid attention to it, they generated bewildering lists of probable causes. Dr. Robertson's flimflammery implicated tropical climates (viewed in the temperate zones as unhealthful, feverish places in general), tea, menopause, and various excesses including, by suggestion, masturbation, which in that century had a nasty reputation as a ravager of healthful minds. A more respectable authority, Dr. Benjamin Rush of the Pennsylvania Hospital, preeminent physician in post-revolutionary America and author of the first American treatise on insanity, opined confidently, "The cause of madness is seated primarily in the blood vessels of the brain and . . . it depends upon the same kind of morbid and irregular actions that constitute other arterial diseases. They are a part of the unity of disease, particularly of fever of which madness is a chronic form . . . affecting that part of the brain which is the seat of the mind." In Rush's formulation, "unrestrained appetite" caused the blood vessels to become overloaded (1). His volume, *Medical Inquiries and Observations upon the Diseases of the Mind*, went through five editions between 1812 and 1835.

Dr. Haslam's experiences as apothecary at London's Bethlehem Hospital—the notorious "Bedlam"—led him to distinguish between "physical" and "moral" causes. The first category included blows to the head, intoxication, fever, and hereditary disposition. Haslam defined moral causes as "the frequent and uncurbed indulgence of any passion or emotion, and any sudden or violent affection of the mind," further warning that "of the causes termed moral, the greatest number may, perhaps, be traced to the errors of education, which often plant in the youthful mind those seeds of madness which the slightest circumstances readily awaken into growth (2). In 1800, Dr. Philippe Pinel, physician at the hospitals at Bicêtre and Salpêtrière in Paris, itemized as "exciting causes" of insanity "very vivid affections of the mind, such as ungovernable or disappointed ambition, religious fanaticism, profound chagrin, and unfortunate love. . . . It is well known that certain professions conduce more than others to insanity, which are chiefly those in which the imagination is unceasingly or ardently engaged. . . ." Pinel remarked upon disproportionate numbers of priests, monks, "country people, terrified to this condition by the anticipation of hell torments," artists, painters, sculptors, musicians, poets, advocates, and attorneys in the registers of Bicêtre. "But," he continued, "there are no instances of persons whose professions require the habitual exercise of the judging faculty; not one naturalist, nor a physician, nor a chemist, and, for the best reason in the world, not one geometrician" (3).

The contemporary reader, ensconced in a post-Freudian armchair and dimly aware of neurotransmitters, may conclude that early nineteenth-century medical theory did not represent much of an improvement over the demonology it aimed to dispel. The fact is that medicine as a whole in 1800 was a primitive science, and the study of mental disease was one of its remote provinces. Thus, Rush, Pinel, Haslam, and a few other physicians who had observed and treated the mentally ill qualified as authorities on the subject of insanity. Although they cannot be said in the long run to have substantially advanced the knowledge of causes or cure of the disease, their work represented the beginning of systematic observation. More importantly, Pinel and Samuel Tuke in particular challenged the conventional view that insanity was incurable and prescribed a mode of treatment which was, as we shall see, quite different from the practices of the times.

As the anonymous doctor's description of the plight of Mr. _____ reveals, people who became mentally ill in early nineteenth-century Boston faced an unhappy fate. There were really only three options. The most expensive, though not necessarily the most humane, was the private "madhouse," usually a boarding arrangement for the mentally ill, though some madhouses claimed to produce cures. In his book *The Mentally Ill in America*, historian Albert Deutsch cited the example of:

> Dr Willard, who, about the beginning of the 19th century, maintained a private establishment for the mentally ill in a little town on the line between Massachusetts and Rhode Island. One of the fundamental tenets in his therapy was to break the patient's will by any means possible. On his premises stood a tank of water, into which a patient, packed into a coffin-like box pierced with holes, was lowered by means of a well-sweep. He was kept under water until the bubbles of air ceased to rise, after which he was taken out, rubbed, and revived—if he had not already passed beyond reviving! (4)

Madhouse entrepreneurs did not have to account to anyone. No inspectors visited the premises or interviewed the boarders; no laws or conventions governed "therapeutic" practices. If family members objected to the conditions, they could only withdraw the boarder; if the family or guardian failed to meet payments, the madhouse ejected the patient. There were instances of physicians or clergymen who accepted mentally ill individuals in their homes and cared for them compassionately within the family. They were, however, exceptions to an ugly rule, and usually very costly. Humane circumstances were too rare to offset the terrible reputation of madhouses. As one man remarked in 1818, "Tender hearted people would not suffer their relations, diseased in mind, to be led to a private Madhouse, and therefore kept them at home, which distressed whole families and probably disturbed whole neighborhoods. This method of keeping the insane was expensive, troublesome and agonizing in the extreme, and after a short time the chances of recovery were nothing" (5).

Thus, the tender hearted, the miserly, or those with limited budgets tried to keep the mentally ill at home. An unruly individual might be locked in an attic or an outhouse, tied in a chair or bed, or overseen by a full-time custodian. Since there was presumed to be no cure for insanity, this way of caring for an afflicted person was morally and socially acceptable. Meanwhile, families hoped the patient would get better. It was known that from time to time people recovered from insanity just as mysteriously as they had fallen into it. These spontaneous cures were interpreted as triumphs of nature over disease. People with ailing friends or relatives tried to stimulate the healing faculties of nature with prayer; judging from the patent medicine advertisements, they also inflicted quantities of foul tasting, sometimes noxious, concoctions upon their unfortunate kinfolk. People who adhered to older concepts of insanity, such as the father of the asylum's first patient, applied more drastic therapeutic regimens.

Sometimes, as in the case of Mr. ——, the family could neither manage the patient at home nor afford a private madhouse. Sometimes the patient escaped and wandered into a strange town. Sometimes an itinerant person, such as a seaman, of whom there were many passing through Boston, fell ill during a voyage or in port. At this point responsibility for care rested with the community where the mentally ill resided or, in the case of a stranger, with the Commonwealth. Legislation to this effect had been on the Massachusetts books since 1676. That statute, the first in the Commonwealth to single out the insane, stated:

> Whereas, there are distracted persons in some tounes, that are unruly, whereby not only the familyes wherein they are, but others suffer much damage by them, it is ordered by this Court and the authoritye thereof, that the selectmen in all tounes where such persons are are hereby impowred & injoyned to take care of all such persons, that they doe not damnify others.

This law was produced by fear rather than compassion. A century later people had stopped worrying so hard about damnation, but they still feared the mentally ill. In short, an insane person who was not locked up somewhere and who could not be controlled by family or friends became a social problem. Small towns often paid for the expense of boarding such a deranged individual with a local family. But in Boston, since 1662, the customary solution to the social problem of insanity had been the almshouse.

Deutsch, writing of the original Boston Almshouse, said:

> As was the custom . . . indigents and petty offenders were herded indiscriminately into this poorhouse—the sick and well, the able-bodied and

> impotent, the law-breaking and law-abiding, young and aged, "worthy" poor and vagrants, sane and insane. (6)

In 1716 Boston built a separate bridewell so as to segregate the lawbreakers and "unworthy" poor from the "worthy." In theory, at least, the insane belonged among the worthy on the assumption that they could not control their behavior. But given the crude standards of assessment in the era, the worthy and unworthy, and the sane and insane frequently got misassigned.

The almshouse in which Dr. X deposited the hapless Mr. _____ in 1815 was a reasonably new structure on Leverett Street, not far from the future site of the Massachusetts General Hospital, having supplanted in 1801 the crowded old almshouse on Park Street. The prolific Charles Bulfinch, architect of so many distinguished buildings of the period that a whole chapter of Boston's developmental history belongs to him, had designed the new almshouse. We may assume that it was a handsome, solid building, a state-of-the-art facility. It contained at least one significant innovation: A small infirmary and some cells for the insane were distinct from, but attached to, the main almshouse. This arrangement was designed principally to protect the healthy inmates from physical infection as well as from the ravings and antics of the insane. The city employed a physician to tend the ill, both physical and mental.

One notes that only eight cells had been provided to house the insane in the new almshouse. The figure suggests that Boston did not consider insanity to constitute a civic problem of serious magnitude. The population of the city stood at around 25,000 in 1800. Since the census data for the time did not include statistics about persons believed to be insane, it is hard to estimate how many deranged individuals were stashed away in attics or in private madhouses. But the number of mentally ill persons roaming the streets and terrorizing the populace appears to have been quite small. This perception of insanity as a relatively trivial social problem, coupled with the belief that the disease was incurable, prevented Bostonians from acting upon three eighteenth-century proposals to provide separate public accommodations for distracted persons. In this respect, Boston lagged behind Philadelphia, where the Pennsylvania Hospital started admitting mental patients for treatment in the 1750s; New York Hospital, which received them in 1792; and Williamsburg, Virginia, which had the first public hospital exclusively for the mentally ill in America in 1773. Meanwhile, except for a quarantine station on Boston Harbor islands, Massachusetts had no hospital whatsoever. Bulfinch's almshouse, with its timid segregation of diseased and healthy, represented Boston's tentative step toward more progressive attitudes about mental illness. But it was still, after all, the almshouse. For all its modernity, the building had been in service less than a decade when its attending chaplain, the Reverend John Bartlett, rebelled against the conditions. "Much of my time was devoted to the sick," he explained later,

> but the portion of the diseased which most interested me was the insane. There were generally from 10 to 20 in the house, and although the care was taken of them, which the circumstances of the house would afford, yet there was no proper place for their confinement and rest; a 20-foot building, with several cells opening into a long entry, in each of which cells was a board cabin or berth, with loose straw, a pail for necessary purposes, was their only accommodation. The violent were confined in strait jackets, and the filth and wretchedness of the place were dreadful. At that time there were no places of refuge for the insane in Massachusetts except a few private houses in the country, owned and managed by Doctors, such as Willard's of Uxbridge, etc., etc., [This would be Willard of the water cure.] The mode of managing the insane then was most cruel, and unfavorable to recovery. . . . The physicians at the Almshouse were humane, good men, but the subject of insanity they did not appear to understand; or rather, no facilities were afforded them for the employment of those moral remedies which Pinel and others had so successfully applied in France. This wretchedness of this class of patients and their miserable condition in the Almshouse moved my feelings exceedingly. I gave my mind intensely to the study of the causes and remedies of mania in its various kinds. I went to Philadelphia, N. York, examined the hospitals there, read Pinel and all the accounts I could procure of the Asylums in France, and England. I became deeply convinced of the importance of a similar Asylum in Massachusetts. What prompted me to action was, several persons of respectability seized suddenly deranged, and brought to the Almshouse were put in these cells. . . .
>
> I sat down to my desk and wrote from 15 to 25 billets addressed to some of the wealthiest and most respectable gentlemen of Boston, requesting them to meet at Conant Hall on the Monday evening following, to take into consideration the importance of adopting some measures for the establishment of a Hospital for the Insane. . . . (7)

The reverend's letter animated the consciences of privileged

Bostonians and opened the way to the establishment not only of the Asylum in Charlestown but also of the Massachusetts General Hospital (MGH) in Boston.

Bartlett aimed his appeals with precision, and they found their marks. His wealthy and respectable gentlemen were, for the most part, merchants or members of merchant families that had made their fortunes in the triangular traffic of the early eighteenth century, in fishing, the fur trade, and, more recently and lucratively, in the China trade which they opened up after the Revolution. Those not directly engaged in shipping nonetheless depended indirectly upon its success for their prosperity as did, indeed, the commercial vitality of the city.

Boston's merchant princes have been portrayed for us in the pages of history books as stern caricatures: ambitious, ruthless, pious, tight-fisted, shrewd, flinty-eyed moralizers. We discover with some surprise that these same cartoon figures were capable of both generosity and a highly refined sense of community responsibility. Social chronicler and wit Cleveland Amory estimated that "at their peak production Boston's First Family merchants were founding not only their Families but also an average of one benevolent institution per year. In the thirty years from 1810 to 1840, for example, exactly thirty such institutions were established" (8). The lists of founders might not have been identical, but the same names kept cropping up, as they still do today on boards of trustees of such venerable institutions as the Boston Symphony, the Athenaeum, the MGH and McLean Hospital, the Massachusetts Historical Society, and of course Harvard University. Colonel Thomas Handasyd Perkins—the "acknowledged king of the merchant princes" according to Amory—was on Bartlett's list. So too were two First Family physicians, Drs. James Jackson and John Collins Warren, who picked up Bartlett's ball and carried it forward with gusto. They, along with Dr. John Gorham, raised the notion of expanding the project and establishing a hospital for both mentally and physically ill. The wealthy and respectable gentlemen adopted this proposal over the objections of a few who feared the double-barreled plan might be too ambitious.

In August 1810, Jackson and Warren drafted the letter that became the cornerstone of the Massachusetts General Hospital and today's McLean Hospital, a document so persuasive that it caused N. I. Bowditch, the first MGH chronicler, to overlook Bartlett's role entirely. The letter, a latter-day model of fund raising, circulated in an enlarged circle of prosperous and influential citizens. It read, in part:

> Sir,—It has appeared very desirable to a number of respectable gentlemen, that a hospital for the reception of lunatics and other sick persons should be established in this town. . . .
>
> It is unnecessary to urge the propriety and even obligation of succoring the poor in sickness. The wealthy inhabitants of the town of Boston always evinced that they consider themselves as "treasurers of God's bounty;" and in Christian countries, in countries where Christianity is practised, it must always be considered the first of duties to visit and to heal the sick. When in distress, every man becomes our neighbour, not only if he be of the household of faith but even though his misfortunes have been induced by transgressing the rules both of reason and religion. It is unnecessary to urge the truth and importance of these sentiments to those who are already in the habit of cherishing them, — to those who indulge in the true luxury of wealth, the pleasures of charity.

Jackson and Warren proceeded from this elevated moral plateau to an itemization of the physically ill people whom the hospital would serve: the poor lodged in garrets and attics, deprived of wholesome food, medicines, and "that first requisite in sickness, a kind and skilful nurse"; the industrious forced out of work by protracted illness; widows; children; journeymen in boarding houses; and servants. In essence, they named the outright poor and people precariously balanced on the economic margins of life.

Turning to the second category of affliction, Jackson and Warren wrote:

> There is one class of sufferers who peculiarly claim all that benevolence can bestow, and for whom a hospital is most especially required. The virtuous and industrious are liable to become objects of public charity, in consequence of diseases of the mind. When those who are unfortunate in this respect are left without proper care, a calamity, which might have been transient, is prolonged through life. The number of such persons, who are rendered unable to provide for themselves, is probably greater than the public imagine; and, of these, a large portion claim the assistance of the affluent. The expense which is attached to the care of the insane in private families is extremely great, and such as to ruin a whole family that is possessed of a competence under ordinary circumstances, when called upon to support one of its members in this situation. Even those who can pay the necessary expenses would perhaps find an institu-

> tion, such as is proposed, the best situation in which they could place their unfortunate friends. It is worthy of the opulent men of this town, and consistent with their general character, to provide an asylum for the insane from every part of the Commonwealth.

Further along—it was a *very* long letter—Jackson and Warren anticipated arguments that the almshouse was supposed to meet these needs: "That it *does not,* is very certain . . . it has become, in some measure, disreputable to live in it; and, not infrequently, those who are the most deserving objects of charity cannot be induced to enter it. To some of them death appears less terrible than residence in the Almshouse." Finally, the authors observed that "a hospital is an institution absolutely essential to a medical school. . . ." Though there was a medical school, the Harvard Medical School, founded in 1783, medical education in New England was, in Jackson's and Warren's words, "very limited" and by later standards a joke. The almshouse did duty as a teaching hospital. The few serious students of medicine who could afford the expense traveled to Europe, as had both authors of the letter, or to Philadelphia for clinical education. Jackson and Warren grasped the potential benefits to the profession and practice of medicine of opening a hospital to students. The dream did even more to propel their efforts than charitable intentions.

The Jackson-Warren letter contains some curious details when reviewed in the light of subsequent events. The facility of their proposal was a single institution; the first sentence, "a hospital for the reception of lunatics and other sick persons," leaves no doubt on that score. They appear to have followed the model of the Pennsylvania Hospital where, after 1796, mental patients occupied a separate wing constructed especially for them. The New York Hospital, which had recently erected a completely detached asylum on hospital grounds, also offered itself as an example. There is no evidence that Jackson and Warren knew anything about Williamsburg; none of the people involved in the hospital proposal either mentioned or visited it. The record does not reveal how or why the concept arose of an asylum geographically removed from the general hospital, but it took hold some time in 1815. This solution was surely more costly than a single facility.

Jackson and Warren never spelled out a treatment regimen for the mentally ill. However, they did express a belief in the curability of insanity when they wrote that "when those who are unfortunate in this respect are left without proper care, a calamity, which might have been transient, is prolonged through life." Moreover, they suggested that prosperous citizens might prefer placing "their unfortunate friends, diseased in mind" in the proposed institution rather than in a private madhouse. By contrast, they did not imagine that the wealthy would wish to send their physically ill friends to the general hospital. This prediction, if that is what it was, proved accurate. By midcentury the asylum treated many well-heeled patients, whereas it was only after World War I that the Massachusetts General Hospital attracted wealthy patients in significant numbers.

Insofar as it implied assumptions about the relative merits of different branches of medicine, the speculation about the social classes of patients likely to use the resources reveals a rather oddly placed confidence in the ability of physicians to treat the mentally ill successfully. This optimism ran counter to the conventional wisdom, indicating that Jackson and Warren were informed about a new approach to mental illness, which went by the name of "moral treatment," and that this enlightened therapy belonged to their program from the outset. Bartlett had studied Pinel. Presumably it was the reverend who alerted Jackson and Warren to the Frenchman's novel theories (9).

Unfortunately, Jackson's and Warren's eloquent circular letter failed to accomplish the most critical business of raising building funds. This was simply a matter of bad historical luck. The New England states and the port of Boston were still reeling from the economic effects of the Jefferson trade embargo, which had prohibited trade with any foreign nation between December 1807 and March 1809. The naval and diplomatic problems entangling the Americans with Britain and Napoleonic France, which had led to the embargo, remained unresolved in 1810. Boston was obsessed with politics, and the local newspapers devoted their pages almost exclusively to threats of a new embargo. In November, President James Madison's administration gained congressional approval to prohibit trade with Britain; like the earlier measure, the new embargo was carried by Southern and Western states over the objections of New England politicians. Friction between the United States and Britain increased, inflamed by Napoleon's mischief behind the scenes. The British blockaded U.S. ports in early June 1812, paralyzing New England shipping. Later that month, the United States and Great Britain went to war. One contemporary witness painted this dismal scene of the port: "Some 250 ships stood stripped and rotting at the Boston wharves, their naked masts and spars outlined against the harbor like so many winter trees" (10).

Such an atmosphere was decidedly hostile to the raising of large sums, particularly from "wealthy and respectable gentlemen" whose wealth was tied up in shipping. Boston's merchant princes had not, for the most part, lost their shirts during the embargoes, but they had suffered reversals and they feared a war. They drew their purse strings tight, hoarded their capital, and did not indulge themselves in the luxury of charitable gestures. This tight money situation persisted to the end of the war of 1812.

Nevertheless, the Jackson-Warren appeal generated sufficient enthusiasm—and, one supposes, sufficient pledges of donation when the ships came in—to permit the founders to obtain a charter from the Massachusetts legislature, form a corporation, elect trustees, design a system of governance, receive a grant from the Commonwealth (contingent on additional private contributions amounting to at least $100,000), and iron out all sorts of bylaws and organizational matters. Former President John Adams moderated the first meeting of the corporation on April 23, 1811, a historical footnote that gives some idea of the caliber of the men backing the enterprise. The original Act of Incorporation named 55 gentlemen as members, including the former president, a future president (John Quincy Adams), a future vice-president (Elbridge Gerry), a future Supreme Court Justice (Joseph Story), a Harvard president (John T. Kirkland), and so on. One remarks, too, upon the serious and time-consuming duties of the 12 trustees who committed themselves to overseeing management of the institution and were responsible to the governor of the Commonwealth and the corporation by an annual election. Deep respect for the concept of "trust," the participation of founding family members on many boards, and the energetic exercise of the office of trustee remain traditions in the late twentieth century and endow old Boston institutions with certain idiosyncrasies, among them the self-confidence of impeccable pedigree.

A second appeal for building funds for the hospital was circulated in 1814, before the war had ended, and once again failed in its objective. By the end of 1816, however, when commercial health had been restored to the region, hospital committees collected almost $79,000 in subscriptions in a mere three days! Although most of the money came from wealthy individuals, a great many people contributed to the fund through church benevolent societies. When asked whether they wanted their dollars to build a general hospital, an insane asylum, or both, donors from the poorer areas were more anxious for an asylum than the wealthier sponsors (11). Accordingly, contributions specifically earmarked for the asylum amounted to less than half of those for the general hospital.

At this point, the name of Dr. George Parkman began to figure somewhat curiously in affairs surrounding the asylum. He was precisely the same George Parkman, physician and member of a prominent family, who acquired notoriety as a dismembered corpse unearthed beneath the floor of a medical school professor of another respected family, John White Webster, in 1849. The murder was the greatest scandal ever to hit Boston society. (Webster protested his innocence throughout the trial. Many distinguished Bostonians believed him, even testified in his behalf, but the jury thought he was a liar. Before his hanging, Webster confessed to the crime.)

Though titillating, this story alone does not justify including Parkman in the current volume. But other aspects of his career command attention. He had studied in Paris with Pinel, an original proponent of moral treatment, and Pinel's successor, J. E. D. Esquirol. This fact made Parkman the only physician in the Boston area who could claim to have "specialized" in the treatment of the mentally ill and to have had clinical experience with the new therapy. From the various overtures he made to the trustees, one infers that he was very eager indeed to head the asylum branch of the proposed hospital. In 1814, he personally offered to build such an accommodation, but he wanted to limit the patients to those who could pay their own way, a condition unacceptable to the trustees. In 1816—by which time he was operating his own private madhouse—Parkman proposed a murky arrangement involving 16 acres of land in Roxbury; the trustees accepted, elected Parkman as provisional superintendent of the asylum, and then discovered that the financial conditions were other than they had been led to believe. They reversed themselves and unseated Parkman as superintendent-designate. In 1817, Parkman published a pamphlet, *Management of Lunatics with Illustrations of Insanity*, in which he championed the cause of moral treatment. Shortly thereafter, he submitted himself as a candidate for physician at the asylum, which by that time the trustees had decided to locate in Charlestown, across the Charles River Bay from Boston. Bowditch recorded that Parkman withdrew his application at some time during the next 12 months, and left us to wonder why. Thus ended the ill-fated Dr. Parkman's involvement with the asylum. One final word: Parkman evidently did not possess those qualities of character well suited to the treatment of the mentally ill. Dr. Webster is reported to have said during his confession: "I am irritable and passionate, and Dr. Parkman was the most provoking of men" (12).

In December 1816, about two months after the second Parkman deal had collapsed, the trustees contracted to purchase 18.36 acres of land situated on Cobble Hill, sometimes known as Miller's Hill, in Charlestown. The parcel was a portion of a 200-acre estate which had been developed in the early 1790s by Joseph Barrell, a Boston merchant of exquisite and extravagant taste. The Barrell place, laid out in the fashion of an English country manor, had enjoyed a brief reputation as the most beautiful country house in New England. Barrell, a horticultural enthusiast, had imported hundreds of ornamental plants and fruit trees from Europe. He had embellished his property with stables and cattle barns, dovecotes, greenhouses, a rose-covered summerhouse, fountains, and exotic fish pools. He had hired Bulfinch (who, incidentally, had labored briefly in a Barrell counting house in downtown Boston before turning to architecture) to design a residence atop the hill, commanding a view to the east of the terraced gardens and, below them, of the private wharf on Miller's River, a small tributary of the Charles, from which one could row across to Boston. Bulfinch worked with a generous budget and incorporated luxurious details in his design, including such modern conveniences as one of the earliest shower baths in New England.

Poor Barrell did not have many years to enjoy his country retreat. His financial fortunes ran afoul, and he fell into debt and died in a snarl of lawsuits in 1804. The hospital trustees purchased their tract, which included the brick Bulfinch mansion, from Barrell's son-in-law and executor, Benjamin Joy. They paid $15,650 for the asylum site, a bargain basement price; the original four acres of unbuilt land in Boston for the general hospital, acquired a few months later, cost $23,000. The trustees issued a public statement about the site in December 1816: "The situation selected appears to unite every practicable advantage; we should say the irreconcilable ones of propinquity and distance, being scarcely separated from the town by water, while its peninsular situation places it at the most desirable distance." This is the only document to suggest a motive for separating the asylum from the general hospital; it implies a certain uneasiness among Bostonians about a hospital for the insane in their midst.

The trustees appear not to have engaged in much discussion concerning the selection of an architect. One trustee, Joseph Coolidge, raised the name of his brother-in-law, Bulfinch, and so it was. Sometimes he seems to have been the only architect in Boston during the period; he must have driven his competitors to tears. Still, it made sense to retain the original architect to adapt and enlarge the Barrell place for use as an asylum. Moreover, as an enterprising professional, Bulfinch kept himself apprised of developments in the field of "domestic economy," namely heating and sanitation (remember Barrell's shower bath) and had a copy of Benjamin Latrobe's plan for a naval hospital in Washington. He was also the architect of the almshouse. So it was appropriate that the trustees should turn to him for proposals for both the asylum and the general hospital. The board sent him to Philadelphia and New York to see what might be learned about the hospitals there. Bulfinch made the trip in early 1817 and submitted two reports. The first, which evidently responded to specific questions raised by the trustees, has not been found if it still exists at all. The second, dated March 15, 1817, was a free-ranging letter in which Bulfinch felt compelled to address a number of issues that would influence his design.

> The first impression on visiting the great institutions of New York & Philadelphia, was that of surprize [sic] at finding the number of patients so small, in comparison with the age & extent of the establishments. . . . In the insane asylums . . . I found only 75 to 80 patients in each, although they receive them from every part of the Union. . . .
>
> Another impression was, that all the sick appeared to be of the poorest classes of society, and, although great order of cleanliness was observable, especially in N York, that there was no provision for discrimination or privacy.
>
> With respect to the insane [in Boston], calculations have been made of the great number who require accommodation. But if the principle is adopted that every insane person is to be a pay patient, I think the number will be very much reduced. . . . I am led to think that a building for 100 will be sufficient for a period of many years.

From Bulfinch's last paragraph it appears that the trustees had not yet completely resolved their admissions policy. This tricky but hardly trivial detail had posed problems from the first days of organization. No need to wade through the swamp of arguments and issues, for they can be neatly summarized: The trustees feared that if the asylum were to accept nonpaying patients, it would degenerate into "a merely pauper establishment," a dumping grounds which private donations could not support (13). Therefore, they successfully resisted attempts, including that by the state legislature, to force the asylum to admit charity cases without payment. The final determination seems to have been made shortly after Bulfinch's report and apparently aroused some public misapprehensions because in May the trustees found it necessary to issue a statement to correct the impression that the asylum would be exclusively for wealthy patients. Ultimately, the asylum failed to deliver completely on Jackson's and Warren's promise to the poor. By contrast with the general hospital, the asylum had no free beds; all patients, or towns sending pauper patients, had to pay something. The trustees made an effort to moderate the financial burden by establishing a sliding fee scale that was based on financial ability, thereby permitting many patients to pay a rate below the actual cost of their board and treatment while being effectively subsidized by those who could afford higher rates.

Elsewhere in his report, Bulfinch estimated the considerable investment of civic pride in the enterprise: "I apprehend that there is a general opinion of the necessity of a provision for a large number of patients, and that the public expect as great, or greater accommodation than can be found in private dwelling houses; that the building[s] shall be spacious, ornamental to the town, and gratifying to the sight and feelings of each one, who may reflect that he has assisted in their endowment."

Bulfinch attached a sketch of a ground plan for the Barrell place to his letter. This initial drawing showed two semidetached single-story wings—one for female and one for male patients—connected to the existing mansion by "covered colonade [sic] or arches" and extending before it at diverging angles in the manner of outstretched, welcoming arms. The unorthodox disposition of the wings was an architectural solution to the severely sloping site as well as to the trustees' conviction that the wings should communicate with the existing building—which would house the superintendent, his family and other staff—while being as distant from one another as possible so as to guarantee separation of the sexes. Bulfinch recommended stone as the building material for the wings, "certainly to be preferred to brick in all situations open to driving storms & sea air. It will be more costly at the beginning, but will be more durable & require fewer repairs . . ." (14). The floor plan showed rooms ranged along a double-loaded corridor, hotel fashion.

Although the trustees accepted Bulfinch's proposal almost immediately, appointed a Building Committee, and moved quickly ahead with the project, the final product showed many modifications. The capacity of the asylum was reduced from 100 to 60; the wings were three stories tall; the building material was brick, which satisfied both the urge to match the new structures with the existing mansion and the trustees' impulses for economy, if not Bulfinch's preference for nobler, more enduring stone.

One can easily underrate the difficulty of this undertaking for all the parties involved. Architect and trustees were trying to invent a building form to accommodate and help a very special class of people (whose opinions it never occurred to anybody to solicit); and the project was all wrapped up in a theory of treatment that nobody in Boston (except Parkman) knew very much about, but which enlisted agreeable surroundings as a therapeutic aid. The ideal of creating a wholesome, pleasant, and secure environment, in which seriously deranged people could be controlled—not to mention cured—without suffering physical abuse or spiritual deprivation involved so many superficial contradictions that it seemed an impossible task. The first superintendent would later observe: "I believe architects have been less successful in providing for the wants in buildings for lunatics, than in those for any other purpose" (15). No wonder discussions of architectural arrangements occupied so much space in the literature on mental illness during the nineteenth century. Since Bulfinch and the trustees could not profit from the mistakes of other institutions, they made mistakes of their own. But, as the trustees wrote in 1814, "If man shall refuse to do any thing, until he can perform what is perfect; if he will put nothing under the care of others, until he finds beings exempt from frailty and error, there is an end to human exertion and of all trust and confidence among men" (16).

The superintendent had not even moved into the old Barrell residence when he started proposing amendments to the architecture. Nevertheless, building construction advanced so rapidly that on September 1, 1818, the trustees announced that the asylum would be "ready for the reception of a few Patients on the first day of October next." The trustees and the public pronounced themselves pleased with the appearance of the buildings. Nine consulting physicians, who inspected the asylum in March 1819, expressed satisfaction with the arrangements, noting that "in the apartments occupied by the patients were all the appearances of neatness and comfort."

CHAPTER

2

Rufus Wyman and the Experiment in Moral Treatment

Bulfinch, who suffered no shortage of self-confidence, advanced opinions on a number of issues that had little to do with architecture; having heard that the resident superintendent of the asylum would be a doctor, he pronounced himself strongly opposed to the plan. "This I think very objectionable," he wrote in his March 15, 1817, report, "both for the hospital and for the asylum. The pay that will be given cannot be an object to a physician of eminence to induce him to devote himself to the charge; and one of little skill would not secure your confidence, and might frequently differ in opinion and treatment from the visiting physicians; being once chosen he would seem fixed for life; for it would be the ruin of his professional character to be dismissed" (1). Perhaps Parkman had entertained such qualms. However, the trustees did not. Precisely a year after Bulfinch's letter, they determined that it was "expedient to unite in one person the offices of Physician and Superintendent of the Asylum" (2). A week later the board acted on a recommendation of the physicians and surgeons of the hospital and selected the man who appears to have been the single remaining applicant to head the asylum: Dr. Rufus Wyman.

The facts about Wyman's life prior to his appointment are

reasonably straightforward. He was born in Woburn, Massachusetts, in 1778, to a family of modest means. He went to Harvard (class of 1799), spent a year as a school teacher, and then took up the study of medicine as a student of Dr. Samuel Brown of Boston. Like other medical students of his time, he attended patients in the Leverett Street almshouse under Brown's supervision as part of his clinical training. But Brown became ill, and Wyman had to find a new mentor. He finished his studies with Dr. John Jeffries, who subsequently invited him into his Boston medical practice. Wyman's own health was delicate, and after a year or so with Jeffries, he retreated to the country and established himself in practice in Chelmsford. He acquired a reputation in that community as an intelligent and compassionate physician. He was appointed a justice of the peace. In 1810 he married Anne Morrill. The couple eventually had four sons and one daughter. In 1816 he produced his first printed paper, an anonymous discourse entitled "Remarks on the Observation of the Lord's Day, as a moral, a positive, and a civil duty. By a Tythingman," which was issued in Cambridge. In January 1817, Benjamin Pickman, about whom nothing is known in this context except that he had contributed $1,000 to the hospital fund, submitted Wyman's name to the trustees. The next time Wyman's name came up in the record was March 1818, the time of his election. He accepted. He was 40 years old.

The threadbare facts frustrate the urge to understand. They fail to illuminate the substance of the man or his motives, save for the strength of his Christian convictions. What possessed him to quit a comfortable, if not prosperous, country practice to run an insane asylum? There is no evidence that he had any particular interest in mental disease or any special experience in treating the mentally ill. The annual salary of $1,500, though a good one for a physician those days and probably more than he earned in the Chelmsford practice, was hardly large enough to arouse suspicions of greed. We do not know why Pickman thought Wyman would be a good candidate, why Wyman permitted his name to be submitted, whether the physicians and surgeons or the trustees discussed the position with him, or why Wyman was willing to relocate his entire family—including, then, three young children—to Charlestown, there to reside in the company of mental patients (which company evidently did them no harm). Had Wyman read George Parkman's tract on *Management of Lunatics* in which he remarked the "Asylums here are so few; their faithful management is full of responsibility, fatigue and danger; needing such patience, resolution, and forbearance; presenting such distress, and disgusting scenes, few follow such objects" (3). What manner of man was this Rufus Wyman?

This is no idle question. After all, Wyman ran the fledgling institution almost single-handedly for 17 years; he established the principles of treatment; and he created the character and reputation of the place. As Philippe Pinel had observed in his famous *Treatise on Insanity*, "The character of a superintendent, who is in the habit of discharging the important duties of his office, with integrity, dignity and humanity, is itself a circumstance of great weight and influence in a lunatic establishment" (4).

The pages of Bowditch's history, asylum records, annual reports, and the casual diary of a young man who served as apothecary at the asylum in 1825–26 offer occasional shards of insight into Wyman, but they cannot be pieced together to form a three-dimensional figure of a man. His early account books reveal him to have been meticulous in financial matters, registering expenses down to fractions of pennies, an accounting practice not at all unusual in his day. More to the point, perhaps, was his refusal in 1830 to accept a $1,000 legacy, in recognition of his "requisite qualities," from the estate of a deceased patient. Bowditch recorded that the trustees received a letter from Wyman "declining the donation of Mr. Lee on the general and high-minded ground of the impropriety of receiving presents from any boarder or his friends" (5). Without wishing to cast shadows upon Wyman's high mindedness, this writer observes that he would have stirred up great consternation among the trustees if he *had* accepted a personal gift. Young William Folsom's diary registered his immediate impression of the Wyman family as "pleasant"—a word that carried more weight in the nineteenth century then it does now. That Folsom developed a friendly and respectful relationship with Wyman is suggested more by the absence of any gripes in his journals than by the presence of affectionate anecdote. Folsom was not a profound or poetic interpreter of the passing human scene (6).

Wyman's dedication to duty achieved legendary proportions in 1832 when the trustees noticed the extraordinary fact that during the first 14 years of his administration he had spent only five nights away from the asylum. Luther Bell, who held Wyman's position from 1837 to 1858, commented on his predecessor's record of residence:

> The last sounds of the closing and the first of the dawning day brought to his ear the presence of his helpless charge and reminded him of duties which never grew wearisome to his spirit. This unexhausted application of course implied, for existence otherwise could hardly have been sustained, an undying devotion to the welfare of the insane; and he never, so far as can be judged, pursued this great end with diminished intensity of interest, amidst the discouragements which all places of trust, and perhaps none more than those connected with the care of those void of reason, occasionally involve. (7)

Wyman could not be intimidated by the patient who told him, "I have you in my power. If you kill me, you'll be hung. But I can kill you with safety; for I am crazy, and therefore not responsible." Nor did Wyman shy away from the wards after another patient bashed him on the skull with a carpenter's hammer (8). He exposed his private life to patients, often inviting those who were well enough to share his family table. The asylum archives testify to Wyman's persistent efforts to improve the quality of life for patients, to promote their cure or, at the very least, to ensure their comfort and security. He gained the respect of his medical peers, who elevated him during the last two years of his life to the presidency of the Massachusetts Medical Society.

Integrity. Justice. Modesty. Patience. Equanimity. Devotion. The words paint an unblemished, not-quite-human portrait. Rufus Wyman disappears in the inflationary prose of obituary writers. There is not a clue to the demons that drove him, to disappointments. Can it be that the weather of his mind never turned stormy? Did he ever tell a joke? There is, possibly, a hint of vulnerability in the frequent episodes of illness that confined Wyman to bed, but knowledge of his history of pulmonary problems prior to coming to the asylum, as well as the general health standards of his day, militates against flamboyant speculations.

Wyman produced only a few published papers, most of them in the form of reports to the trustees. According to Bell, Wyman's reluctance to publish arose from

> a hatred of ostentation, an avoidance of anything which could be construed as self-laudation, which perhaps was carried to an extreme actually prejudicial to the interests of this institution and thus to the insane generally. He had such a dislike of newspaper notoriety, such distrust of any form of reputation higher with the public at large than with his professional brethren, the sole adequate judges of character in a medical man, that perhaps the light of his good works was too much hidden under a bushel to serve its proper end as an example. (9)

Given Wyman's double duties as doctor and administrator, he had little energy to spare for writing. As he once wrote to the governor of Massachusetts in response to a request for his expert opinion, "My duties at this Asylum . . . require so much of my time, that I have very little for other pursuits" (10). However, that he failed to act as a medical *scientist,* as opposed to a publicist, and seize the opportunity for systematic observation of his patients and their responses to treatment was a great loss. Both Pinel and Tuke had emphasized the desperate need for gathering and dispensing information about mental illness. But Wyman had the instincts of a medical practitioner, not of a researcher. More than 100 years later, Cecil Drinker, reviewing Wyman's career, was moved to comment, "It seems there is but poor recognition of the fact, that these early explorers of mental disease were in a peculiarly difficult position. They were housekeepers, architects, doctors, legal advisors, almost anything except men with time to think and to record their views" (11).

Among the few documents that Wyman published, one in particular tells of the quality and character of intelligence that he brought to his work. In 1830 the Massachusetts Medical Society asked him to deliver its annual address, an invitation that was a great honor. Wyman chose as his subject "Mental Philosophy as Connected with Mental Disease." He began by discussing the practices of moral treatment at the asylum and then continued:

> Each individual being himself conscious, that he is at different times in different states, is so constituted as to infer from this fact that others have a similar experience in regard to themselves. These different states, such

> as perceiving, remembering, comparing, and discerning, and also the different states in anger, joy, hatred, etc., constitute the phenomena which are called mental. . . . They are as distinct in their character from the organic phenomena of vegetables and animals as the organic are from the physical. Nor are the organic actions more interesting to the physician than should be the mental operations. There is a natural and fixed course of each, which is denominated perfect health. *'Mens sana in corpore sano.'* There is a difficulty, and perhaps an impossibility of defining disease of mind; yet the difficulty seems not to be greater, than in disease of the body. The state of perfect health is taken as the standard for each. Each deviation from this state is, strictly speaking, a disease. The deviations in the organic functions, however, are not usually considered diseases, unless they should be attended with pain, uneasiness, or other inconvenience. Neither are the deviations in the mental states or operations of one man to be considered as amounting to disease, unless they be obviously inconsistent with the feelings, judgement, or belief of other men who are competent judges; so that the mutual adaptation, by which one mind is fitted to act in concert with others, is destroyed. (12)

Wyman's definition was based on a dozen years of cohabitation with the mentally ill. The originality of expression, rather than of substance, strikes the modern reader. The statement is such a gentle mix of humanism, generosity, and common sense that it still resonates across a century and a half of more precise, scientific formulations. Wyman revealed himself here as a man profoundly involved with his fellow creatures—the healthy and the sick and the infinite permutations in between—a man who moved thoughtfully through experience, attending carefully to other humans, who valued kinship and communication, and was not afraid to search within himself. He might have said with the Roman dramatist Terence, "I am a man. Nothing human is alien to me."

Shortly after Wyman's election as superintendent and physician of the asylum, the trustees packed him off to inspect facilities in Philadelphia and New York, as Bulfinch had done before him. Characteristically, Wyman delivered an oral rather than a written report of his travels, once again leaving future historians in the dark about what he saw, let alone what he *thought* about what he saw. In addition to the hospitals in Philadelphia and New York, he almost certainly visited the Friends' Asylum at Frankfort, Pennsylvania, near Philadelphia, which had opened in 1817. This Quaker establishment, modeled on the Quaker Retreat at York, England, was the first institution for the mentally ill in the United States explicitly built and operated on the principles of moral treatment and, as such, provided a singular opportunity to observe the theory in practice. Wyman did attend, in May, the laying of the cornerstone for the Asylum at Bloomingdale, a new branch of the New York Hospital geographically removed from the general hospital. He contributed two 50-cent pieces to the coins deposited under the cornerstone. In exchange, Thomas Eddy presented him with the original architectural plan for Bloomingdale's, along with an inscribed copy of Samuel Tuke's *Description of the Retreat* at York, published in 1813, a gift which indicated how swiftly the idea of moral treatment was catching on in the United States. Wyman's marginal annotations prove that he studied Tuke with close attention. He also took meticulous notes on his journey, particularly about administrative and architectural matters. He returned to Boston, reported to the trustees, and in July 1818 moved his family into the Charlestown Asylum mansion. Bulfinch's wings for patients were not quite completed, and Wyman's recommendations no doubt influenced some of the interior arrangements. But the project was so far advanced by the time he arrived that his opinions cannot have made a significant difference in the final form of the buildings.

On September 1, the trustees announced to the public that the asylum would be ready to receive patients in a month's time. The notice listed the rules of admission, which, one observes, were considerably more detailed than the rules then in force for admission to the medical college. Most of the regulations concerned finances. The application had to state whether the patient "be a pauper, or whether he or she has property in his or her right, or whether his or her friends (liable by law for his or her support) are in good circumstances, or unable to support such Patients. . . ." The trustees explained the sliding fee scale, noting that though "compensation will be demanded for the board of all patients . . . the price for board will, in all cases, be proportioned to the circumstances of the Patient or of his or her friends. . . ." Paupers dependent on towns for support would be charged the lowest rate, which was initially set at $2.50 per week. The trustees further required a general description of the patient's case and suggested that a friend or physician supply information concerning "previous habits and occupations, age, usual health, former disease, accidents (if any), peculiar propensities, or traits of character, the time of first appearance of the disease, and of its intermission (if any), as well as the probable or supposed cause of the complaint—whether the Patient had at any time shown a disposition to injure him or herself or others. . . ." The object of this document was to "enable the Physician to decide on the most proper mode of treatment. . . ." The descriptive letter had to be accompanied by a certificate, signed by a magistrate, clergyman "or other person of known respectability" testifying to the accuracy of the facts. The trustees reserved the right to show preference for patients who belonged to donors' families or sent by towns which had contributed to the hospital fund. They further announced a prejudice in favor of patients "where there is strong ground to hope for speedy relief, over those in which the cure shall seem hopeless." This provision made unambiguous the asylum's mission to cure the mentally ill and not to become a receptacle for chronic cases. Oddly enough, the trustees' notice said nothing about philosophy of treatment, and those who sought reassurances that patients would not be abused looked in vain, although earlier circulars and the reputations of the trustees probably inspired some confidence in that respect (13).

Applications trickled in slowly. The initial feeble show of public enthusiasm suited Wyman and the trustees because they planned to admit only a few patients for the time being so as to acquaint the inexperienced attendants, and a relatively inexperienced superintendent, with conditions of work. This was an emphatically sensible approach. One can easily imagine the chaos let loose if 50 or so mentally ill individuals had been assigned all at one time to green caretakers. Accordingly, the first patient was selected with extravagant care. Bowditch wrote that:

> a father asked to have his son received as an inmate; and the [Visiting] Committee spent three hours in conversing with him, in order to learn all the particulars of the case. He informed them that he believed his son to be one of those spoken of in the Bible as "possessed with a devil;" and, when asked what remedial measures he had adopted, replied that he was in the habit of whipping him. The young man was entirely cured, and

> became subsequently a peddler, in which vocation he displayed so much Yankee shrewdness that he acquired a property of Ten or Twelve Thousand dollars. (14)

Patient Number One might have come straight from central casting: a victim of medieval superstitions, he had been salvaged from intractable disease by enlightened, humane treatment. Not only that, he went on to amass a small fortune (what better proof of sanity) and thus endear himself forever to asylum chroniclers. If one is tempted to read Bowditch's story skeptically two centuries later, it bears repeating that Patient Number One's father was beating him, that a private madhouse would most likely have submitted him to some other medium of torture, and he would have rotted in the almshouse. Rufus Wyman and the staff at the Charlestown Asylum treated him kindly and he improved.*

Nine patients had been received by November 23, thirteen by December 17. Of those, four had been discharged "cured" and four "by request," which ordinarily meant that family or sponsors were unwilling to pay further board and withdrew a patient before Wyman felt treatment had taken hold. Even when the patient appeared much improved, Wyman advised strongly against premature discharge because he believed longer residence in the asylum could effect a complete cure.

On April 2, 1819, 15 patients were in residence: six females and nine males. The Visiting Committee passed on all admissions and set the rate of board for each patient. The committee consisted of three trustees responsible for the affairs of the asylum and was called "visiting" because of its obligation to visit and inspect the premises every Tuesday afternoon, and that of one member to visit some other, random, day of the week. As time passed and the numbers of patients increased, the committee could not afford to spend three hours mulling over the individual merits of every application. Nevertheless, they scrutinized the documents thoroughly. The patient population multiplied slowly as Wyman and his staff accumulated experience and the public yielded its confidence. By December 31, 1821, after slightly more than three years of operation, 146 patients (plus 3

*In keeping with the McLean Hospital's policy of protecting the privacy of its patients, no patient, past or present, will be identified by name in this history, except in instances where hospitalization is already in the public domain by virtue of previous publications.

"unfit subjects") had entered the asylum. Of these, 118 had left: there had been six "elopements," as escapes were so fetchingly called in those days; nine deaths; and 29 removals by request. A total of 23 patients had been discharged "improved," 19 "much improved," and 32 "cured." In another three years, the patient population had doubled. The asylum was occupied almost to capacity, and Wyman began to press for expansion.

A random page from the admissions and discharge register for 1826 listed 18 patients, 16 of them with occupations: four housewives, two mariners, two merchants, two tradesmen, one scrivener, one grocer, one farmer, one student, one shipwright, and one counselor-at-law; two women were registered without occupation. This particular group contained no paupers. In fact, though towns sent patients from their jails and almshouses at this time, indigents represented a minority in the asylum. The register further recorded the name, age, home town, sex, rate of board, name of financially responsible person or township, time of onset and duration of illness, and the "probable cause" of disease for each patient. Under the last heading were advanced such explanations as heredity, fever, disappointment in expectations, amenorrhea, masturbation, family troubles, vegetable diet, intemperance, religious perplexity, death of husband, and—my personal favorite—"excitement of elections" in the case of a lawyer.

Statistics and lists disclose nothing of the anguish of the patients or the severity of their afflictions. Take Patient Number Forty-Nine, for instance. He was a native of Westbrook, Massachusetts, 27 years old, single, and employed as a mariner. He was admitted to the asylum on October 6, 1819, by his brother, who stated that the patient had become ill for the first time about 14 months earlier. According to the case record, the first thing the admitting person (probably Wyman) noticed about Forty-Nine was that he was infested with "vermin," apparently lice. Accordingly, he was "shorn immediately." It was also observed that his eyes were black and very inflamed, and that he had callous ridges on both arms above the elbow. Forty-Nine volunteered the information that he had been confined by cords while he was at sea. An examination the next morning revealed a pulse rate of 84 and a slightly coated tongue—in short nothing to explain the eye inflammation. Forty-Nine's temperature was not taken: The thermometer would not become a standard instrument in the medical armamentarium until much later in the century.

During his first two weeks in the asylum, Forty-Nine resisted the attendant, dashed his chamber pot against the window, smashed four panes of glass, and repeatedly fouled his room with excrement. After having been placed in a darkened room with the object of becalming him, Forty-Nine was found with eyes and temples bruised and inflamed. He said he had beaten his head against the wall to relieve the disagreeable sensation he felt in it and that his head now felt much better. He persisted in his attacks on attendants, battering one, and in bashing his head against walls until Wyman ordered him placed in restraints. The attendants strapped him into a chair by day and confined him in the sleeping crib by night.

The chronicle of foul rooms, assaults on attendants, punitive shower baths, confinement in the "dark room," and strapping into chairs continued through the months of October and November. On December 4, Forty-Nine raised some hopes when he emerged from his room "and saluted his fellow boarders, bidding them 'good morning' with apparent civility." No sooner done than he aimed a "violent blow" at another patient. Fortunately, Forty-Nine missed his mark. By December 6, he was strapped into the chair again. Two days later he fouled his room, tore off his clothes, and threw them into the hall. The next day, upon finding the room filthy yet again, Wyman ordered Forty-Nine isolated in a cell. He refused to put on his clothes and sat there naked.

Two more months went by in much the same fashion, but the level of Forty-Nine's agitation subsided a bit. From time to time he passed a few days without incident, and once he promised to behave better. On February 12, the record reads: "For the past week has been improving. Walks much in the gallery and in the yard when the weather permits. Keeps his room neat and treats his fellows with civility. . . ." Forty-Nine continued to improve during March and into April—with the exception of one incident, of which more anon. However, on April 17 he showed signs of mounting excitement: "Not often talks to himself, but frequently bursts into an idiot laugh when alone. Says he never shall be well enough to work hard again for a living. Intends to preach. Talks to himself more than formerly, especially when alone." Forty-Nine's subsequent outburst never equaled the violence and disorder of the fall of 1819.

The last real episode occurred on May 24: "it appears he beat his head against the wall of his room last eveg. Also bruised the belly in several places." Thereafter, he settled down to harmless pursuits: "July 8: continues as usual, writes incoherent nonsensical letters to his friends, quotes scripture at random, talks of preaching, solicits friends to discharge him from the asylum." The last entry to suggest an approaching crisis appeared on July 15; fortunately, Forty-Nine's "wildness"—as they put it—dissipated quickly. He spent the next six weeks among his fellow patients, calm, courteous, and rational. He was discharged on September 2, 1820, "in an improved state." Upon taking his leave, Forty-Nine politely thanked the asylum personnel for their attentions.

The early case records were neither systematic nor thorough, and three or four days often elapsed without an entry. Thus, many details of Forty-Nine's therapeutic regimen are missing from the account. His pharmaceutical diet consisted principally of magnesium sulfate—epsom salts—which acted as a gentle cathartic. From time to time, he received more powerful cathartics, calomel and cochineal. On at least one occasion, during a period when he seems to have been acting calmly, Forty-Nine was heavily dosed with both strong cathartics and an emetic. Another time, when agitated and complaining of abdominal pains following an administration of antimony salts (an emetic which sometimes produces symptoms resembling arsenic poisoning), he received tincture of opium. And in March 1820, after a spell of delusions, he got the full treatment: venesection, cathartics, and emetics all on the same day. However, the total number of entries referring to medicinal remedies does not exceed two dozen—not much for a patient who spent nearly 11 months in the asylum. Even assuming that an equal number of routine purgings were omitted from the case book as too insignificant to mention, the record of medical intervention was still a conservative one, ancillary to that treatment form called "moral" which the records do not reveal.

Wyman explained moral treatment in his 1830 address to the Massachusetts Medical Society as follows:

> The treatment of insanity chiefly depends upon the connection between the mind and body. If there be inflammation of the brain, or its membranes, it is to be treated as inflammation of those parts. If there be other organic disease, whether of structure or of function, in any part of the body, medical treatment will be required. But in mental disorders, without symptoms of organic disease, a judicious moral management is more successful. It should afford agreeable occupation. It should engage the mind, and exercise the body; as swinging, riding, walking, sewing, embroidery, bowling, gardening, mechanic arts; to which may be added reading, writing, conversation, &c., the whole to be performed with order and regularity. Even the taking of food, retiring to bed, rising in the morning, &c., at stated times, and conforming to stated rules in almost everything, is a most salutary discipline. It requires, however, constant attention and vigilance, with the greatest kindness in the attendants upon a lunatic. Moral treatment is indispensable, even in cases rising from organic diseases.
>
> In regard to medical treatment, I believe that purging, bleeding, low diet, &c., have been adopted with little discrimination. They are to be resorted to only when there is organic disease, which requires the "reducing plan." But these remedies, especially in debilitated subjects, are seldom useful in relieving mental disease. They are usually injurious and frequently fatal. It is undoubtedly true, that impressions upon the alimentary canal by purging or vomiting, and upon the skin of the extremities by blistering, are useful in chronic cases of mental disorders. But these remedies must be suited to the strength and general health of the patient. (15)

Presented with such a statement, the twentieth-century mind tends to stumble into the potholes of nineteenth-century medical theory—the fuzzy, inconsistent connection between mind and body (a biological/philosophical dilemma that has never been satisfactorily resolved); the obsession with purgatives and emetics; the infernal blisters—at the risk of underestimating the genuine reforms effected by moral treatment. The system entailed a great deal more than throwing away the whips and chains of yesteryear and being nice to patients. Moral treatment was an active therapy and implied an assumption that everyone and everything in the patient's environment influenced the condition of mind and therefore possessed therapeutic potential. The patient played an active role in treatment by participation in occupations, adherence to a rigorous schedule, and engagement with the community.

By now, of course, the basic elements of moral treatment have graduated to the taken-for-granted category and, in new verbal disguises (structured programs, social interaction, occupational and recreational therapy) and with variations, are standard features of all well-run mental institutions in the Western world. But in the early nineteenth century, moral treatment stood as the first systematic psychological approach to mental disease, a remarkable innovation in an age before psychology had defined itself as a discipline. Moreover, moral treatment conflicted with the fundamental tenets of physical medicine. As Luther Bell remarked later, the idea of a regimen that did not depend on medicine but nonetheless resulted in recovery injured "the pride of medical science" (16). Wyman required intellectual courage to stand before an audience of physicians, most of whom revered the works of Benjamin Rush (an energetic bloodletter and purger), and question the validity of medical intervention.

Though the remote origins of the moral treatment movement do not reveal themselves clearly, common sense suggests that its sources can be found in simple human compassion. As Europe passed from the superstitions of the Middle Ages to the Renaissance celebration of man, a few brave and conscience-stricken individuals liberated the insane from their torture chambers and handled them gently. Edward Tyson, physician and later governor to Bethlehem Hospital at the end of the seventeenth century, tried to humanize treatment of the insane by introducing women nurses, restricting spectators, and clothing indigent patients. His most remarkable innovation, follow-up treatment of discharged patients with periodic calls to their homes, unfortunately failed to be passed on to later generations of reformers (17). Those elements of care that were observed to benefit the mentally ill gradually evolved into a system. The rough outline of moral treatment was known in eighteenth-century England, but its practitioners had failed to study and report their experiences. Therefore it fell to a Frenchman, Philippe Pinel, to gain fame as the "Father of Moral Treatment." Pinel was appointed physician to the infamous Parisian asylum for male lunatics, Bicêtre, in 1792, during the French Revolution; three years later his services were extended to the female asylum, the

Salpêtrière. He achieved immortality through the efforts of a painter, Robert Fleury, who portrayed him striking the chains from a female patient while a woman who had just been freed kisses his hand in gratitude. Some historians believe Fleury committed an injustice and that it was really Pussin, superintendent at Bicêtre before Pinel became the physician, who struck the first chains; and, in fact, the Italian reformer Vincenzo Chiarugi of Florence disposed of chains before either Pussin or Pinel! But the fact remains that it was Pinel who produced the first disciplined study of moral treatment and became its publicist, so one does not begrudge him a bonus of unearned recognition.

Pinel approached the problem of mental illness with a scientific rigor unusual in his day. He tested the prevailing theory that insanity resulted from organic disease of the brain, and was therefore incurable, by studying the brains of people who had died with mental illness. He could find few consistent patterns of organic disease; in fact, the tissues he examined usually showed no anomalies at all. Although he did observe irregularities in people who had been born with mental defects, he concluded that "lesions or deformities of the skulls of maniacs which cannot be acquired in adult age . . . are very rare, if ever occurring causes of accidental insanity" (18). He reasoned that much mental illness was a functional rather than a structural disturbance and that its causes were psychological. Hence the logic of moral treatment: a psychological remedy for a psychological disease. Yet even Pinel was not quite prepared to abandon the occasional bleeding or purging.

Pinel's *Treatise on Insanity*, printed in 1800, described the practices of moral treatment in detail. Haslam's *Observations on Madness*, published nine years later, belonged to the same stream of thought as did Tuke's 1813 description of the Quaker retreat at York. Tuke captured the essence of moral treatment in a quotation from Aeschylus: "Soft speech is to distemper'd wrath, medicinal." All three gentlemen countered the presumption of incurability of insanity by reporting high incidences of recovery, especially among patients suffering their first attack of mental illness. Pinel and Haslam used the term "cure," while Tuke, the most understated of these authors, preferred the word "recovery" because cure implied an active outside medicinal agent and, he confessed, "we have not discovered any anti maniacal specific and profess to do little more than assist Nature in the performance of her own cure" (19).

Wyman read Pinel, Haslam, and Tuke and adapted their recommendations in designing the treatment plan for the Asylum at Charlestown. Wyman's version of moral treatment went pretty much by the book—the book being Tuke, in particular—and refrained from experimentation. But since moral treatment was in itself experimental in the United States, Wyman had plenty on his hands. Among the earliest documents in the McLean Hospital archives is a page called "General Rules, without minute details," in Wyman's hand. The first sentence reads: "Every thing and place, from the Cellar to the Garret, to be kept as clean and neat as the nature of the Place will possibly admit." Visitors would be admitted by permission only, "with strict segregation of sexes," a provision intended to protect patients against voyeurism and disruption of treatment.

The most extensive set of regulations governed the attendants. In this area before the advent of a nursing profession, the problem of hiring intelligent, unflappable attendants, training them, and keeping them on the staff preoccupied Wyman. He recognized that patients would pass most of their waking hours in the company of the attendants and that improvement depended to some extent on the quality of their attention. As he explained in his 1826 annual report, "Attendants are selected with utmost care and circumspection. The principle being to employ mild, gentle, and most especially a uniform course of conduct, it being particularly important that those who have the constant and immediate care of the patients should possess amiable dispositions and soundness and maturity of judgement. Attendants have been persons from the country whose characters were well known and in general have been employed in keeping schools."

Anyone who wonders why a school teacher would apply for a job as an attendant in an asylum might ponder Justin Kaplan's account of poet Walt Whitman's teaching "career" in the late 1830s: "The customary rewards of countryschool teaching, [Whitman] said, were 'poor pay', 'coarse fare'—sometimes a pickled hog's head with an olla-podrida of fried turnips, potatoes, and cabbage—and a straw mattress with little privacy in the homes of his pupils' parents; he was once invited to bed down with a sick cow" (20). Unfortunately, however, Wyman had to deal with a turnover rate comparable to that of a contemporary administrator.

Strict segregation of the sexes was observed in the deployment of attendants as in everything else at the asylum; women were assigned to the female wing, men to the male wing. The regulations provided that the attendants were never to leave the patients alone during the day, save for a half hour after each mealtime when patients were supposed to remain quietly in their rooms. When the patients retired in the evening, the attendants collected all their clothing and inspected, brushed, and otherwise cleaned every item; naturally, attendants were not allowed to appropriate any patient property for their own use. Most emphatic was the injunction that "the attendants shall *not* on any occasion strike a boarder," nor was it within their power to place a patient in restraints without the order of the superintendent.

Restraints were a sensitive issue. The word never occurred in the full Rules and Regulations, a 10-page document printed in 1821, although there was a reference to "strong rooms" in each wing. Obviously, the use of mechanical restraints conflicted with the ideals of moral treatment. They were nonetheless practical necessities at the Asylum in Charlestown as well as in Tuke's, Pinel's, and Haslam's respective establishments. Wyman stated truthfully in his 1833 annual report that "chains or strait jackets have never been used or provided in this asylum." But his account book showed purchases of chair straps, hemp webbing, cast brass buckles, bed straps, and a crib during the summer of 1818, before the asylum opened (21). The chair and the crib figured in Forty-Nine's case history; the dark room or "cell" in which he was confined was one of the strong rooms located in the wings and mentioned in the rules. Other casebook entries reveal the use of muffs (or mittens), wrist straps, and sleeves that restrained the use of arms. But the records also show that Wyman resorted to mechanical restraint reluctantly and used it for as short as possible periods of time, suggesting that he viewed it as a means of pacification and control rather than of punishment or coercion. That patients sometimes interpreted his intentions otherwise is another matter.

Wyman's responsibilities were enormous. As superintendent he had to purchase all "articles necessary for the Asylum, and shall be responsible for the safe-keeping and economical use and expenditure of the same." He hired, managed, and, when necessary, fired all personnel. As physician he was required to see every patient at least once a day, direct all treatment, and submit various oral and written reports to the trustees. He had some help in the person of a medical student who doubled as apothecary and clerk and who was required to visit all male patients twice a day, along with such female patients as the superintendent designated as in "a suitable condition." "But," the regulations continued in the throes of Puritan prudery, "his visits to the female apartments shall not be prolonged for the purpose of conversation either with the Boarders or Attendants, and his deportment must be free from even the appearance of familiarity with either."

The Visiting Committee appeared weekly, decided upon admissions and discharges, set fees for each new patient, reviewed overall financial status, and visited "the wards and rooms in every building belonging to the Asylum." This tour brought the Visiting Committee members in contact with patients and inevitably led to incidents, some of them amusing. Bowditch related that one patient cornered a trustee who tried to evade a story he had heard many times before. "Don't tell *me* about your not having time to hear my story," the patient retorted. "If you haven't you ought to have. It is the very thing you were sent here for" (22).

The regulations spelled out the duties of all domestic employees, including the porter, the outdoor laborers, cooks, laundresses and washerwomen, and the superintendent's chambermaid. The rules governed meal times, established the weekly menu with monotonous predictability, and even gave the recipe for "the drink for the asylum" (an odious concoction of water, molasses, and small beer) and the grain content of asylum bread.

Wyman shared Pinel's and Tuke's view that the primary condition for treatment of the mentally ill was the removal of the patient from customary surroundings, "that absence from home is always indispensable—that a lunatic at home perceives he is watched and followed in every movement and deems every restraint to be an act of tyranny and usurpation, inducing hatred towards nearest relatives and dearest friends. . . ." Within the asylum the methodical activities of attendants, routine visitations of physician, medical student, and Visiting Committee, the rhythmic wakings, mealtimes, and bedtimes, and the expected food on the table supplied structure to the patient's life, and this structure was the second fundamental of therapy. Wyman believed that regularity, "living under a system of rules and regulations for everything, [has] a powerful effect in tranquilizing the mind, breaking up wrong associations of ideas, and inducing correct habits of thinking as well as acting" (23). After a few years of experience at the asylum, Wyman came to consider duration of treatment crucial to effecting a recovery. In 1823, at his insistence, the trustees adopted a rule that patients who quit the asylum against the physician's advice within three months of admission would still be charged for the full three months. Various recreations and liberties, a list which expanded during Wyman's tenure, constituted the third element of treatment in that they "divert the attention from unpleasant subjects of thought, and afford exercise both of body and mind."

Wyman's son Morrill wrote down these memories of life at the asylum:

> Some of the boarders were quite at liberty to come and go as they pleased. These found their own occupation and amusement; one was a frequent visitor at the reading-room of the Boston Athenaeum, and might have been seen daily among the literary gentlemen who associated there. A constant effort was made to increase the means of occupation and amusement for all. Walking in the airing courts or in the country with attendants, going to church on Sunday, visiting places of interest on other days, were the most common, or riding in open wagons in pleasant weather. Soon afterwards [in 1823] the physician was "authorized to procure a carriage and pair of horses to be used . . . for the purpose of giving air and exercise to the borders. . . ." A rowboat upon Charles River, then attractive and unpolluted, was in frequent use, affording an amusement particularly relished by those who had been sailors, of whom the Asylum usually contained several.
>
> In summer, excursions in the harbor in large boats gave a pleasant sail, a run upon the islands, a chowder on board, and all the enjoyment of a day from home. There was bowling, gardening, the exercise of the mechanic arts, books, papers, and various games. Chess was a favorite

> with some; the physician was an excellent player, and not unfrequently met with a worthy antagonist among his boarders. (24)

Wyman appeared in Folsom's journals entertaining the women on the third floor of the south wing by throwing shadow rabbits on the wall. Thus, the severe framework of regulations enclosed warm, informal moments, hardly any of which showed up in the case records. No wonder Folsom was surprised by his first encounter with the asylum in February 1825: "Find crazy people much more pleasant than I expected," he wrote, "—& easily managed by attendants" (25). The administration of medicinal remedies played a subsidiary role in this system. Since most medicines employed at the asylum acted upon the digestive system, they seem more like agents of regularity than of medicine. (It is interesting to note that Folsom, who suffered from some digestive ailment, submitted himself to treatment very much like that of the asylum patients; he was constantly ingesting purgatives and emetics. Unfortunately, his illness was severe, and he died in 1827, at the age of 24.)

As a psychological approach to mental illness, moral treatment differed from twentieth-century therapies in one important respect: it did not directly engage disordered mental processes—hallucinations, phobias, delusions, or whatever. Tuke had written that "no advantage has been found to arise from reasoning with [the insane], on their particular hallucinations. ... In regard to melancholics, conversation on the subject of their despondency is to be found highly injudicious. The very opposite method is pursued" (26). Indeed, moral treatment was aimed at deflecting the patient's attention, "breaking up" irrational thoughts, as though they would shrivel up from sheer lack of exercise; that is, curing the disease by altering the content of thought.

Wyman also discovered the futility of arguing with deranged individuals but was occasionally willing to resort to trickery. Bowditch told a story of one patient who believed himself to be a convict under a death sentence and suffered so terribly from the delusion that Wyman thought he might be relieved by a full pardon. A bogus document was prepared, complete with a large seal, and delivered to the patient with appropriate ceremony.

The ruse worked for a few days, but the patient then claimed to have repeated his crime, "and nobody ever heard of a person being twice pardoned" (27). This is a fascinating little episode because, while it reveals Wyman's readiness to try unorthodox remedies, it also exposes his naivete with respect to the dynamics of delusion. Many decades would pass before Freud would begin his patient study of the psychological content of mental illness and peel back the layers of consciousness. Meanwhile, moral treatment studiously ignored aberrant thought and tried to shift the focus of attention.

To the extent that Wyman made mistakes in developing the moral treatment program, he erred in the direction of the humane and progressive. He underestimated the problem of security from the start. Patient Number Three eloped. The casebooks and Folsom's diary recorded numerous escapes; the attendants usually fetched the wayward patients back, although a few, like Three, eluded them. These unauthorized flights do not seem to have bothered Wyman very much, for he adopted no drastic measures to prevent them. Violence, however, was more troublesome. Wyman disliked mechanical restraints; he ordered them only as a last resort. Forty-Nine, who committed a whole string of misdeeds against himself and the attendants before he was placed in restraints, was a representative case in this respect. Wyman trusted patients with all manner of potentially lethal instruments: tableware, garden tools, billiard cues, and knitting and sewing needles; glass window panes were frequently shattered. Wyman got cracked on the head with a carpenter's hammer. Yet, when he balanced the risks against the therapeutic value of activities and windows that admitted light, the advantages always weighed in heavier. He observed, however, that very violent patients upset more tranquil boarders, sometimes causing a reversal in improvement. Therefore, in 1822 he prevailed upon the trustees to build a facility for isolating "raging female" patients. Strong rooms for violent male patients were constructed in 1826.

The quarters for women must have been unsatisfactory in some respect because they were razed and supplanted by a new structure in 1836; we know only that they contained five rooms. However, the "lodge" or "retreat" for males received quite a bit of attention, and Wyman's son Morrill left a detailed description of the building. Erected according to Wyman's specifications, it was a 54- × 23-foot two-story brick structure containing four strong rooms on the upper floor. The lower story, a below-grade cellar, held heating stoves. The rooms were built as islands, each of two rooms, surrounded and separated by a continuous corridor some four or five feet in width. Light entered the corridor through ordinary glazed windows in the exterior walls and penetrated the strong rooms through unglazed openings. Wyman and the builders adapted the ingenious method of heating and ventilation that had been used by the Romans in Pompeii; they also included many thoughtful details such as rounded corners in the rooms, as well as inclined floors with drainage systems that enabled the attendants to keep the quarters clean with a minimum of fuss and discomfort to the patients. For, as Wyman had discovered, "what can not be done easily, is not likely to be done at all" (28).

Morrill Wyman wrote that "By strict rule of the Asylum these rooms were the first visited in the morning. Every morning before breakfast the patient was bathed and placed in a similar adjoining room. Everything which had become soiled was removed, the room well washed, and the walls and floor carefully cleaned with transparent lime-water, which left the walls free from odor and visible lime deposit" (29). Altogether, Wyman considered assigning a violent patient to the lodge preferable to placing him or her in mechanical restraints for several days. The solution was easier on the attendants and healthier for the other patients. Isolation was also believed to becalm the violent person by reducing sensory stimulation. As soon as the violence abated, the patient returned to the company in the wing.

Wyman's 1822 annual report, though characteristically modest in language, was an optimistic document. As noted earlier, his figures showed a cure rate of approximately 24 percent; cured patients plus those "improved" and "much improved" accounted for 56 percent. (Three unfit subjects, six elopements, and nine deaths are not part of these calculations.) To a public which had given up hope for treating mental illness, these statistics were positively inspiring. Therefore, the trustees printed Wyman's report and included it in a 34-page fund-raising appeal circulated in 1823. The bottom line of this long-winded pamphlet was the gloomy financial fact that "the debts of the institution [hospital and asylum] being $19,850, and the income of its property not enough to pay the salaries" (30).

The trustees' effort may or may not have influenced the next major financial event in the asylum's history; it does, however, document the institution's unstable fiscal condition. For whatever reasons, some months after this appeal, on November 2, 1823, the trustees discovered, much to their delight, that a Boston merchant, one John McLean, had named the asylum in his will. McLean had made the asylum his residuary legatee; that residue would yield almost $95,000 over the next three years. He had further provided that the asylum would receive an additional $25,000 upon the death of his widow.

According to Bowditch, John McLean was a "truly noble specimen of a Boston merchant" (31). He had inherited a great deal of money, increased his fortune, then lost the whole bundle and had to settle his affairs in bankruptcy court. However, he had the luck of Antonio in *The Merchant of Venice*: A ship that had been presumed lost sailed into Boston harbor with McLean's valuable cargo intact. He promptly invited his former creditors, who had been shortchanged in the bankruptcy proceedings, to dine at a Boston hotel and slipped a check for the balance due, principal plus interest, under each plate. Of such stuff is the Boston legend made!

It is not clear why McLean chose to favor the asylum in his will, for he had shown no interest in it before and was not among the original subscribers. However, he was childless and therefore probably more thoughtful than average in planning the disposition of his estate. That his wife's family, the Amorys, were strong supporters of the hospital may have borne on his decision. He may have acted on the advice of friends or lawyers, or he may have had some private reason to care about the mentally ill.

Whatever McLean's motives, the trustees happily accepted his legacy which, as Bowditch pointed out, "served to relieve the institution from embarrassments" (32). A committee was immediately appointed to commission McLean's portrait—the customary tribute to big benefactors. Gilbert Stuart produced a likeness of the well-fed McLean seated at a writing desk. It is a handsome painting, on today's market worth nearly as much as the McLean legacy. Meanwhile, the widow McLean expressed her wish that her late husband's name be perpetuated by changing the name of the hospital corporation in his honor. Though she pressed her case aggressively, the trustees were not prepared to go that far. They compromised by agreeing to rename the asylum. Thus, in 1826, the Asylum in Charlestown became the McLean Asylum for the Insane.

Wyman felt the effects on the McLean legacy almost instantly, in a manner which must have warmed his heart. Three weeks after they had learned about the will, the trustees created the position of steward at the asylum and elected John M. Goodwin to fill it, thereby relieving Wyman of a set of routine, time-consuming, nonmedical tasks. At their next meeting on December 7, 1823, the trustees had to turn down several applications for admission because the asylum was full. Accordingly, Wyman began to advance arguments and plans for expansion to which, given McLean's money, the trustees listened sympathetically.

A major building program finally got under way in 1826, and over the next three years the trustees spent nearly $100,000 to enlarge the asylum and update the existing facilities. Two new buildings for patients were erected: the "north building," an addition to the male wing, three stories in height with a five-story dome; and the aforementioned lodge, which while adding square footage did not increase asylum capacity, since when a violent patient was assigned to the strong rooms his regular quarters in the wings were kept vacant, awaiting his return. Other items in the building program were a new laundry, new kitchen, improvements and repairs in existing patient wings, extensive repairs and additions to the mansion, and landscaping. Pending the completion of new patient quarters, Wyman and the trustees opened up space for new admissions by discharging some patients considered incurable.

McLean's expanded quarters added more patients to the register and enabled Wyman to group them according to a system he believed therapeutically beneficial. He made a series of divisions, separating first the sexes, then the quiet from "the noisy and violent, the clean from the dirty, the clothed from the naked and the latter from each other, that one patient should in the least possible degree disturb or offend another. Each division should form a little family, producing the greatest degree of comfort and happiness of which its members are susceptible."

Wyman distinguished four classes of patients, based primarily on degrees of agitation and habits of personal hygiene and ranging from those who were "generally tranquil, harmless, susceptible of much enjoyment, capable of walking abroad without an attendant, and violent." The broad categories were further subdivided into "families," each one consisting of the patients on one floor of a wing. Social and economic origins acted as secondary ordering elements in Wyman's scheme. Except for the "very noisy, dirty, and violent," whose money and breeding carried no weight, patients who paid more got better accommodations, and, if quiet, they occasionally even got small apartments with servants' quarters in the front part of the physician's mansion. Wyman opposed the indiscriminate mingling of social classes on the grounds that they differed in "habits and feelings." Of course, his attitudes conformed to the mores of his era. Wyman's classification had nothing to do with differential diagnosis. It developed from his effort to create the healthiest possible environment for each patient and, in his administration, approached something like individual treatment.

On May 17, 1832, Wyman startled the trustees with his resignation, which cited reasons of health. He had long suffered from a pulmonary condition which often laid him low in the family apartment in the mansion and which by that time had become quite debilitating. It was on this occasion that it was observed that Wyman, during 14 years of service, had never taken a vacation and had spent all but five nights at the asylum. Rather than accept his resignation, the trustees offered him a leave of absence plus a $500 bonus "for his extra services" (33). Wyman thanked them for their kindness, took the money, and set off for a leisurely journey in New England with his wife and daughter. But he was a working man to the core. When he learned of an outbreak of Asiatic cholera in Canada, he left his family and rushed to Montreal to pursue investigations concerning the question of contagion of that disease. Unfortunately, he contracted violent diarrhea—not cholera, but a typhoid-like illness—returned to McLean quickly, and grew progressively worse.

On August 1, feeling frail and no doubt guilty about neglecting his duties, Wyman again asked the trustees to accept his resignation. They pretended to agree, telling him he could keep his residence at the asylum. Meanwhile, the doctor who had been assigned to McLean during Wyman's absence and illness continued to tend the patients. Then, in mid-September, the trustees voted to separate the offices of superintendent and physician at the asylum (just as Bulfinch had recommended) and begged Wyman to accept the physician's office at the same salary he had received with the dual responsibilities. Wyman relented. Administrative aides were enlisted. One Captain Luke Bigelow became superintendent in October, at $700 per year; Mary Sawyer was appointed "Supervisor of the female department." Feminists take note: In January 1834, the trustees raised Sawyer's pay to $200!

The new arrangement of officers displeased the trustees for reasons now lost. In March 1834, they recombined the superintendent and physician—namely, Wyman—made Bigelow the "Steward," and hired Dr. Thomas G. Lee as assistant physician. For the first time in nearly 16 years, Wyman had full-time, full-fledged medical help. But Wyman, by then in his late fifties, had worn out and kept renewing his appeals to the trustees to find a replacement for him. They finally gave in on January 9, 1835, the resignation to take effect on May 1. They could at last release Wyman because they had identified his successor in the person of young Lee, who had gained their confidence during his few months at McLean.

In promoting Lee, the trustees tried to protect him against the erosion of physical health, and perhaps of spirit, that had brought Wyman's term to an end. Lee was requested "not to confine himself too strictly to his duties, or debar himself from the enjoyment of social intercourse with his friends, or to neglect that occasional relaxation by which his health may be improved and preserved" (34). As for Wyman, the trustees voted him a departing gift of $1,000 and the corporation elected him a trustee, but he declined the role. Having served the asylum with absolute attention for 16 years, he surrendered it completely.

He retired to rural Roxbury and lived there quietly, reflectively, until June 1842, when he died of a lung infection.

Wyman's last major report to the trustees, printed in 1834, consisted largely of statistical analyses of all the patients who had passed through McLean during the first 15 years of operation. A total of 1,015 cases had been admitted, including one male child, age 10, and nine persons between ages 70 and 80. "The most prominent of the predisposing and exciting causes of insanity, in the cases admitted, are intemperance, insane ancestors, pregnancy and the succeeding states of parturition and lactation. To these I ought to add masturbation by both sexes, as a frequent cause of insanity." Of the 1,015 total, 12 were unfit, 89 had died, and 21 eloped; 140 were considered improved, 144 much improved, and 362 recovered, leaving only 180 removed in a "not improved" condition and another 67 remaining in the asylum. Wyman noted that the recovery rate for the first five years had been only 28.5 percent, whereas it jumped to 43 percent during the second five and 40 percent during the last five. He attributed the dramatic change to the 1823 regulation stipulating full payment of board for a three-month period. Even so, patients who might have benefited from still longer treatment had been withdrawn before they could achieve a complete recovery. Nevertheless, this was a happy set of figures.

Wyman's reporting system had some huge gaps, lacunae that went unremarked upon at the time when people were still flushed with the success of achieving any progress at all with the mentally ill. Wyman never offered precise definitions of improved, much improved, recovered, or cured, nor did anyone demand them. This omission becomes statistically significant when Wyman's figures are compared with McLean casebooks and registers. The 1,015 "boarders received" in his 1833 report were not 1,015 different women and men; a number of them were readmissions, and some individuals had been readmitted more than once. Wyman's only allusion to this situation was his remark that "those readmitted received new numbers in the Books." Relapses occurred with notable frequency among patients who would now be diagnosed as schizophrenics or manic-depressives. Many of the readmitted patients had previously been discharged improved, much improved, and in a few instances, recovered. Wyman, the Visiting Committee, and the trustees knew these facts, but the reports did not engage them. Wyman was not being dishonest; he merely used the standard bookkeeping and reporting practices of similar institutions of the time. Still, he surely recognized that his figures concealed as much as they revealed.

Therefore, having told the happy stories of Patients Number One and Number Forty-Nine, this chapter ends with the cautionary tale of Patient Number Three, whose tenure at McLean outlasted Wyman's. Luther Bell, who became superintendent and physician in 1837, took inventory of the patients bequeathed to him by his predecessors and discovered among them a man who

> was the third patient received in the Asylum; his first entry having been October 16, 1818, at 32, disease having then been four years in standing and having been occasioned by "loss of property and disappointment in matrimony." No history of the case is on file or on record. His mother recently told me that about embargo and war times he was engaged in commerce to various parts of the globe as a supercargo, was active, enterprising, and successful which latter fact is proved by the circumstances of a property having been acquired before his derangement on which he has been supported to the present day. His derangement came during some of his voyages, and he continued to go to sea even after his mind was deemed much insane and even ran risks of capture &c. which no rational man would have done. He remained at home, traveling and roaming until this Institution was opened. He remained here only until November 11, 1818 when he is recorded as "eloped, improved." June 12, 1819 he was returned and remained till July 1, 1820, when he was again at the request of his friends discharged improved. January 12, 1824, he was again admitted and in the record it is stated that "of late he has been violent; was once on the point of throwing a flatiron at a female; once attempted to cudgel a man; now is brought from the public jail at Ipswich, somewhat dirty in appearance—wants to take lodgings in the center house [i.e., physician's residence]—holds long arguments on the impropriety of his being kept under lock and key &c." Stated that he plays draughts &c.
>
> During his preceding residence the only facts reported as to him are his irritability and his once or twice going without food—once for four days and then voluntarily ate. In tracing his history through the case books to the present time little occurs worth mentioning, except his irritability—quarrels with other patients, habit of jumping from spot to spot into the airflues with his feet sometimes falling and injuring the back of his head, and evidence of his gradually falling into state of dementia; was removed to the lower story some ten years since.
>
> Since my residence, his mind is almost entirely gone, yet he will sometimes recollect and speak freely of parts of the globe he has visited; he is

not very irascible though occasionally will have fits of passion when he will break glass, and tear his clothes. The points most worthy of note are the perfect manner in which his erect gentlemanly bearing and address on first being saluted are maintained. When dressed up to walk out, he presents a countenance of more intelligence and character than nine out of ten in State Street. Another peculiarity is his disposition to injure himself. . . . So he has frequently put tight rings on his fingers, producing pain and suppuration; yet so fond is he of the excitement of suffering that he must be held while they are cut off. If he can get a sore on his shin he will torture it, so that month after month will pass before it is allowed to get well. He will open his window on the coldest nights, is much and long given to masturbation, which perhaps is the first and perpetuating cause of his insanity. . . . His demency is yearly augmenting and bids fair to end in complete fatuity. General health good. Never married. (35)

CHAPTER

3

Luther V. Bell: The Golden Age of Moral Treatment

Moral treatment made a substantial impact in a relatively short time. Wyman and superintendents of other institutions practicing the therapy advanced statistics proving its effectiveness. Wyman's claims were humble by some standards; the Hartford Retreat reported a recovery rate of over 91 percent during the year 1827. Never mind that the numbers had been arrived at by measuring "recovery" only among discharged patients rather than as a fraction of the whole number treated. These figures, along with sympathetic descriptions of the Hartford establishment, received widespread newspaper coverage. Presented with such evidence, the public willingly exchanged its belief in the incurability of insanity for what Pliny Earle would later call the "curability delusion." Circulation of the Hartford cure rate also stimulated the competitive juices of certain other asylum superintendents who adopted perverse methods of statistical manipulation to arrive at comparable results. Whatever the flaws of his own figures, Wyman had not deliberately participated in this inflationary spiral. No wonder he was wary of publicity.

Confidence in curability as well as in the decency of therapeutic methods led to the building of more mental hospitals. Public sympathy and funds could be engaged by an image of institutions which treated the mentally ill with dignity and discharged them as productive members of society. In 1828 young Horace Mann, a state representative in Massachusetts, stood before the legislature and delivered a passionate appeal based on the principle that "the insane are the wards of the state." That speech gave rise to the committee that recommended the construction of a state hospital for the mentally ill. Worcester was selected as its site; Wyman was invited to offer his professional opinion on architectural matters; and the State Asylum opened in 1833 with Dr. Samuel B. Woodward as its superintendent.

The Worcester asylum drew its first patients from Massachusetts jails and almshouses. It was supposed to care for the mentally ill who could not afford even the modest rates of McLean or those for whom McLean did not have any space. The McLean trustees discussed, a little apprehensively, the likelihood that their own census would drop off sharply. Although McLean had never had large numbers of paupers, it was assumed that they, along with patients whose families had to strain to pay charges, would use Worcester. But the anticipated population decline never occurred. Instead, the existence of the state facility produced changes in the social configuration at McLean. Towns sent their paupers to Worcester while wealthier families showed more eagerness to refer mentally ill relatives to McLean, where they would no longer have to fraternize with the destitute. Only six years after Worcester had opened, McLean had more applicants than it could accommodate. Rather than refuse admission to a patient, which had never been done and which, moreover, violated their principles, the trustees simply decided to raise the rate of board to no less than $3.00 per week for Massachusetts residents and $4.50 for out-of-staters, who constituted roughly one-third of the boarders. The trustees took this step with clear consciences, reassuring themselves that the local poor had a refuge in Worcester, while any out-of-stater who could afford the trip to Massachusetts could also afford higher rates. Thus did the socioeconomic level of McLean patients begin its upward creep.

But the story has gotten a little ahead of itself, and it is time to go back and pick up the reins handed over in May 1835 to Dr. Thomas G. Lee. Lee was a mere 26 years old when he became the McLean superintendent. Adulthood and its responsibilities arrived much earlier in those days of shorter life spans. Before coming to McLean as first assistant physician in 1834, Lee had worked as an assistant physician at the Hartford Retreat—they of the 91 percent cure rate—with Dr. Eli Todd, and therefore had direct experience of moral treatment and asylums.

Lee found Wyman's regimen somewhat stuffy. Before the end of 1835 he introduced a number of new diversions. The trustees were induced to purchase a piano, a billiard table, books for a library, and materials for a carpentry shop for male patients. In Wyman's tenure, well-behaved patients had been permitted to attend religious services outside the asylum; Lee arranged for them to be conducted at McLean on Sundays. He encouraged female patients to occupy themselves with sewing, and they formed a group that they called the "Belknap Sewing Society." Firmly convinced that "useful labor is the best employment," Lee put male patients to work on the asylum farm and gardens, females in the laundry and kitchen.

On the recreational side, Lee reported that "the better class [in this context a medical, not a social, distinction] of patients are now invited once a week to a dancing party in the oval room, the evening is spent in dancing, marching, and cheerful conversation. The presence of all the officers, and as many of the nurses and attendants as can be spared from the wings . . . is security" (1). After 18 years of rigid segregation, the sexes were permitted to mingle. At least 40 patients regularly dined with Lee's family. He hired more attendants, increasing their numbers from 11 to an average of 14.5, or one for every six patients. Suicidal boarders always had individual attendants, and the extra expense was charged to their accounts.

Lee also experimented a little with medical remedies; his successor noted that "In 1836 Dr. Lee placed most of the old and hopeless cases on the 'opium treatment,' but without any change resulting therefrom, and it being very difficult subsequently to abandon its use" (2). One observes the efforts of these pioneer physicians with admiration. The becalming effects of opium were well known, and the substance was easy to obtain. Its indiscriminate employment would have made the management of asylums much simpler. But the doctors also knew about opium addiction and were therefore extremely careful about administering the drug. They did not take the easy way out.

The energetic, articulate, and resourceful young superintendent pleased everyone, from McLean patients and staff to the trustees, with both his performance and "the cheerfulness and gentleness of his deportment, and the piety which was the habitual guide of his life" (3). Though no less devoted to duty than Wyman, Lee did from time to time seek a change of scenery. Toward the end of October 1836, feeling slightly under the weather, he called on his friend and colleague Woodward at the Worcester asylum. Lee's symptoms, presumably of typhus, immediately grew worse. Woodward put him to bed and notified Mrs. Lee, who in turn informed the trustees. The latter convened a special session on October 23 and dispatched two of their members plus the venerable Dr. Jackson to Lee's bedside. Unfortunately, they could do nothing for him, and he died six days later, at the tender age of 28.

The trustees hastened to find yet another superintendent. Jackson submitted the name of Dr. Edward Jarvis, a physician then practicing out in Concord, Massachusetts. Jarvis's candidacy was further supported by a strong letter from Ralph Waldo Emerson. Jarvis wanted the position badly, and with recommendations like these, it is hard to understand how he failed to get it, though perhaps Emerson's opinion did not count for much in medical circles. When Jarvis learned the job had gone to someone else, he packed up in a huff and moved to Louisville, Kentucky.

The someone else was Dr. Luther V. Bell, of Derry, New Hampshire, who recalled the circumstances of his appointment as follows:

> While attending the winter session of the New Hampshire Legislature, of which I was a member and had taken some interest in stirring up the people to the foundation of an insane Asylum, I received an intimation from Mr. Cowes of Portsmouth by letter, very obscurely, that my name had been mentioned as a candidate for the vacant office at Charlestown and advising me to present myself at Boston, which after some hesitation thinking the chance so small, I did carrying a line of introduction from him to the Rev. Louis Dwight. There I saw one or two of the Trustees and the next day returned home. Not hearing anything for a week or two, the expectation of receiving the appointment rested so little on my

> mind that I commenced making preparations to remove to Concord [New Hampshire] to engage in practice at the conclusion of the session. . . . I accordingly advertised my property at Derry, and notified my townsmen of my proposed removal. Toward the close of Dec. I received a letter of appointment from . . . the Trustees, and requesting my attendance to meet them forthwith. (4)

By the time he wrote this account, Bell's memory was a little off. His appointment actually occurred on December 11, and he accepted it on December 16.

Bell is one of the most fascinating and capable men who ever had charge of McLean. Fortunately, there is an ample record of his life, both in his own words and in the writings of others, so he can be delineated with more assurance than Wyman.

Bell was born on December 20, 1806, in Francestown, New Hampshire, into a distinguished family of Scotch-Irish Presbyterian ancestry. His paternal grandfather had fought in the Revolutionary War and later became a state senator. His father, Samuel, a lawyer, served as governor of New Hampshire for one term and as a U.S. senator for two terms. Samuel married twice. Luther was the youngest of four boys, among six children from the first marriage. His mother died before he was four years old. He was said to have been a very bright and lovable child. He was certainly an enterprising one. Feeling handicapped by the lack of a middle initial, he inserted a "V." in his name, "so that he might show as many initials in his signature as other boys" (5). He kept the "V." throughout his life, leading some people to think it stood for "Virgil." Posterity, in the form of the *Dictionary of American Biography*, decided it stood for "Vose." It didn't.

Luther moved quickly through private schooling and entered Bowdoin College in 1819, when he was only 12, young even by the standards of his times. Among his friends there was Franklin Pierce, two years older but one year behind him in the college, who was a distant relative—their mothers were cousins and they both came from political families—and who one day would be a somewhat inept American president. Bell also befriended Pierce's chum, Nathaniel Hawthorne, and knew Henry Wadsworth Longfellow, who, like Pierce, entered Bowdoin at the age of 14. (Colleges of the early nineteenth century were obviously very different from our contemporary institutions.)

The record of Bell's conduct as a student is almost unblemished; one infraction, some trivial misdemeanor, rescues it from monotonous perfection. His academic achievement was respectable, and he graduated on schedule in 1823.

The tall, skinny, 16-year-old headed directly for New York to begin his study of medicine under the tutelage of his older brother John. Later he attended medical lectures at Dartmouth College and obtained a professional degree in September 1826, before he had turned 20. He returned to New York and cast around for opportunities to practice his new profession. Convinced by family and friends that he was too young to practice, he occupied himself for a year in the counting house of his brother-in-law's mercantile establishment and, after that, in the care of his consumptive sister. When she died, Bell returned to New Hampshire and in 1831 set up medical practice in Derry. Three years later he married a Derry woman, Frances Clark Pinkerton.

Bell's memorialists maintained that he was a first-rate country doctor. That is to be expected. Memorialists are not in the habit of saying "so-and-so was a rotten doctor, lawyer, or whatever"; that is the dirty work of more remote historians. Still, in Bell's case, there is no evidence to contradict the claims of excellence, and much to support them. As an example, there is the story of young Bell's having been summoned several miles from his office to the aid of an overweight, hard-drinking farmer whose leg had been crushed and required amputation. Realizing that delay would be fatal, Bell improvised instruments from farmhouse tools, performed the surgery, and later carved a wooden leg for his patient, who lived on many years working as a bricklayer. While making his daily rounds through the agricultural precincts of New Hampshire, Bell distinguished himself from the run-of-the-mill country doctor by displaying an active interest in medical research. In 1834 and 1835 he produced dissertations on vegetarianism (he argued against it, and this paper earned him the Boylston Medical Prize for 1834), diagnostic procedures (principally of respiratory ailments), and the epidemiology of smallpox and related diseases.

Around this time New Hampshire became embroiled in public debates about a state institution for the mentally ill, a cause which interested Bell greatly. Apparently he had inherited the political instincts of his grandfather and father, for he chose to wage the debate on political turf. With the singular objective of arousing public sentiment for the foundation of an insane asylum, Bell offered himself as a candidate for the seat representing his town in the state legislature. He won the election handily, no doubt aided by confidence in the Bell name.

Once in office, Bell succeeded in getting himself assigned to the special committee which had been designated to investigate the number and condition of the mentally ill in the state. He prepared the committee report that proposed the establishment of a state institution modeled on the Massachusetts asylum at Worcester. In the words of George E. Ellis's charming memoir, that report "terrified the representatives of the people, as involving an immediate outlay equal to half the annual expenses of the State Government." The politicians, therefore, returned the question to the voters. Bell worked furiously on behalf of a state institution, firing off articles to the press, charging around the state to make public speeches, collecting every iota of data he could about existing cases of mental illness. It was that campaign that brought him to the attention of the McLean trustees. Their invitation caught him more or less *in medias res.* (The New Hampshire Asylum for the Insane was formally established in 1838 and erected in Concord four years later.)

Bell's enterprises as physician, researcher, and politician, all in the decade of his twenties, foreshadowed his energetic career in maturity. Unlike Wyman, who had led an almost cloistered existence within asylum walls attending to his patients with religious devotion, Bell engaged in numerous activities outside McLean. Many of them, such as his research and organizational efforts, concerned problems of mental illness and will be discussed later in this chapter. But Bell's enthusiasms extended well beyond professional boundaries. Encouraged by his success in the New Hampshire legislature, and by force of family habit, he kept alive his political ties. In the early 1850s, Bell campaigned vigorously in behalf of the moribund Whig party, much to the distress of certain friends who thought a man of his professional stature ought not be mucking about in anything so vulgar and who further disapproved of Whig compromise politics. He became their candidate, by acclaim, for the Seventh Congressional District in Massachusetts while he was still superintendent at McLean. He won a plurality of the vote on the first ballot but lost in the run-off election. In 1853 he was a working member of the State Convention for revising the Constitution. In 1856 the Massachusetts Whigs fielded him as their candidate for governor, presumably against his will.

Bell's restless, inquisitive mind went off in yet other directions. Columbus Tyler, for many years the steward at McLean, who saw a great deal of Bell, described some of his other talents:

> He was fond of architecture and the mechanic arts. With an eye quick to perceive, he had a wonderful power in the adaptation of means to ends. He had great skill in the rough drawing of beasts, birds, and men; and, to please the children, by a few strokes of the pen would make otherwise natural figures most grotesquely ridiculous. . . . I have no doubt that he was the first person who passed communications over the electric telegraph. He declared such to be the fact. The communications were fully and accurately established; but owing to some difficulty in the machinery for expressing the thoughts conveyed, with funds failing, the labor was for the time suspended; and, in the interim, his friend and associate died. He petitioned Congress for remuneration, and claimed himself to be the inventor. At the same time he was interested in a loom, or gin, for the manufacture of flax; which, I understood from him, was perfected, and is now in successful operation abroad. I was quite interested in a bed he made with his own hands to keep himself dry while in or out of camp. Taking two India-rubber sheets, he sewed them together on the sides and at one end, with blankets intervening,—leaving one end open like a great bag, into which he slipped; reposing dry and warm, however damp the ground or atmosphere might be. (6)

Tyler's account, particularly of Bell's claims to invention of the telegraph, ought to be taken with a grain of salt and the passing comment that patent squabbles in the nineteenth century were Byzantine events; from time to time legitimate inventors did indeed fail to collect the credit, let alone the royalties, they deserved. Whatever the truth in this instance, schoolchildren are left with Samuel F. B. Morse's immortal "What hath God wrought?" instead of a *bon mot* from Bell.

Bell's adventures in spiritualism form a spooky chapter in his life. Spiritualism was that movement based on the belief that spirits of the dead communicate with the living, usually through a medium—a world of seances, mysterious rappings, and levitating furniture. Spiritualism enjoyed measurable popularity in mid-nineteenth-century America, a fact that profoundly distressed American scientists. Bell estimated that there were over two million devotees; some other estimates were higher. Since science had not yet gained a secure foothold in public confidence, quasi-scientific or off-the-wall movements presented real competition. Phrenology, for example, was also very much in vogue. So proximate were the domains of science and superstition in the age that Johann Kaspar Spurzheim, an apostle of phrenology, had actually been giving a course in brain anatomy at the medical college when he died in 1832; the Massachusetts Medical Society mourned his passing. That such educated rational individuals as John Roebling, engineer of the Brooklyn Bridge, were attracted to spiritualism suggested that it was a competitor of some power. Scientists customarily dismissed it as humbug and refused to confront it, though physicist Joseph Henry confidently offered a substantial sum to anyone who could make *his* tables move in the Smithsonian Institution.

In the early 1850s, after a number of supposedly well-balanced acquaintances, not to mention patients at McLean, insisted that they had found a channel of communication with the dead, Bell attended some seances in what he explained as a scientific investigation. He made no secret of his visits to mediums. In fact, he often invited skeptical friends to accompany him to sittings. Consequently, rumors began to circulate that the eminent Dr. Bell was dabbling in spiritualism. The gossip alarmed and embarrassed his colleagues and must have caused a few furrowed brows among the McLean trustees. Bell, however, could not be dissuaded from his "research." Dr. Isaac Ray, another asylum superintendent who knew Bell, later justified his friend's interest as a proper one. Bell, Ray explained,

> believed it to be within the limits of legitimate scientific inquiry, and well worth the attention of those whose special province is to study the mind, both in the normal and the abnormal state. It is not strange that one who, for so many years, had been devoted to this study, should have been strongly moved by the accounts which daily came to his ears, of performances among his neighbors, some of whom were his most respected and intelligent friends, that indicated apparently some psychological agency which, if not new and original, was strange and curious. Indeed, he felt that he would be false to his professional trust if he neglected to improve

> the opportunity thus placed before him, for the good of science and humanity.

Still, something about Bell made Ray remark upon "his peculiar turn of mind" (7).

On two occasions Bell discussed spiritualism at meetings of the Association of Medical Superintendents of American Institutions for the Insane, of which he was a cofounder and which will be described in greater detail later. The subject made the audience acutely uncomfortable. Bell's first paper was neither published nor reported in the pages of the *American Journal of Insanity*, where association papers customarily appeared, "by request of several members. They considered that the whole subject was then too immature, and so much connected in the public mind with the ridiculous, as to make it inexpedient that it should be more than generally announced as among the topics discussed by the Association." However, the journal did print an extensive summary of Bell's second presentation. He opened with detailed descriptions of the antics of one extremely lively table along with the steps he took to assure himself that concealed wires or other mechanisms had not been used during the performance. He gave an astonishing account. The summary concludes:

> Dr. B. was understood to say that this made five or six times in which he had seen the table move without human contact, and all under circumstances apparently as free from suspicion as this just related. He also stated that the Rev. Mr. P., a clergyman of extraordinary sagacious perceptions and mechanical skill, took this same medium to his own house, without previous thought, where she never before had been, and where his own table, in the presence of his own family alone, went through the fullest locomotion without human touch. Dr. B. mentioned that, in his last experiment—that just narrated—the entire space moved through was over fifty feet.

Bell turned without further elaboration to the matter of conversation with spirits of the dead.

> The result of the inquiries of Dr. B. and his friends—for several gentlemen of eminently fitting talents pursued the investigation with him—was briefly this: *that what the questioner knows, the spirits know; what the questioner does not know, the spirits are entirely ignorant of.* In other words, that there are really no superhuman agencies in the matter at all—no connection with another state of existence; but that it bears certain strong analogies to some of the experiences of *clairvoyance*, in that mys-

> terious science of animal magnetism, as it has been protruding and receding for the last hundred years. . . . Dr. B. concluded by the expression of his full conviction that, while a faith in spirits must be given up, as connected with these facts, it was a topic, whether regarded as a psychical novelty or even as a delusion, cutting deeply into the very religious nature of our people, which was worth our fullest examination. (8)

Though relieved by Bell's conclusions about spirits of the dead, association members were disturbed by his failure to account for the perambulations of tables and the rapping noises through which the so-called spirits telegraphed their messages. The summary leaves the impression that while Bell discredited the existence of spirits, he was satisfied that the medium could indeed move tables without muscular or mechanical intervention. He seems never to have qualified his account by saying "well, I suspect there is some hocus-pocus going on here, but I can't for the life of me make out what it is," or words to that effect. Therefore, it is not surprising that many people in the audience suspected that Bell was more of a believer than not. Perhaps it was his inability to explain those phenomena scientifically that prevented Bell from publishing any papers on spiritualism. As he confessed to his friend, Dorothea Dix, "If I can believe anything, I must believe that there are new and before unknown *influences* or whatever you may choose to term them brought into relation between mind and matter" (9). Rumors concerning his convictions continued to dog him long after he had quit attending seances, despite his assertions that "I never was a believer in Spiritualism; on the contrary, I always supposed I did as much as any man in New England to put a stop to that gigantic epidemic, by demonstrating that its facts were only those of old Mesmerism, &c., and that the mediums never told what the inquirer did not know before" (10).

Bell was a long, lean man. At six feet two inches, he towered over most of his contemporaries. He was a handsome figure whose grace of carriage was accentuated by a certain negligence in his dress. He had a full head of dark hair and bushy eyebrows. A portrait in oil finds him clean shaven; a photograph captures him with a well-trimmed beard, looking something like Abraham Lincoln. His personality is described variously as urbane, just, aloof, warm, patient, humorous, moody, gentle—in short, a variegated man who eluded capsule definitions. Ray wrote that "With all his ability he manifested the gentleness of a child, and, contrary to the usual course, I apprehend, the older he grew, the more gentle, the more patient, the more forbearing, the more tender he became." Bell was apparently absolutely unflappable, a characteristic that came in handy in dealing with the mentally ill. Ellis, who often visited McLean, remembered one incident in particular.

> As I approach the entrance door of the Asylum . . . a carriage drew up, from which issued the most distressing and heart-piercing screams, as of one in the intensest agony of body and mind. Three men, friendly, but not professional, attendants, had alighted from the carriage; thus wholly disabling themselves from any power of control over their charge, whom they left in it. That charge was a woman suffering from extreme mania. She thought herself surrounded by flames, and blazing in torture. She threw herself wildly about in the carriage, lacerating herself with the broken glass, beating her dress as if to extinguish the fire, and screaming most piteously for "water! water!" Surrounded by a group of paralyzed observers, who knew not what it was wise or safe to do, the sufferer was left to herself for a few minutes that seemed hours. Dr. Bell, summoned from some inner apartment, appeared, to give us all sweet relief; for we felt that we shared it with the patient. He approached the door of the carriage, fixed his gentle eye upon her, and, with mild tones of ordinary speech, said, "Madam, come with me, and you shall have water." She smiled pleasantly, took the proffered arm, and passed into the Asylum as if bent on a stroll through its beautiful gardens.

In December 1836, when Bell accepted the trustees' offer to become superintendent and physician at McLean, he asked their permission to inspect other institutions before assuming his post. They granted him leave until March 1, 1837. He went first to Worcester where the hospitable Woodward took him under his wing and spent nearly two weeks sharing his institutional experience. Bell proceeded to the Hartford Retreat, intending to spend a few days there, but for some undisclosed reason was "not . . . particularly pleased," and left after a few hours; he did, however, hire an assistant physician for McLean. He quickly surveyed the Bloomingdale Asylum in New York, then decided not to bother with Philadelphia because the weather was foul and he did not feel well. So he returned to New Hampshire to tidy up his personal affairs. He makes no mention of having consulted Wyman, still very much alive in Roxbury—an omission that probably says more about Wyman's determination to have nothing to do with McLean than it does about Bell's motives. While he was preparing his household for removal to Massachusetts, Bell received a message from the trustees urging him to hasten to Charlestown because Columbus Tyler, the steward, was gravely ill and McLean desperately needed some leadership. Bell complied in haste and arrived at the asylum on February 11, a Saturday.

Bell found a slightly diminished patient census. There were only around 70 people in residence, largely because, given Tyler's sickness and the lack of a superintendent, the trustees had been refusing some admissions. A new building, begun during Lee's administration (known as the Belknap Ward in honor of its benefactor, Mary Belknap, who left nearly $90,000 to the asylum in her will in 1832) had been erected, closed in, and stood empty, awaiting further instructions. Bell moved swiftly and decisively. The building, for 50 female patients, was completed during 1837. That same year the admissions rate began a steep upwards climb. During 1837 the average number of patients on any given day was 80; during 1838 the figure increased to 95; in 1839 it was 112; and so on until 1850 when the average daily census reached 201, where it came to rest when Bell insisted, and the trustees agreed, that a larger institution would be unmanageable.

Meanwhile, there was a great clamor for entrance into McLean. Bell looked for ways to make room for those recently afflicted patients who were considered most likely to benefit from a course of moral treatment. His initial impulse upon arrival was to clean house. He reviewed the old cases and discharged some long-term patients who showed no improvement, among them a 70-year-old man, first admitted to McLean in 1823 and at that time a patient for the seventh time (11). The removal of "incurable," often elderly, patients in favor of promising candidates emphasized the asylum's therapeutic as opposed to custodial mission. But external circumstances soon enforced some modifications of attitude. In 1839, anticipating a day when patients would have to be turned away for lack of space, Bell hit upon the solution of discouraging applications by raising the rate of board. Nevertheless, by 1844 patients had to be refused for want of a room, and in 1852 more applicants were turned away than admitted.

Thus, in about a dozen years the McLean patient population nearly tripled. The physical plant strained to keep apace. Twelve rooms were added to the male patient wing in 1838; in 1839, scarcely two years after it had opened, Belknap House was enlarged. Two houses, one for men and the other for women, each accommodating eight patients and providing a suite of sitting room, bedroom, and bath for every boarder, were begun in 1850 and completed in 1853; they were named after William Appleton, president of the MGH Corporation, who had donated $20,000 toward their construction. Simultaneously, heating, water, and ventilation systems throughout the asylum were improved—the mechanically minded Bell being much interested in modern domestic comforts. Hot water heating was introduced in 1848. McLean tapped the Boston water supply in 1851. Gas was installed in 1854. Despite all this building activity, in 1852 when the average daily census stood at 200, McLean only had comfortable accommodations for 160. On some days as many as 210 patients crowded into attics and dormitories. Having already complained in his 1848 report that "the architecture is hopelessly inadequate" for such numbers, Bell in 1852 began to press for a second asylum, one to be used for women, the other for men. The trustees sympathized with his plan but did not think they would be able to promote it, so it never amounted to anything.

Of considerable satisfaction to the trustees and the corporation was the financial phenomenon at McLean. Beginning in 1842, the asylum began to defray its operating costs. In 1846 receipts exceeded expenses by approximately $1,300. Evidence of competent financial management made a good impression on benefactors, whose gifts enabled construction and renovation projects. Furthermore, by reflecting positively on the trustees, McLean's economic well being benefited the general hospital which for numerous reasons—not the least of which were the crude state of the medical arts and the utter terror with which educated people regarded hospitals—did not enjoy similar fiscal health.

The improvement in the asylum's accounts occurred not as a

consequence of the total increase in patient population but rather because a greater percentage of the patients came from financially sound families willing to pay charges well above the minimum rate of board. As mentioned at the outset of this chapter, the opening of the State Asylum at Worcester had relieved McLean of some obligation to paupers and lower-income patients. When the Boston Lunatic Hospital, a municipal institution, began receiving patients in 1839, McLean's responsibility to the financially less fortunate members of society diminished even further. (Incidentally, the Boston Lunatic Hospital was the asylum immortalized by Charles Dickens's tender description in his *American Notes*; it was one of the few things he admired in the United States.)

Bell's first annual report, of 1837, already noted that because of the Worcester facility McLean had become host to "an improved class of sufferers" and that the population was becoming more uniform "as respects external condition and position in society." "This increasing absence of patients from the pauper and humbler ranks of society has rendered the classification, especially of convalescents, far less embarrassing and difficult" —meaning *social* classification which, of course, was thought to have medical implications.

The trend continued, and Bell began to press for more luxurious patient accommodations. "In this asylum a large proportion of the inmates are from those classes of society whose artificial wants are many. They have become accustomed to a thousand minor comforts and attentions, which they peculiarly need when their minds are enfeebled by disease" (12). Carpeting, wallpaper, mirrors, open fireplaces, and more elegant furniture were introduced into patient quarters during the 1840s, on therapeutic grounds. The two Appleton houses, with suites that might lodge a private servant, represented yet another level of gentrification. By the end of Bell's administration in the late 1850s, McLean had evolved into an institution tilted in the direction of the privileged classes, and so it would remain. Accordingly, after the 1850s McLean and a handful of similar establishments traveled along a historical path parallel to, but distinct from, that of tax-supported mental hospitals. McLean, for instance, never had to cope with large numbers of mentally ill, impoverished immigrants who packed the wards of state institutions.

As the socioeconomic status of the McLean patient population followed an ascending curve, admissions policies gradually shifted. The Visiting Committee began to welcome long-term, "incurable" patients whose families were willing to pay high rates of board. The same Bell who discharged long-term, hopeless patients in 1838 wrote in 1843 that

> no hospital could receive its inmates with less discrimination, or with more unpromising cases. The epileptic, the demented, the paralytic, in every form of exhaustion, and complicated with every form of bodily malady, are alike welcomed as the curable forms of mania and delusion. Believing that one of the great ends of the institution as determined by its founders, was not only the recovery of the cūrable and the custodial comfort of the violent and troublesome, but also the relief of friends from the painful and anxious guardianship of the helpless and hopeless insane, we have never declined or avoided receiving any case, when the requisite evidences of insanity have been furnished.

Bell might have added that this policy was in tandem with adequate demonstration of financial ability to support the patient indefinitely. Here Bell was second-guessing the founders in much the same way that the Supreme Court reinterprets the intentions of the framers of the Constitution with reference to altered circumstances. The evidence shows that the founders had definitely not conceived of a guardian role for the asylum; but the founders had not foreseen the building of state hospitals or the day when affluent patients would constitute a significant portion of the asylum population. The hospitable policy toward "incurable" patients, which was humane, economically sensible, and unproblematic in Bell's time, would lead to difficulties later down the line.

Pauper patients became the exception at McLean. Those admitted, usually in some emergency, were soon transferred to a less costly facility. There were, however, many middle- or working-class patients, particularly people afflicted with those forms of mental illness that had a favorable prognosis. As Bell observed, "The records of this Asylum justify the declaration that *all cases certainly recent*, that is, whose origin does not either directly or obscurely run back more than a year, recover under a fair trial. This is the general law; the occasional instances to the contrary are the exception" (13). Bell, like Wyman, noticed that many of these patients were removed for want of funds before "fair trial" permitted cure to be effected. He encouraged William Appleton to establish a fund enabling these individuals to prolong treatment and allowing McLean to admit "desirable" patients for whom the $3.00 rate presented a hardship. Appleton donated $10,000 to this end in 1843; the following year McLean had around 30 patients paying only $1.50 per week. (Samuel Appleton added another $10,000 to this fund in 1854.) So, while the principle of no free beds prevailed, there existed a sort of scholarship fund available for financially pressed, promising cases, "affording aid to such patients. . . . as from straitened means might be compelled to leave the institution without a perfect cure" (14).

Creature comforts improved enormously. Admissions policies changed. Therapy, however, remained faithful to the principles of moral treatment. Bell did make some alterations in practice. He eliminated Lee's aggressive program of mechanical and agricultural labor in deference to the change in the social class of patients. Proper Victorian ladies and gentlemen did not soil their hands, and this was a Victorian society. Another of Lee's innovations, the mingling of sexes at religious services and dances, created numerous, unspecified "inconveniences," and Bell put an end to it. He also stopped the practice of permitting patients to be absent on "parole" because he discovered that, although the patients nearly always honored their promises to return, they usually came back more, rather than less, distraught. He concluded that "almost every patient, who was so far disordered in mind as to justify detention at all, was too much disordered for even a qualified liberty" (15). Whereas Lee had moved in the direction of flexibility, Bell tended toward discipline and control, administrative attitudes to some extent indicated by the vastly increased number of patients under his care, to some extent dictated by the social prejudices of mid-nineteenth-century New England.

Life at McLean, though more regimented than in earlier days, appeared to one eyewitness to be civilized and pacific, at least for the quieter patients. Marianne Finch, an Englishwoman who toured the United States in the early 1850s, reported visiting female wards at McLean with a friend from Cambridge:

> The steward and matron are man and wife and work together admirably —as man and wife always do when they are perfectly united. Some twenty years ago the matron entered the place as a patient, was cured, and has remained ever since in her present capacity. [This is more or less accurate. The steward, Tyler, was working as an attendant when Mary Sawyer was a patient. She stayed at McLean as an attendant after her recovery, and later married Tyler. He moved up the career ladder to Steward while she became first a "Supervisor" and later the "Matron." The Tylers remained at the asylum until 1863.] She is an excellent person, and much liked by the patients. She is firm and kind, and never known to lose her temper. . . .
>
> Those who have a private parlour and an attendant to themselves pay about one hundred and fifty pounds per annum; others, who cannot afford this, live in families of six or seven, having an attendant always with them. Each group has a sitting-room and a dining-room (opening into each other); a bedroom is provided for each person. The matron took me through five or six of these wards, occupied by women, introducing me to each person. Some of them were friendly—hoped I would come again and make a longer stay; others took little notice of me. They looked very comfortable, most of them either sewing or doing fancy work; in the latter they seemed much interested. (16)

Bell's term of office coincided with the beginning of a long international debate over the use of mechanical restraints as an adjunct to moral treatment. A vigorous nonrestraint crusade developed in England, where it was systematized by Dr. John Conolly, who upon becoming medical superintendent of the Middlesex Asylum at Hanwell in 1840, banished straitjackets, arm straps, confining chairs, and other devices from his premises. Other English institutions followed Conolly's example and adopted nonrestraint practices. Reports of their success quickly reached the United States, where most asylum superintendents greeted them resentfully. Which is not to say that American superintendents liked using restraints—nobody *liked* them, in principle—but, rather, that they could not see any practical, affordable alternative for managing violent patients. Since nonrestraint sounded attractive and humane, that portion of the American public that concerned itself with mental institutions argued the cause. Bell, for one, approached the debate sensibly. He had visited Hanwell during a European vacation in 1840. Conolly made a good impression on him—Bell remarked on his "urbanity" and the quality of his hospitality—and after his return to McLean Bell followed the Hanwell experiment closely. He observed that according to Conolly's reports, while devices restraining the torso and limbs had indeed been eliminated, various contrivances were employed to prevent patients from removing their clothing, as was a "stuffed glove without a division for the thumbs and fingers" for patients who tried to tear their garments or strike others. Remarked Bell:

> Any gentleman, familiar with the management of this, or I believe any other of the New England institutions, from their origin, will at once declare, if this is all that is meant by an absolute disuse of restraining means. . . . our experience for years may encourage them to go on freely.
>
> An amount of restraint less than is intimated in [Hanwell's] exceptions has long proved adequate in this institution. . . . But to lay down the broad absolute rule of disusing all the mild forms of restraint, would not comport with the best good of an institution. . . . [As to McLean,] for some years the average number of patients under the restraint of leather mittens has not exceeded one percent, and often week after week elapses without a single instance. (17)

Bell's claim in his 1854 annual report, namely that "the trial was made here, for several years, of the entire disuse of all forms of muscular restraint," must therefore be read carefully. Bell always allowed the use of leather mittens. Strong rooms, which did not count as restraints because the patient was physically free within them, confined the dangerously violent. Perhaps the statement means that Bell tried to do without restraining chairs or bed straps for a while but came to distinguish situations when he believed them preferable to the strong room. Unfortunately, the records from the period are haphazard, to say the least. But it does appear as though restraints of any kind were employed even less during Bell's administration than they had been in Wyman's.

When it came to medicinal remedies for mental disease, Bell was even more skeptical than Wyman.

> Each year that I have passed in this extensive field has served to diminish my confidence in an active medical treatment of almost every form of disease of the mind, and to increase my reliance on moral means. No individual at the head of an insane institution would now think of combatting any form of insanity, with the depletory and reducing means once regarded as indispensable. The practice of bleedings, violent purga-

> tions, emetics, vesicatories [blistering agents] and derivatives, has passed away before the light of experience. . . . A *wise expectation* and a cautious use of medical agents to meet symptoms, comprise most of the aids that the pharmacopoeia is capable of affording.

Nevertheless, Bell had an open mind and would not offhandedly dismiss any highly touted medical agent without trial. More than anything else he believed treatment of mental illness to be "peculiarly dependent upon experience and direct observation, and not upon theory or transmitted information" (18). Thus, in October 1845 he could have been found mixing a tincture of hashish from ingredients sent to Boston by a physician in Calcutta and received in the form of an "apparently pure and perfect extract." Bell tried the stuff on five women patients, four of whom had suffered manic attacks and a fifth who had paranoid delusions. The experiment failed (19).

In describing Bell's attitude toward medical intervention, Isaac Ray reflected that "he had no theory on the subject. His views were the result of observation, for at first he resorted freely to the medication then in vogue. The hackneyed argument, that insanity being a disease of a bodily organ, is therefore a proper subject of medication as any other disease, did not convince him. . . ." Said Bell: "My experience has long since convinced me that the curative and custodial treatment of the insane was essentially moral treatment; that while constant regard was to be had to physical symptoms and medical agents were of use in assisting nature to restore the mind by regulating the body, there was no specific treatment for insanity *per se*" (20).

Although there is at least one recorded incident of a patient's attack upon Bell (a woman, on her second day at McLean, broke a window and concealed a piece of glass in her hand; as Bell and the trustees passed through her hall on their rounds, she aimed the weapon at Bell's eye, but only inflicted a slight cut on his cheek), his manner with patients was remarked upon by those who chanced to witness it. Said Ray:

> In his intercourse with his patients, the great variety of his knowledge, both of men and things, always furnished him with some topic of conversation which engaged their attention and rendered his visits agreeable. With no arts of address to strike the fancy, yet his easy and courte-

> ous demeanor, and his frank, good-natured manner, secured, in no ordinary degree, their esteem and confidence. With the most perfect control of his feelings, even under the severest provocations, he always maintained that happy blending of firmness and gentleness which is essential to the superintendent of the insane. With inexhaustible patience he listened to their long stories, and manifested an unaffected interest in their troubles. . . .

Bell was uncommonly sensitive to a patient's dignity, masked though it might be by illness. There were no laws protecting patients' privacy—anyone certified insane at that time had very few rights indeed—yet Bell respected it. He refused to include any titillating "Bedlam sketches" in his annual reports, though he was aware of an element of prurient public interest. He thought such case stories would do an injustice to his patients while further distorting the general perception of insanity and asylums.

Some patients inevitably failed to appreciate Bell or his efforts. Bell accepted this fact with weary resignation. Among his papers in the McLean archives is an undated draft of a letter, beginning "Dear Madam," and continuing halfway down the page, "if I allowed myself to be distracted for a moment by the reports of non-recovered patients who leave us, my situation like that of any other head of an insane hospital would be intolerable." He must have written dozens of variations on this letter. In his 1851 annual report he cautioned the public to be wary of "*tittle-tattle* arising against asylums for the insane, mostly from unrecovered patients and servants discharged for mal-conduct."

Families and friends, not patients, caused the truly unpleasant moments in Bell's days. This passage from the 1856 annual report evokes images of some of the scenes that must have taken place in his office.

> The interdiction of the visits and correspondence of friends is ever one of the severest trials of those in charge of hospitals. As the indispensable necessity of such separation was one of the earliest of the recorded facts of medical observation, so it remains true and prominent in every day's experience of every asylum. If the head of an institution can be tempted in any point to yield or evade his convictions of duty, it will be here; for such convictions he must have with his first practical lessons, and they will keep strengthening with each year of experience. He will be pressed to abandon his duty by those who must be assumed to have a far nearer interest in the sufferer than he can have. After earnest and prolonged

> expositions of his grounds of action and the results of his often-repeated experimentings, and after the most earnest appeals that the welfare, and perhaps recovery of his patient shall not be put in jeopardy by any feelings or false reasonings or capricious suspicions of friends, he will find fathers and mothers, husbands and wives, brothers and sisters, whose whole knowledge of the subject is bounded by the case in hand, willing and anxious to assume all responsibilities, and take all risks, for obtaining this strange gratification. The hospital superintendent who will the most readily yield to such importunities, backed by perhaps the most degrading intimations as to the grounds of refusal, will be the most popular. . . . After a life devoted thus far almost exclusively to this specialty, were there any one counsel which I would impress on any one who may be called to this trust, it would be to stand firm in his convictions on this greatest item of moral treatment.

The descriptions of Bell by friends and colleagues, along with his own reflections, confirm his intelligence, integrity, and humanity. Through them one begins to piece together the pattern of his days at McLean. As a form of medical practice, it was a far cry from amputating the leg of a New Hampshire farmer. He passed among his asylum patients, a benign but remote figure, symbol of order and authority. A routine inspection tour of the premises lasting, say, three hours, would have allowed him about a minute with each patient. Bell could not carve up his time into thin slices; he had to concentrate on those patients who raised questions—the newly admitted, those close to discharge, those who presented physical symptoms, the violent and disorderly, instances of sudden behavioral changes. Only when he examined an individual complaining of aches and pains, prescribed some medicine, or patched up a wound did he behave as a conventional physician.

The remedy for mental illness was moral treatment, not some elixir meted out in greater or lesser doses and substituted with something else when the symptoms persisted. Wyman had to a certain extent fashioned occupational programs to suit individual inclinations. By Bell's time McLean had grown too large to sustain irregularities in routine, and the practice of moral treatment had to be tailored to institutional needs, with the conviction that a smoothly functioning institution helped the patient. The classic doctor-patient relationship had no place in this scheme.

The concept of the role of physicians at McLean in the mid-nineteenth-century is suggested by the fact that in 1854, the year the asylum finally acquired a second assistant physician, the daily census was about 200. Three doctors plus one medical student-apothecary constituted the entire medically trained staff. Attendants bore the brunt of the caretaking duties; the ratio of one attendant to every six patients, plus especially assigned individual attendants for suicidal patients, held during Bell's tenure. Meanwhile, at Massachusetts General Hospital, the average in-patient census was 133; a staff of a dozen or so attending physicians and surgeons, plus a chemist, an apothecary, a pathologist, and six medical students, tended the patients, though the nurse-patient ratio was lower than at McLean. At the asylum, one casualty of increased patient population and small professional staff was the keeping of case records, work which was never assigned to attendants. By the mid-1850s the writing of records had become very sporadic indeed, with entries in a record often lapsing for several weeks, then quickly brought up to date with sketchy observations. Visiting Committee inspections and reports became equally perfunctory. July 19, 1853, when there were 93 males and 102 females in residence, was a characteristic entry: "Mr. S---- visited, saw all the patients & found the house in proper order." There followed names of patients discharged and their condition, and of those admitted with the rate of board and name of the person who would pay it.

Bell served chiefly as administrator. He made the rules of moral treatment, saw to their implementation, and authorized such measures as forced feedings, restraints, or confinement in strong rooms. He had overall fiscal responsibility, while the steward handled day-to-day purchases and disbursements. Bell hired, fired, ran the staff, and reported to the trustees. He pacified patients' families and friends. In the normal course of his duties, medical expertise came into play in evaluating the mental status of the patients for the purposes of admission, placement within the asylum, and discharge. But it cannot be said that Bell *treated* patients. Perhaps his most articulate expression of what he thought he accomplished for them was contained in a letter to Dorothea Dix:

> My experience . . . convinced me . . . that a state of mind reacting on the physical cause was attained mainly by moral influences, and that in application of these moral influences, much depended on the head to whom the patient is referred in his trials; upon the personal exact acquaintance which that head possessed of the mental conditions, circumstances, habits, associations, domestic relations, and in fact every thing touching the individual. Tuke well observes that the success of any man in curing insanity will depend upon his power of inspiring hope. (21)

A man of lesser imagination and energy might have settled into the superintendent's role—not that it was exactly an easy one—run a clean, orderly institution, and kept the trustees happy with balanced budgets. But Bell's restless intelligence would not be the captive of small quarters. He mastered administrative essentials quickly and instinctively turned to broader problems of mental illness. He realized that McLean patients represented a body of data from which much might be learned—what would now be called a research opportunity.

Looking back over his work, one gets the feeling that he recognized the potential early in his career but did not quite know what to do with it. In March 1838, a little more than a year after assuming his position, he started an inventory, originally intended to cover all patients admitted before his arrival and still in residence along with those who had arrived under his supervision. He studied the casebooks from Wyman's and Lee's days, added his own observations, and worked systematically, beginning with long-term patients whom he personally reviewed with Wyman. Bell's early entries were detailed, often running several pages. Later they got shorter. After two years he had barely progressed beyond Lee's patients. The last entry came on June 20, 1840, when he wrote wearily, "Finding it impracticable in my numerous avocations to detail the history of every case, I have concluded to insert only those of peculiar interest, and in such order as my convenience dictates" (22). If Bell was searching for common denominators he failed to find any. Yet the aborted exercise furnished a much better education about mental illness than he could have obtained from any literature of the period because he could study the living patient as well as the case history.

Ellis's memoir notes that Bell initially identified absolutely with the welfare of McLean. "He had not served many years, however, before he found it essential to the healthfulness, cheerfulness, and vigor of his own frame and thoughts, while exposed to so many morbid and exhausting influences, to keep open some channel of intercourse with the outside world, and to interest himself in some wider converse with human improvement." Therefore, in the early 1840s, Bell began to tackle generic problems of mental illness and the institutions of treatment. In the opinion of one historian—and as a clue to the condition of research at midcentury—for the next few decades Bell and two other asylum superintendents, Isaac Ray and Amariah Brigham, were responsible for nearly all of the research on mental illness that occurred in the United States (23).

Although Bell produced a number of publications, they do not constitute a coherent body of research as such things are defined today. The topics are too diffuse, and only the broad subject heading of mental illness binds them together. Bell wrote about the architecture of asylums, their heating and ventilating systems, about statistics on mental illness, the classification of patients, the use of restraints, the coercive administration of food to patients, and various aspects of medical jurisprudence as related to mental illness. One of his papers, a more traditional medical effort, described a new disease: "On a form of disease resembling some advanced states of mania and fever, but so contradistinguished from an ordinarily observed or described combination of symptoms as to render it probable that it may be an overlooked and hitherto unrecorded malady." "Bell's Disease," as it was called, faded away in later taxonomic systems. From a twentieth-century perspective, Bell's research lacked focus and discipline, the compulsion to understand that drives original, fruitful study. Among the several reasons for this, perhaps the key one is that Bell did not work with a hypothesis that he tested or stretched in search of new solutions. He was by nature an observer rather than an explorer, a pragmatist rather than a theorist. He was less concerned with discovery than with enlightenment of the public and his professional brethren. He drew generalizations from his experience, common sense, intelligent observation, and unwillingness to accept without question the received wisdom of the profession. It must also be noted that the concept of research had not yet been integrated in the structure of the medical profession. Franklin B. Sanborn, writing at the end of the nineteenth century, reflected on the pre-Civil War years in which Bell worked:

> The asylums were few and small, receiving but a portion of the insane, and had no means of determining the exact physical condition of the patients they treated. The microscope had hardly begun to do its work in revolutionizing medicine. The localization of function in the brain was in its rudiments, and was obscured by the charlatanry of phrenology. The classification of insanity by its external manifestations was very little advanced, and had to be the study of each alienest in his own narrow field of observation. They experimented with medical and moral treatment; and, like Dr. Rush, they formed singular notions of what treatment was applicable to the mass of the insane. Still, knowledge advanced under their isolated experiences. They communicated facts to each other and to the public. (24)

Deutsch made the intriguing and, I think, accurate observation that progress in Bell's era "took the negative form of *discarding* therapeutics shown by experience to be unavailing or even injurious, rather than of discovering *better* methods of treatment" (25). Bell's work can only be fairly evaluated in that context.

Bell at first used the pages of his annual reports, which the trustees customarily had printed and circulated in large numbers for public relations purposes, as his place of publication. Two or three years after he came to McLean he adopted the habit of embellishing the *pro forma* account of the institution with an essay on a single topic. In the 1841 report, for example—perhaps driven to distraction by the duty to compile yet another set of numbers—he attacked the infatuation with statistical manipulation of most asylums, including his own. "There are but few circumstances touching the history, causes, type or results of the cases of insane persons which are capable of being stated numerically," he wrote.

> Of these few, it unfortunately is true, that their importance is almost too insignificant as matters of curiosity or of science, to render their communication of much more value than the fashion of their dress or the aspect of the planets. I presume that the ages of patients, their civil state as married, widowed or single, the color of the hair and eyes, the complexion and the like, might be recorded and conveyed with a tolerable degree of exactness but beyond this any thing of the ordinary tabular statistics requires so many explanations and qualifications on account of their

> complexity, uncertainty and changeableness, as to deprive them entirely of the character to which they seem to aspire.

Bell elaborated the difficulties of expressing almost every aspect of a case with precision—cause, duration, type of disease, cause of death, and so on. The terms improved and much improved applied to patients upon discharge were, he observed, "obviously mere expressions of opinion" for which asylum superintendents had never developed objective standards. "[A]nd the term *recovered*, apparently sufficiently plain and intelligible, is far from conveying an exact unqualified idea. . . . The register . . . of any institution will not fail to present many instances of 'recovery' which have 'recovered' before, and that perhaps repeatedly. . . ." He warned that "as things are now progressing, there is infinite danger that the public mind may arrive at such views and expectations as to the curability of insanity as will eventually react most unfavorably on our successors in these holy though arduous avocations, if not upon ourselves."

That is pretty strong stuff for an annual report. Bell's remarks were tantamount to saying "we've been handing you these statistics year after year, and they weren't worth a damn" (while reporting 75 of the 141 patients discharged from McLean during 1841 as recovered). That the trustees printed his statement and circulated it publicly speaks well of them.

As one of the earliest, respected, and most vocal of critics, Bell helped cut through the statistical fog of reporting procedures and make way for sounder, standardized techniques. Unfortunately, however, numerical reform was a long way off, and Bell's prophecy would come true before it happened. Meanwhile, Bell was fed up with numbers. He knew they had political value; he had run all over New Hampshire collecting data in the 1830s. But numbers did not accomplish anything for the mental health of his patients. In 1849 he wrote: "We have vast accumulations of facts and observations, laid aside in the records of each case admitted, but until the veil of mystery and darkness is more withdrawn from the functions of the nervous system, it is hardly to be expected that any more collections of facts lying around the distant periphery of the circle can aid in solving the obscurity of its centre."

Bell's dissertations on statistics, as well as some papers on heating/ventilating systems, were the most influential of his publications. Yet the others make good reading because Bell had a nice touch with the English language, producing articulate, sometimes poetic prose, and because they convey so well the medical and moral flavor of his age. Although space does not permit a careful review of all his work, it is worth pausing over his annual report for 1843, in which he set down some thoughts about forms of mental illness and treatment. He objected to the customary reduction of mental disturbance to four classes of insanity; namely, mania, melancholy, monomania, and dementia. The patients he saw simply did not manifest such clear-cut symptoms; rather, the symptoms were complicated and mixed.

> This classification appears to me unsound therefore; . . . it also will not bear the test of accuracy as regards the cause of disease, or the pathological condition of the sufferer, since there is every reason to believe that the peculiar affection called insanity, whether the sequence of primary affection of the cerebrospinal system, or merely the reflex action of more distant irritations upon that system, is a unit, and these forms are merely the changing external symptoms, often having scarcely a diurnal continuance, before passing from one to another. It is a division useless, as regards moral or medical treatment. . . .

Bell, the relentless pragmatist, did not try to develop a scientifically or philosophically satisfying nomenclature. Instead, he suggested two classification systems, each useful in different circumstances. For the purposes of treatment he recognized insanity "connected with the puerperal state," "with suicidal propensity," "accompanied with strong suspicions of personal injury threatened," "connected with the abuse of stimulants," "of hereditary disposition," and "that terrible complication, . . . *paralysie generale.*" He advanced ideas of treatment and prognosis for each category. Patients suffering mental illness connected with pregnancy or childbirth were, for example "ordinarily the most pleasant and satisfactory, as far as results are concerned, of any that ever enter an Asylum"; cases of hereditary disposition might "be looked upon as affording a most favorable prospect as regards recovery, although the danger of a recurrence of attacks at periods of greater or less distance, is more probable than in cases recovered with no such predisposition," and so forth.

Bell believed another classification scheme would be helpful in cases of medical jurisprudence. He proceeded to divide insanity along different lines, distinguishing one form that affected only the intellect (including mania, delusions, incoherence, and imbecility); a second, called "moral insanity," involving perversions of emotions and moral attitudes, but not of reasoning faculties and without hallucinations; and a third "consisting in deranged or perverted sensibilities . . . where both the understanding and the moral sense alike appear to be undisturbed," such as deep depression with suicidal tendencies. Bell pursued his argument in a historical account of legal doctrines concerning the insane, presenting a powerful case for overhauling the laws of insanity in New England to afford protection for the mentally ill.

Overall, the 1843 annual report was quintessential Bell, at least his professional persona: commonsensical, compassionate, observing, not very original in a scientific sense, active, concerned—and frustrated by the problems of mental illness.

According to the 1840 census, of a total American population of approximately 17,070,000, 17,457—or 1 in every 977 persons—was thought to be insane or "feebleminded." Only 2,561 individuals were patients in mental institutions, which were widely believed to be the only cure for mental illness. It matters little that these figures cannot have been accurate or that there was no standard definition of insanity, because these were the statistics placed before the public and their elected representatives.* Despite the establishment of mental hospitals here and there, most people afflicted with mental illness in the 1840s still suffered under conditions similar to those in the eighteenth century.

Dorothea Lynde Dix, a Boston schoolteacher who was asked in 1841 to begin a Sunday school class in the East Cambridge House of Correction, observed the inhumane treatment of insane and disturbed inmates there, practically in the shadow of McLean upon its manicured hilltop. Those who destroyed their clothing were left naked in unheated, unwashed facilities; some

*Times change. In October 1984, the National Institute of Mental Health estimated that approximately one in every *five* Americans was subject to mental health disorders, and caused a certain amount of speculation about the accuracy of *their* figures. Newspaper columnists had a grand time for themselves.

were chained to the walls and flogged. Shocked and morally offended, Dix set out on a two-year inspection tour of Massachusetts and discovered all manner of wretchedness in treatment of the insane throughout the Commonwealth. In 1843 she submitted a detailed report of her findings to the state legislature, which responded by expanding the Worcester asylum. Dix then took her case to the nation at large in a 40-year, passionate, personal crusade for the construction of mental hospitals.

Early in her work, Dix naturally turned to Bell, unquestionably the local authority, for information and advice, and the two became friends. She often used his publications, particularly the annual reports, to document her arguments. Once, when she asked him about figures on the number of insane in the United States as well as the number in hospitals, Bell responded that it was all a matter of "guesses, especially in the former case," which shows that he did not put any faith in the census figures (26).

Dix often visited McLean, and it became her model of what an institution for the insane ought to be. Bell furnished documents, letters of introduction, advice, and endless encouragement. He honored Dix at McLean by getting the north building, the male patient wing, named in her honor. He regarded her as "one of the extraordinary women of the age," and indeed she was, in the American tradition of great social reformers (27). Almost single-handedly she made mental illness and, more specifically, the provision of institutional care for the mentally ill, items of national concern. She was a first-rate propagandist, in the best sense of the word: She put the issue on the front page and kept it there. Even then, publicity made things happen. As Walt Whitman noted, "The public is a thick-skinned beast, and you have to keep whacking away on its hide to let it know you're there" (28).

Bell had been born with that knowledge in his bones, but he chose a different channel for his political energies. At 10 o'clock Wednesday morning, October 16, 1844, he became a founding member of the Association of Medical Superintendents of American Institutions for the Insane, grandparent organization to the current American Psychiatric* Association, having weath-

*Alert readers will note that this is the first time the word *psychiatry* in any form appears in this book. Physicians who specialized in mental illness in Bell's era and well into the twentieth century usually referred to themselves as "alienists." The expression

ered an intermediate phase as the American Medico-Psychological Association.

By virtue of his presence in the Jones Hotel in Philadelphia that morning, Bell is an official founding father of American psychiatry, one of the "Original Thirteen" enumerated with reverence in histories of the specialty. The other 12 were: Samuel B. Woodward of the Worcester State Asylum, who originated the idea of a professional association and set it in motion; Isaac Ray of the Maine State Asylum; Charles E. Stedman of the Boston Lunatic Asylum; Nehemiah Cutter of the Pepperell Private Asylum in Massachusetts, one of the rare, respectable private proprietary institutions in the country; John S. Butler of the Hartford Retreat; Amariah Brigham of the New York State Lunatic Asylum at Utica, who had just found the *American Journal of Insanity*; Samuel White of the Hudson Lunatic Asylum in New York State, another well-run private establishment; Pliny Earle of the Bloomingdale Asylum; Thomas S. Kirkbride of the Pennsylvania Hospital; William M. Awl (sometimes called Dr. Cure-Awl) of the Ohio Lunatic Asylum; Francis T. Stribling of the Western Lunatic Asylum in Staunton, Virginia; and John M. Galt of the Eastern Lunatic Asylum at Williamsburg, Virginia. Together, these men represented just about everything that was known about mental disease in the United States. All but three of them were under the age of 45. Galt, a man of renaissance scholarship and talents, was only 25 and had been an asylum superintendent since the age of 22, a record of early achievement surpassing even Bell's.

The objective of the association was to set up communication lines among the superintendents in the interest of translating individual experiences into a more systematic body of knowledge and, thereby, to improve treatment of the insane. Nothing suggests the usefulness of such a society more obviously than the tours of other institutions that both Wyman and Bell had felt obliged to make before starting at McLean, or the avidity with

was adopted from the French, whose word for the insane was *aliené* or alienated, which term I confess I find more evocative of the conditions now customarily called mental illness than any other, past or present; it has no social stigma, at least in English. Following the terms of the times, I shall not refer to psychiatrists until the term becomes part of the language. By the same logic, I have used the word "insanity" as freely as it was employed in the nineteenth century in this section of the manuscript.

which superintendents read each other's annual reports, scouring the contents for applicable information.

At the initial gathering, the Original Thirteen voted to extend membership in the association to the superintendents of all legally constituted institutions—about 20 in all at that time—as well as new ones that might be established before the next meeting. In 1848 the association voted to invite trustees, managers, and official visitors of insane asylums to its meetings. The *American Journal of Insanity*, which Brigham had started four months before the Philadelphia decision, became the association's unofficial vehicle of communication. (The association did not take over publication of the journal until the end of the century.)

The association was the first national society of medical men in the United States. The *American Journal of Insanity*, now the *American Journal of Psychiatry*, was not only the first American periodical devoted to mental disease and its treatment but also the first specialized medical journal of any kind. Gradually, the same impulses that had driven asylum superintendents into a discrete organization caused them to drift gently away from the mainstream of medicine, which was beginning to record some impressive progress. (The most noteworthy medical event of mid-century occurred in 1846 at McLean's sister institution, the Massachusetts General Hospital, in the form of a demonstration of the efficacy of ether as an anesthetic during surgery.)

Asylum management and moral treatment posed very different problems from the practice of conventional medicine or surgery; accordingly, asylum superintendents looked to each other, not to physicians treating physical ailments, for help. The pages of the *American Journal of Insanity* reflect their preoccupation with institutional mechanics as opposed to scientific medicine. During the first 25 years of publication, the journal is filled with plans and descriptions of existing mental hospitals, with discourses on asylum architecture, construction, amenities (Bell's work on heating and ventilation, for example), and administrative arrangements. The subject of mechanical restraints took up a lot of space during the debate on nonrestraint. Medical jurisprudence was another favorite topic. Speculation on the nature and cause of insanity was also to be found in the journal, but if numbers of pages are taken as a measure of the importance of an issue, this one fell far behind the others, particularly in the early years.

Just as mental hospitals were geographically removed from general hospitals, so would the association of their superintendents contribute to the isolation of alienists from medicine. However, this separation did not become visible until later in the century. During its early years, when Bell was a leading figure, the association did much to advance the public comprehension of mental illness, to demystify the practices of well-run asylums (thus relieving people of some of their fears), to modify asylum architecture and statistical reporting, and most importantly, to encourage the exchange of ideas among physicians treating the mentally ill in asylums. It was an ideal forum for Bell, because it drew on both his professional and political talents, and he viewed it as the best instrument for improving institutional conditions. He supported it enthusiastically, serving as vice-president from 1850 to 1851 and president from 1851 to 1855. Meanwhile he kept one foot in the conventional medical camp as a member of the Massachusetts Medical Society, of which he was elected president in 1857.

The list of Bell's activities is by no means exhausted. In December 1844, the trustees of the Butler Hospital in Providence, Rhode Island, who were in the process of establishing their own asylum, asked the McLean trustees if they might borrow Bell to advise them on a building program. Bell was granted a leave of absence. In 1845 he sailed to England and France to investigate hospitals there. He submitted recommendations on architectural arrangements, complete with plans and diagrams, most of which were incorporated into the Butler design. But he refused a handsome offer to head the new institution and stayed on at McLean.

Bell also made a name for himself as an expert witness in court cases involving insanity. He was forever being summoned to jail cells to interview suspects and to courthouses to testify before juries. In the absence of soap operas and other immediate forms of entertainment, the public followed newspaper accounts of criminal trials with rapt attention, and Bell was sometimes in the limelight. In 1850 he was appointed to the Massachusetts Executive Council, which, along with other duties, was supposed to advise the governor in cases of pardon for criminals under sentence.

Almost immediately, Bell was obliged to decide the fate of Dr. John White Webster, mentioned earlier. Despite Webster's protestations of innocence, in November 1849 a jury pronounced him guilty of the murder of Dr. George Parkman—he who had once so eagerly sought to run the asylum—and a judge had sentenced Webster to death. Webster's loyal supporters made a last-ditch effort to get him a pardon. The case could not have been an easy one for Bell. In the social circles he frequented, Webster was an object of sympathy. Among the prominent people who had testified as character witnesses on Webster's behalf were Dr. Oliver Wendell Holmes and Nathanial Bowditch, for many years a McLean-MGH trustee and at that moment chairman of the trustees. But Bell reviewed the material with a clear head and concluded that there was no good reason for the governor to overturn the verdict. Webster's 11th-hour confession appeared to confirm the correctness of Bell's opinion.

In 1853 Bell was appointed to a Board of Commissioners who examined convicts in the state penitentiary for signs of mental illness. His task was largely one of distinguishing those who suffered genuine mental illness from cunning deceivers who simulated symptoms in hopes of exchanging a long prison sentence for a shorter term in a mental hospital. It was said that Bell never let a faker slip through, while rescuing many mentally disturbed people from inappropriate incarceration. In the latter 1850s, after he had retired from McLean, Bell spent much of his time in courtrooms, rendering his professional opinion concerning the mental competence of various persons involved in criminal and civil proceedings. State supreme court Chief Justice Lemuel Shaw (better known for decisions that established the "separate-but-equal" doctrine and legalized the trade unions), who frequently listened to Bell's testimony, gave him high marks for performance under oath.

One of the nightmares of an asylum superintendent was the appearance of contagious disease within his precinct. The summer of 1847 was a bad season for dysentery in the Boston area, and despite precautions, the illness infiltrated McLean at the end of July. Within an eight-week period, 70 of the 170 patients in residence came down with dysentery; 12 of them died. There were 10 cases among the staff, including Tyler the steward, who suffered a particularly debilitating attack. The disease hit the Bell family hard: Bell's charming 10-year-old daughter died in the epidemic on August 22. Then, six weeks later, his five-year-old son died of consumption. Bell apparently felt the losses keenly. Yet it is important to remember that people in the era before the great medical developments of the twentieth century were more accustomed to the death of infants and children and accepted it more philosophically than we do now. The patterns of Bell's professional and extracurricular life continued uninterrupted.

But the death in November 1853 of his eldest son, Samuel John, a promising Harvard student, seems to have exacted a severe toll on Bell. It is probably not accidental that his research on spiritualism began shortly after this death. The next loss, the most devastating of all, came in March 1855, when Bell's wife Frances died during her confinement at the age of 42. Bell advised the McLean trustees almost immediately that he would not be a candidate for reappointment to another term of office, and they accepted his resignation. On an early April day that year, about a month after his wife had died, Bell had an unsettling experience of another sort. He recorded it in a confidential letter, composed in 1858 and opened after his death, quoted in Ellis's memoir.

> By the wish of the children, we went out upon Monument Square with one of them [Clara] in my hand, and Fannie in my arms. We walked around the Monument. As I was wearily and heavily turning across the path parallel to High Street, . . . I felt an irritation and tickling about my throat, which resulted in the ejection of a small quantity of bloody expectoration. Having had no previous symptoms of pulmonary trouble, I tried to make myself believe that it was consequent upon some small exudition of blood in the nasal or pharyngeal passages. Yet, in the recollection of my brother John's first symptoms and my general acquaintance with the subject, I could not shut my eyes to the probability of its having come from the lungs, and of its being the indication of tubercular disease awakened into action.

Though shaken, Bell continued at McLean through the end of 1855 and departed with a graceful annual report, reflecting upon 19 years of experience. Unlike Wyman, he did not flee the neighborhood but moved to a house he had just built on the north side of Monument Square in Charlestown, in the shadow of the Bunker Hill Monument and within easy walking distance of the asylum. He planned to devote himself to the care of his four small surviving children for as long as his disease allowed him life. Meanwhile, he did not talk about his health.

The trustees, with Bell's blessing, appointed Dr. Chauncy Booth, who had been first assistant physician at McLean for 13 years, as his successor. After a promising first year, Booth's health declined, and he resigned in November 1857. A few months later he was dead of the same disease that afflicted Bell, tuberculosis. The latter, conveniently close by, agreed to fill the gap as acting superintendent until a new man could be found. He returned to duty for four months and then left McLean for good.

Bell's disease caused him some discomfort and took the edge off his stamina but did not incapacitate him. He retained positions on various commissions, remained active in the Massachusetts Medical Society, testified in numerous court cases, and counseled patients and friends who called at his home. Ellis wrote that "the image in which he is most likely to rise before the minds of his fellow citizens, during the last five years of his life in Charlestown, is as a pensive, serious, and dignified man, leading two or three little children through the streets, or stopping with them to gaze at any thing that attracted them in the shop windows or the highways. His tall form did not prevent his coming down to their familiarity in all things. At congenial seasons, he was seen with them, or alone, training or weeding the flowers in the garden-patch adjoining his house." It was as if he were a doomed, kindly character from a Dickens tale.

Bell's final chapter came from some other novel. The United States tore apart in civil war. On April 19, 1861, the day Abraham Lincoln proclaimed a blockade of Southern ports, Bell defied medical reason by volunteering for military service. He was no longer a young man. He knew he was ill. He was father to four motherless children. Yet in the letter he wrote applying for duty, Bell described himself as "in health so good as not to have been confined to my house a day in the past three years, and entirely removed from all cares by easy personal circumstances," surely a bending if not a breaking of the truth (29). When informed that the militia staff was already full, Bell presented himself in the office of the surgeon-general, in the state house, who pressed his case with the governor, who relented and gave Bell a commission as surgeon of the Eleventh Regiment of Massachusetts Volunteers, dated June 10, 1861. It was, of course, a death warrant.

Bell served with General Hooker's division. He returned to the practice of medicine as he had once known it in rural New Hampshire, but on a massive, horrifying scale. He wrote spirited, detailed, illustrated letters home bragging that his lungs were stronger than ever. He seemed to relish the adventure and action of war. On February 5, 1862, during a cold, wet spell at Camp Baker on the Potomac, he complained to his attendant of a strong pain in the lumbar region and ordered him to administer chloroform. Bell lingered on for six more days, suffering severely but refusing to be moved to a proper hospital. He died in the evening of February 11, at the age of 54.

One final note: Many years later, Pliny Earle quoted Bell as having said, some time after he had left McLean, "I have come to the conclusion that when a man once becomes insane, he is about used up for this world" (30).

CHAPTER

4

Drifting Through the Doldrums

Institutions, like people, have their ups and downs. Seasons of fertile energy and innovation alternate irregularly with those that are fallow or that yield undistinguished harvests. Following Bell's departure, McLean entered a phase most succinctly describable as the "blahs." For about 20 years, little remarkable can be said to have happened at the asylum—or, for that matter, in the increasingly introverted world of American mental institutions, save for the building and filling of more establishments. Medicine's honeymoon with moral treatment came to an end. The excitement of experiment subsided, and the promise faded. McLean lapsed into a complacent holding pattern.

Although this trend is obvious to any thoughtful student looking at the situation through the corrective lens of history, it was not evident to McLean patients or their families, superintendents, personnel, or trustees upon the scene. The asylum continued to submit its patients to a humane, ever-more-opulent regimen of moral treatment, to return a portion of them to the world recovered or much improved, to make life as comfortable as possible for those who did not respond to therapy, to maintain a sound financial status, and to have an excellent reputation. McLean was as good as any asylum in the United States, better than most. The extent to which it had relinquished a leadership role in the effort to understand and treat mental illness—had neglected to pursue important questions raised by Bell, let alone pressing issues suggested by more recent developments in medicine, biology, and the emerging social sciences—only became apparent in the early 1880s when a dynamic superintendent started making heroic changes.

In 1861 Dr. Oliver Wendell Holmes, champion of scientific medicine, faced a new class of Harvard Medical School students and told them that "Science is the topography of ignorance. From a few elevated points we triangulate vast spaces enclosing infinite unknown details. We cast the lead, and draw up a little sand from abysses we may never reach with our dredges" (1). In no province of medicine was the scientific terrain more obscure and treacherous than in that of mental illness. Yet with few exceptions, asylum superintendents during the post Civil War decades buried their heads in administrative problems and engaged in parochial dialog; intellectually, they were as isolated in the asylum as were their patients.

Meanwhile, outside the asylum a number of scientific and scholarly developments ought to have attracted the alienists' curiosity by virtue of their implications for the understanding of brain, mind, and human behavior. The list might begin with the publication of Charles Darwin's *Origin of Species* in 1859. Darwin's startling theories were placed before the American public in Boston by Harvard botanist Asa Gray in a series of heated debates with naturalist Louis Agassiz. Asylum superintendents, ostensibly concerned with treating hereditary mental illness, paid little attention. But a Viennese university student, Sigmund Freud, read Darwin with fascination in the early 1870s.

Of more obvious and immediate relevance to people in the business of ministering to the mentally ill was the rapid rise of neurology as a medical specialty. The Civil War had presented numerous cases of injury and disorders of the nervous system, and some physicians had sharpened the focus of their attention and started to call themselves neurologists. The new specialists claimed the entire nervous system as their domain, and since the brain belonged to that system, they expressed interest in mental disease. Neurologist George M. Beard wrote about neurasthenia. During the Civil War, Dr. S. Weir Mitchell invented the "rest cure," a regimen of seclusion, rest, massage, electricity, and hyperalimentation in the treatment of "nervous exhaustion." In Boston, the Massachusetts General Hospital appointed Dr. James Jackson Putnam as physician to outpatients with diseases of the nervous system in 1873.

The new specialists organized themselves as the New York Neurological Association in 1872. Two years later their scholarly vehicle, the *Journal of Nervous and Mental Disease*, proclaimed the scope of their interest in its title and declared war on asylum superintendents. Leading the list of neurologists' gripes were the absence of scientific research in mental institutions and the unwillingness of the superintendents to admit them, or pathologists, to their sanctuaries. The singular presence since 1869 of a pathologist at the New York State Lunatic Asylum at Utica was hardly enough to pacify them. Neurologists further charged the Association of Medical Superintendents of American Institutions for the Insane with running a private club from which it barred noninstitutional physicians interested in mental illness as well as junior members of asylum medical staffs, and of operating asylums more like boarding houses than hospitals.

The neurologists' chief reproof—namely, that asylum physicians ignored scientific research—represented a gravitation within the medical profession at large toward a more deliberately rigorous approach to what was still commonly viewed as the "art" of medicine. Experiences in field hospitals during the Civil War had underlined the necessity for disciplined study. The work of Rudolf Virchow in cellular pathology, of Koch, Pasteur, and Lister on microorganisms, improving techniques for analyzing the chemical composition of blood and urine, and an increasingly powerful armamentarium of research instruments all suggested promising avenues of exploration. At the same time, competition from nonmedical practitioners such as homeopaths and purveyors of patent medicines challenged the medical profession to demonstrate more effectiveness. It was not, after all, doing a very good job of healing.

Charles William Eliot, once a professor of analytical chemistry at Massachusetts Institute of Technology, became president of Harvard in 1869 and immediately launched a bold program of educational innovation. Among his prime candidates for overhaul was the medical school. "The ignorance and general incompetency of the average graduate of American Medical Schools, at the time when he receives the degree which turns him loose upon the community, is something horrible to contemplate," he wrote in his annual report for 1869–70 (2).

Along with major structural changes in administration, Eliot's reforms at the Harvard Medical School extended the curriculum to include compulsory laboratory work in physiology, chemistry, and pathological anatomy. The subject of mental disease, however, remained peripheral to the curriculum and outside the laboratory. The quotable Dr. Holmes, with his pleas for scientific study, was a lone voice. Even he recognized the peculiar problems of such research. "The scientific study of man is the most difficult branch of all knowledge," he wrote in 1872. "It requires, in the first place, an entire new terminology to get rid of that enormous load of prejudices with which every term applied to the malformations, the functional disturbances, and the organic diseases of the moral nature is at present burdened" (3). To lay the ancient superstitions to rest, the brain had to be studied "microscopically, chemically, experimentally, in the lower animals, in individuals and races, in health and in disease, in every aspect of external observation, as well as by internal consciousness" (4). To the extent that Holmes himself explored the brain, it was largely through the last approach on his list. His examination of "internal consciousness" led him, for instance, to speculate in his 1871 essay, "Mechanisms in Thought and Morals," that in dreams "we do battle with ourselves, unconscious that we are our own antagonists."

During this period—roughly 1860 to 1880—some of the most original and imaginative studies of mind and brain were under way in Europe. Hermann von Helmholtz, a Berlin physiologist, investigated the sensations of vision and hearing. His three volumes on optics, published between 1856 and 1867, along with his monograph on hearing (1863), helped demonstrate the neurological bases of mental functions. Helmholtz laid down the axiom that "No other forces than the common physical-chemical ones are active within the organism." Another German physiologist, Wilhelm Wundt of Leipzig, designed laboratory experiments to explore the mechanisms of thinking, memory, and cognition. His was the first systematic effort to put the study of psychology on a scientific footing.

Wundt's 1873 volume, *Grundzüge der Physiologischen Psychologie* (outline of physiological psychology) attracted immediate attention in the United States, but not among asylum alienists, for whom Pinel, Tuke, and the *American Journal of Insanity* still represented authoritative literature. Wundt's work caught the eye of William James, then assistant professor of Physiology at the Harvard Medical School. He persuaded the Harvard authorities to allow him to introduce a course in physiological psychology into the *philosophy* department. By 1880, James had drifted permanently out of medicine and into philosophy, taking experimental psychology with him. One of his graduate students was Granville Stanley Hall, who had studied in Germany in 1869–70 and was also acquainted with the work of French neurologist J. M. Charcot with hypnosis. In 1879 Hall earned the first American doctorate ever awarded in psychology. There was probably not a single asylum superintendent in the United States who remarked upon the birth of a new discipline or who had read Wundt's work.

The latter half of the nineteenth century also saw the germination of other social sciences. In a matter of a few decades, new breeds of researchers opened up territories of human consciousness, behavior, and institutions that had for centuries been the private provinces of theologians and metaphysicians. (Artists, of course, had been trespassing at least as far back as the Greek dramatists. Haslam, Bethlehem's apothecary, wrote in 1809 that William Shakespeare was the "highest authority on everything relating to the human mind and its affections" [5]. And it would be hard to find a more penetrating study of the human mind than Herman Melville's *Moby Dick*, published in 1851.) Anthropology developed through the efforts of such individuals as Lewis Henry Morgan and Edward Burnett Tylor, whose stories Daniel J. Boorstin tells so lovingly in *The Discoverers*. Sociology slowly emerged from statistical analyses and the social work of charity organizations. During its fledgling stage in the United States, sociology was a reform movement rather than a science. Social workers were especially concerned with mental illness because they saw its victims in settlement houses, poor-houses, and homes and witnessed its devastating consequences for both the ill and their families. Having encountered so many examples of failure, social workers became increasingly critical of mental institutions and began to attack them publicly.

The asylums presented a broad target, especially the tax-supported institutions. The days when conditions at state asylums did not differ significantly from those at McLean had passed. Many if not most state hospitals had become overcrowded and understaffed, an imbalance that led to brutality and neglect of patients as well as to quick resort to severe forms of mechanical restraint. Social workers also began to agitate in behalf of educating the public in matters of "mental hygiene" as a means of preventing mental illness—a subject that asylum alienists did not address with any vigor (6). It was the neurologists, not the asylum superintendents, who joined the social workers' cause. In 1880 the two groups created the National Association for the Protection of the Insane and the Prevention of Insanity. The association had a short life. It faded from the scene around 1884 and seems to have vanished altogether by 1886. Nevertheless, during its few years of aggressive activity, it put asylum superintendents on the defensive.

Though McLean and the few privately financed, well-run institutions were exempt from charges of patient abuse, their superintendents indirectly shared the blame by virtue of membership in the Association of Medical Superintendents of American Institutions for the Insane. They were undeniably guilty, as charged by the neurologists, of delinquency in scientific matters. But throughout the 1860s and 1870s, as the clamor for reforms in mental health care got noisier, the association behaved in the traditional manner of good professional clubs: It closed ranks and protected its own.

At McLean the principal focus of administrative attention during the humdrum decades was not what happened within the asylum—where, to all appearances, things went along reasonably smoothly—but what transpired immediately beyond its borders. The proper telling of that story requires a brief retreat into Bell's era. First, to keep the record straight, McLean had been located in Somerville since 1842, when the inhabitants of the section of Charlestown in which the asylum was located succeeded in incorporating a separate township. This political realignment was of little consequence to McLean. However, the ambitious development of railroads and industrialization in the vicinity became a source of abundant aggravation. The railroad made its appearance in 1835 in the form of the Boston & Lowell Railroad; by 1854 there were four other lines. Railroad building in Somerville made sound geographic sense: The lines served the local brickyards and acted as a distribution center from Boston towards the northeast.

Unfortunately for McLean, however, the tracks encroached upon its territory, merged and switched at the base of Cobble Hill, and terminated in unsightly, noisy yards. The screaming of train whistles and clanging of metal drove Luther Bell absolutely wild. He claimed the noise was bad for his patients, that they required a quiet, pastoral environment. Although someone suggested that McLean patients really enjoyed the distractions of the trains, Bell and subsequent superintendents were quite sure that they didn't. Bell became obsessed by the racket and started collecting newspaper clippings detailing train collisions and other evils of rail transportation to support his conviction that railroads would ruin America, or at least McLean. The trustees responded to the threats of encroachment by buying up bits and pieces of land adjacent to the asylum properties in an effort to give it some extra breathing room, as well as a few trump cards to play at a later date. They also initiated a series of lawsuits from which the asylum gained some financial compensation but not the removal of railroad tracks (7).

Industry followed the railroads with economic inevitability. Metalworks, bleaching and dying, lumber, meat packing, distilling, and rope-making enterprises moved into an area that had formerly been devoted to brick making and agriculture. Nearby East Cambridge was also an industrial mecca; John P. Squire & Company occupied 22 acres of land across Miller's River, employed 1,000 people, and slaughtered 2,500 hogs per day. The rural landscape that had attracted the asylum founders was slowly transformed into an industrial terrain, offensive to the senses. A Somerville newspaper remarked in 1870 that "While the corporation [Asylum] has been building up and beautifying within, the opposite has been going on without. What, with slaughter houses, miasmatic swamps, dirty habitations, and the railroads, the area may be said to be slightly unpleasant if it [is] not very unhealthy." As to the river, in Wyman's time the scene of asylum picnics and boating parties, the pollution was disgusting. "Miller's River! faugh!" exclaimed an observer in 1875, "it smells to heaven; not even the Rhine at Cologne could surpass it. Such draughts of air as are wafted to your nostrils from the slaughterhouses, where whole hecatombs of squealing victims are daily sacrificed, are not of the chameleon's dish" (8).

In 1871 the Boston & Lowell Railroad expropriated a strip through the front of McLean grounds, slicing across the main access road and completing the encirclement of asylum properties with railroad tracks. Bulfinch's handsome old buildings, the attractive newer structures, and the carefully tended grounds were marooned in an industrial wasteland, as though absent-mindedly misplaced by a drunken urban planner. The trustees finally gave up whatever residual hopes they may have entertained that McLean could be adequately defended against the advancing armies of industrialization. They decided that the asylum had to be moved. In 1872 they hired Frederick Law Olmsted, the landscape designer, to advise upon the selection of a new site. They acted on his recommendation in 1875 by purchasing more than 100 wooded acres on Wellington Hill in Waverly (now Belmont), Massachusetts for $75,000.

Although these external conditions made administering McLean more troublesome and living there less desirable than in the past, they were not to blame for the lackluster period in the asylum's evolution.

While Bell temporarily filled the void left by Chauncy Booth's abrupt withdrawal from office, McLean's trustees searched for a new superintendent. They chose Dr. John Eugene Tyler, superintendent of the New Hampshire Insane Asylum and otherwise equipped with excellent credentials. Tyler, a Massachusetts man, had studied at Dartmouth and the University of Pennsylvania Medical School and practiced successfully in New Hampshire before being selected to direct the state mental institution. When he accepted the offer to come to McLean in 1858, he was 38 years old and married for a second time, his first wife and an infant having died. Tyler arrived in Somerville in March and established himself in the superintendent's quarters in the Barrell mansion.

Tyler, though lacking the intensity of Wyman and the insatiable curiosity of Bell, seems to have combined administrative efficiency with common sense, compassion, and a more lenient attitude than had prevailed at McLean during his predecessor's tenure. His first assistant physician, Dr. George F. Jelly, characterized him as "conservative, but cautiously progressive" and a man of great warmth (9). The Civil War disrupted the staff because several men were drafted. Tyler took the situation in stride and quickly hired replacements. In 1862, when state institutions were feeling the wartime pinch, McLean succeeded in raising $45,000 in four weeks for the building of a new "cottage" for excited patients. However, there were no building projects that increased the asylum's capacity, and by deliberate design, the average daily census gradually declined. The peak number of 201 remained approximately steady from 1850 to 1866; it decreased to 186 in 1867 and fluctuated thereafter between 150 and 180 for several years. In this manner the trustees relieved the crowded conditions without constructing new wards—the possibility of moving out of the unfriendly neighborhood being much in their minds—and ended the practice of using the large rooms under the domes to warehouse quiet demented patients.

Tyler expanded the range of diversions available to the patients, whom he called "boarders." After almost 20 years of segregation, men and women were again permitted to mingle. There were games and lectures. A dozen or so male patients formed an orchestra and performed concerts. There were classes in singing, drawing, and French. The staff arranged sleigh rides and regattas in appropriate weather conditions. A library was established for the patients. There were billiards, bowling alleys, saddle ponies, carriages, chess sets, cards, backgammon boards, and bagatelle. At Christmas, New Year's, Washington's birthday, and the Fourth of July, there were parties with dancing, ventriloquists, and the stereopticon. A better-equipped resort hotel would have been hard to find. A devotee of the sound body-sound mind school of thought, Tyler hired Dr. Dio Lewis, who taught his personal system of gymnastics to both men and women patients and, according to the authorized account, aroused "great delight for both the practitioners and the bystanders." (Lewis, a physician and lecturer on hygiene and physiology, had his own theories of human behavior, among them that spicy foods such as mustard and Worcestershire sauce stimulated carnal appetites.) In 1867 Tyler succeeded in persuading the trustees to appoint the Reverend David G. Haskins as chaplain to the asylum. However, the evidence does not quite justify the remark of an earlier historian that Tyler was of "an extremely religious temperament himself [and] encouraged the wave of religious revival which swept over the institution . . ." (10). Tyler does not seem to have been extreme in his religiosity, nor would an impartial observer have noticed anything so dramatic as a "wave" of revival at McLean during his administration.

The patients in Tyler's charge enjoyed more liberties than had been admitted by Bell. It is not at all unusual to find in the case records entries such as the following, concerning a young woman patient who had been in residence for several months: "She has been to Boston with Mrs. Tyler to attend concerts several times. Engages in all the games of the house, attends chapel, parties, and concerts, eats and sleeps well, and is becoming more established mentally and physically." The patient was discharged four weeks after this entry, appearing "quite well. Is very happy, kind, and ever ready to help others." Near the end of his administration, Tyler cautiously began the practice of leaving the doors of four or five of the women's wards unlocked during the day, allowing the women to move freely from one ward to another or out into a large enclosed garden reserved for their use.

Tyler also relaxed Bell's stringent rules about allowing friends to visit the patients. Historian Ellis, writing around 1871, noted that "Recently, of the whole number of patients in the Asylum—being 167—the friends of 142 of them could and did visit them at their pleasure. . . . Only 25 of the whole number of the patients were pronounced by the Superintendent as in a condition to render visits from friends, for the time, unadvisable. In no single case, and under no circumstances, is the nearest friend or guardian, having personal rights, precluded from an interview with a patient . . ." (11). Perhaps Tyler lacked Bell's steely temperament and simply caved in before pathetic entreaties; more likely, however, he did not take the principle of separation of the mentally ill from family and friends literally as a therapeutic agent. At the same time the regular traffic of visitors protected McLean against rumors that popped up from time to time concerning awful things going on in the asylum.

Tyler earned a modest niche in the history of psychiatry in the United States when he was appointed "lecturer on Mental Diseases" at the Harvard Medical School in 1863. Though a few other medical schools had extended token recognition of mental disease as a distinct field of medicine by inviting an occasional alienist to deliver lectures on the subject, Harvard had the first medical faculty to introduce it on a permanent basis, a gesture applauded by the Association of Medical Superintendents of American Institutions for the Insane. However, an editorial in the *American Journal of Insanity* immediately noted that "it was but a partial measure, inasmuch as attendance upon the lectures delivered by Dr. Tyler of Somerville was optional with the student, and not essential to the conferment of his degree" (12).

Tyler, a kind, amiable man with a hearty laugh, may have been an engaging lecturer. But he did not have anything to say that Harvard medical students could not have learned by reading random issues of the *American Journal of Insanity*, the books of Tuke and Pinel, or Bell's annual reports. Tyler delivered the shopworn message: Insanity was a disease, not a disgrace or diabolic possession; insanity was curable under proper conditions, more curable if the sufferer was submitted to specific treatment early in its manifestations. He described moral treatment. He recited the litany of causes of insanity: improper training and education in childhood, unrestrained appetites, intemperance (in particular, Tyler was especially concerned with alcoholism), masturbation, and overexertion of any one of the moral, physical, or intellectual faculties at the expense of the others. Tyler's lectures are lost to posterity, so one can only surmise the drift of his argument from his published annual reports on McLean, which if not as original or thoughtful as Bell's, were reasoned, straightforward, and humane. Nor do we know how well his lectures were attended, although it would have been remarkable if he drew a crowd during the 1860s, because "Mental Diseases" was not a required course and the students had to pay per lecture. However, he did survive Eliot's reforms of the medical school, became professor of Mental Diseases in 1871, and retained that title until 1878. But Tyler's influence was so trivial that Henry K. Beecher and Mark Altschule did not mention him at all in their history of the Harvard Medical School; instead, they began the history of psychiatric education there with Putnam, the neurologist (13).

In 1867, pleading fatigue, Tyler requested a leave of absence from McLean and traveled abroad, where he spent part of the time visiting asylums in Britain and on the continent. Whatever health benefits he may have derived from the journey were temporary. Early in 1871 he submitted his resignation on medical grounds. The trustees accepted it with reluctance and the customary declarations of gratitude. Tyler left and opened up a practice as a consulting physician in Boston. The withdrawal of Dr. J. Whittemore, the first assistant physician, a month after Tyler's resignation—Whittemore, too, cited ill health and a desire to study in Europe—left McLean in an administrative lurch (14). The trustees prevailed upon Isaac Ray, Luther Bell's old friend and one of the Original Thirteen, to interrupt his retirement in Philadelphia and hold the fort in Somerville until a permanent superintendent could be found. Ray by then had passed from "young turk" through 20 years of progressive leadership of the Butler Hospital in Providence to grand old man among the American alienists. Now, at age 64, he ventured forth to serve for three months as acting superintendent at McLean, for which he received the extremely handsome sum of $1,500, along with the impression that McLean had an extraordinarily high percentage of suicidal patients (15). He was relieved by Dr. George F. Jelly, promoted from his post as second assistant physician. Jelly's salary was set at $3,000 per year, a figure that demonstrates the generosity of the fee paid to Ray.

By the time Jelly moved into the superintendent's office, in October 1871, the trustees had already decided to move McLean; the Committee on Improvements at the Asylum had been disbanded and supplanted by a committee to inquire into a new site. The trustees' vision and financial energies focused on some imagined point in the future, leaving the existing asylum as a lame duck. Although McLean in Somerville was not permitted to fall into a condition of neglect, the standards of building maintenance declined. Certain modernizations were introduced, notably, a "magnetic annunciator" that connected all wards to the apothecary's office. But aside from two cottages for "excited" patients, the trustees authorized no substantial building or renovation programs for several years. This state of suspended animation in Somerville, coupled with a lack of activity on the new site in Belmont, may have discouraged young Jelly, who was only 29 when he became superintendent, from attempting ambitious programs. He more or less followed the patterns of Tyler's administration.

Two reforms initiated during Jelly's eight years in office appear to have originated with the trustees. The assignment of one female nurse to take charge of the dining room on the male ward, in 1877—an enlightened idea on the surface—seems to have been driven by motives beyond the well being of male patients. According to the Committee on Admitting Patients, "If women nurses were substituted for men on the gentlemen's side, perhaps 20 out of the 33 male attendants could be discharged, at a saving of $2,500 per annum, and the Committee believes that such a change would also be greatly for the benefit of the patients" (16). (Small wonder that Louisa May Alcott and Susan B. Anthony were on the warpath!) It was also in Jelly's administration that McLean staff—physicians, attendants, cooks, etc.—were permitted, for the very first time, to take vacations: two weeks every year. Toward the end of his administration, Jelly decided patients might enjoy ordering their own meals more than the predictable fare of a regulated diet. Apparently they did, but the new privilege raised havoc with the trustees when the household expenditures rose precipitously. The board ordered the controlled menu reinstated.

There isn't much more to say about Jelly. His reports were perfunctory, lacking in imagination. He and McLean parted company in 1879. He was the first superintendent whose resignation did not cite poor health as a factor. In the absence of verbal flourishes from the trustees, one may suppose the departure was mutually agreeable. Jelly left office in June and opened a private practice in Boston. He went on to a public service career in his specialty: He was appointed examiner of the insane for the city of Boston in 1880 and was chairman of the State Board of Insanity from 1898 to 1908. He died in 1911, at a ripe old age. People reciting the list of nineteenth-century McLean superintendents often overlooked his name.

The asylum records for the Tyler-Jelly period reveal some subtle alterations in the patient population, consequences of changes in social perceptions and unanticipated aftermaths of admitting practices rather than of deliberate policies. The number of quiet, withdrawn patients gradually increased in proportion to the violent and dangerous. The trend suggests that the message of institutional treatment had filtered through to some portion of the public. Families became more willing to commit a quiet, melancholic victim of mental illness—who might have been kept at home without serious disruption to the household—to the care of the asylum, with the hope of cure. At the same time, a backlog of chronic, "incurable" patients, many admitted under policies adopted during Bell's administration, began to make itself noticeable. The presence of "incurable" patients in significant numbers undermined McLean's curative mission by demoralizing other patients and occupying space that might have been used for recent, "curable" cases. Tyler's strong assertion in his report for 1869 that the cases of insanity appropriate for admission were the "violent and dangerous, and the recent and curable" amounted to a criticism of the practice of admitting the chronic cases, a subject which he no doubt discussed more frankly with the trustees.

> The Trustees recognized a problem of sufficient magnitude to justify a committee. In 1871 they assigned some of their members to secure the removal of at least ten incurable female patients from the Asylum, who could be removed without injury to them. It was well known and well understood by the Trustees, in their constant visits, that there were such patients within the walls whose condition was hopeless, who would be as well provided for in some other institutions, who would not suffer from a change of place and surroundings. . . . But very slender results followed of the nature desired. It was found very difficult in any case, and impossible in most cases, to induce the friends of such patients to consent to their removal. In one point of view the incidental measures brought into action called out gratifying evidence of the high consideration in which the Asylum was held by the parties concerned, of their full confidence in

> and grateful appreciation of the kind and faithful care bestowed upon the afflicted objects of their solicitude.

Having acknowledged the problem of long-term patients, tried to address it, and failed, the trustees did not revise admissions policies. Historian and former trustee Ellis's account continues: "The Asylum would best reward the hopes and labors of its friends by receiving almost exclusively curable patients, and by discharging them on the earliest day on which their restoration is assured. But it must meet the wishes and needs of the community as a merciful refuge for many incurables" (17). In short, people were committing hopelessly ill relatives to McLean. Fifty years earlier, when madhouses were the only option, many families would have suffered the presences of the severely deranged or disabled at home; the asylum represented a humane alternative to a desperate situation. One can scarcely fault the families for wanting a safe and sympathetic refuge or blame the trustees for responding to a legitimate need. But as the number of chronic patients rose, their presence increasingly obscured the original primary purpose of the asylum, which had been to cure.

The McLean patient register for 1875 listed 76 patients admitted before 1871; since the average weekly census for 1875 was 156, patients who had been in the asylum four or more years accounted for nearly half the population. One man, Patient Number 1488, had been in residence since 1838. Both he and the other two patients of longest duration paid the princely sum of $50.00 per week, at a time when the average weekly cost per patient was $21.07, and thereby subsidized some less-affluent boarders. During 1878, cases believed to be chronic or incurable accounted for 32 percent of admissions. Families who could afford to support their mentally disabled relatives at McLean indefinitely were also the same people likely to respond to fundraising appeals, a fact the trustees could not easily ignore. Thus, mercy and money sometimes became entangled with one another.

Rising numbers of chronically ill patients were inhabiting all mental institutions in the latter decades of the nineteenth century, presenting a dilemma, especially for tax-supported asylums. At least privately endowed places like McLean, which could pick and choose their patients, derived some economic rewards. But even at McLean this class of patient began to transform the character of the place from a medically active institution to a passive, caretaking one. The energy and optimism that had animated the early days of moral treatment evaporated as patients became permanent residents or returned time after time after time to weather another spell of illness.

One McLean patient, a 49-year-old civil engineer who suffered from "chronic mania," was admitted in late November 1879 for the fifteenth time, his last previous admission having occurred less than a year earlier. His brother, who had learned to read the signs of an approaching attack, alerted the asylum. Two attendants were dispatched in the evening to the Parker House in Boston. The prospective patient, already in bed, was surprised to see them and said that he felt sure there was no need for his removal but that he was willing to go along and stay until the doctors were satisfied with his mental health. By morning the patient was "raving as only an insane man can." He passed the next few weeks in a state of acute agitation—breaking pottery, striking attendants, and committing other acts of violence. Then, his excitement subsided, and after two weeks of calm, he was discharged as recovered. He was back at McLean again before another year had passed. This went on for years; the patient's 32nd admission occurred in 1895 at the new McLean in Belmont. There is no indication that the physicians tried to treat him. They protected him from injuring himself or others until his mania abated, observed when his behavior stabilized, and discharged him. This is one of those instances that raises doubts about use of the term "recovered." Since each admission was entered into the records as a separate case, then it might have been fair to say that the man recovered, because he apparently negotiated the outside world reasonably well in the intervals between attacks. Thus recovery referred to individual disease episodes rather than to a continuum of illness.

While the proportions of chronic and incurable patients rose, recovery rates dropped off sharply. Taking recovery as a percentage of admissions, one finds the McLean rate sliding from the 50 percent mark of the 1850s down to 20 or 25 percent in the 1870s and hitting an all-time low in 1878 when only 9.5 percent of the patients admitted (the civil engineer among them) were considered to have recovered. This last figure prompted Jelly's observation that

> no one can examine, carefully, the statistics published by the various Hospitals in this country, and note the diminished percentage of reported recoveries without being convinced that this diminution must be owing to a change in the curability of the cases themselves; from alteration in the constitution, habits of life and the ways of business of our people, and, very often, to too long delay in being placed under proper treatment, rather than to the peculiarities of temperament in those making up the statistics. (18)

Jelly's remarks pointed to the fact that McLean's figures were pieces of a larger pattern, for other institutions had, indeed, also been reporting declining recovery rates.

There are two conventional explanations for this change in the statistical curve. First, the venerable Pliny Earle, of the Original Thirteen, exploded the "myth" of the curability of insanity by exposing the numerical monkey business that had given rise to what he called the "curability delusion." His volume, *The Curability of Insanity*, published in 1877, picked up the gauntlet thrown down by Bell in the 1840s. Earle analyzed the statistics of dozens of American and British asylums and demonstrated how abuse of the term "recovery," as well as failure to distinguish between the case and the patient, had presented a distorted picture of the efficacy of asylum treatment. The second explanation concerns the accumulation of incurable patients. Yet even if recoveries are figured as percentages of patients discharged, rather than of those admitted or of the whole number treated, the rates still fall off. The place to look for the effect of the chronic patients is not, I think, in the statistics but in the attitudes of asylum staff.

I believe Jelly was wrong in his assertion that "peculiarities of temperament" had nothing to do with diminished cure ratios. The asylum superintendents of his generation *were* of a different temperament than those who had preceded them. By the post Civil War period, they had moved beyond the era of progressive pioneering in the style of Wyman and the youthful optimism of the Original Thirteen. Those early alienists had worked in an information vacuum and with relatively small numbers of patients. By the 1870s, however, they communicated through a professional association and their journal. They reviewed the cumulative records of institutions—the increasing numbers of chronic patients (some of whom had been thought curable at the time of first admission), patients like McLean's civil engineer, who were admitted, discharged, and readmitted through the asylum's revolving door. Confidence in the curability of insanity began to collapse under the weight of 50 years of evidence and experience.

The figures started their downward trend long before Earle's studies went into print; in fact, he calculated that reported recoveries in 20 American asylums had decreased from 46 to 34 percent (annually, of cases admitted) over a 25-year period. He also observed that the statistical decline had occurred simultaneously in both tax-supported institutions and expensive institutions like McLean and that, therefore, the amount of money spent on asylum treatment did not have anything to do with the rate of cure. Some superintendents, like Earle, ran the entire gamut from optimism to despair in a single career. Luther Bell has already been heard uttering his tragic, private belief that, once insane, a man was "used up for this world." Such denunciations did not initially sit well with asylum superintendents, but by the end of the century professional opinion about the curability of insanity wound up approximately where it had been 100 years earlier, before Pinel and the Tukes had raised hope. Moral treatment, the principle upon which the institutional system had been founded, lost credibility as a medical regimen if not as a humanist ideal.

That leaves this question: Had moral treatment ever cured anybody at all? There is reason to believe that many patients discharged as "recovered" from nineteenth-century asylums practicing moral treatment actually did regain mental health. Between 1882 and 1893 the Worcester State Hospital conducted an unusual follow-up survey of more than 1,000 individuals who had been patients between 1833 and 1846—during Woodward's administration—and found that 54 percent had remained well or died in sound mind. Although the methods of collecting and manipulating data would be suspect by current standards, it is reasonable to suppose that a good proportion of Worcester's 54 percent would indeed meet contemporary psychiatric criteria for health. Based on what is known about mental illness today, it is probable that some of those patients would have gotten well without institutionalization through the mysterious process of spontaneous remission. However, asylums protected the insane from undernourishment, infection, and social ostracism; people who might have committed suicide or died of starvation in society survived in institutions and went on to regain psychological stability. For others, whose distress had been precipitated by troubles at home or in business, removal to the asylum and the compassionate, supportive course of moral treatment were effective, more so in the early years before institutions became crowded with chronic patients and the medical forecast turned gloomy. Thus, the answer to the original question—did moral treatment cure anybody at all?—is technically "no." But the evidence supports Tuke's original contention that moral treatment did "assist Nature in the performance of her own cure" (19).

The application of moral treatment evolved after the Civil War under the influence of increased numbers of incurable patients and gathering doubts about the efficacy of the therapeutic program. While continuing to pay lip service to moral treatment, Tyler and Jelly relaxed some of its more repressive rules, such as minimum duration of stay and the prohibition of visitors, and administered the recreations and diversions in a manner that suggested that they did not take them seriously as medical therapy. Games and concerts and sewing circles might, indeed, amuse, engage, or fill up empty time for some anguished souls but were not viewed as curative measures. This is a subtle point, I know, and one difficult to prove. Yet the inference is inescapable that as the chronic population increased and the recovery rate decreased, physicians and attendants held diminished expectations for their patients and unintentionally expressed those attitudes in the performance of routine duties. Jelly's apologia in his report for 1878, that miserable year of the 9.5 percent recovery rate, effectively acknowledged McLean's revised role: "While we can but regret that the year has been productive of no greater results," he wrote, "I believe that the

Asylum has not been unsuccessful in the broad field of its work, the amelioration of the condition, and the proper care of all the patients committed to its trust."

Dr. Charles F. Folsom, who had been first assistant physician for a year during Jelly's administration, wrote a chapter on mental diseases for the fifth volume of the *American System of Medicine*. His remarks on mental institutions were not complimentary.

> The character of the asylums . . . has changed from being small, easily managed institutions to overgrown affairs, crowded with so many incurables that the duties of the superintendents have become largely administrative, and the medical treatment of the sick has been driven to a subordinate position. Medical officers, too, are more cautious in using the word cured after experience has shown them how many reported cures are only remissions. . . . [I]n enlarging our asylums, as we have been compelled to do, we have lost something in personal care of patients, and . . . we have increased the depressing influences of large masses of sick people to such an extent as to involve serious disadvantages in their treatment. (20)

Folsom admitted that in his private practice he sometimes "acted contrary to the usually accepted views" and advised against removal of a patient to an asylum but, instead, supervised treatment at home, usually with happy results. For a mainline alienist to have advanced such views in the 1850s or 1860s would have been downright heresy. Not so in the 1880s. Folsom's chapter was reprinted and bound for the use of Harvard Medical School students. The new McLean superintendent, Edward A. Cowles, had it in his personal library.

CHAPTER

5

Edward A. Cowles: "The only way to begin is to begin . . ."

Jelly submitted his resignation on February 28, 1879, in a letter that did not specify a reason for leaving. Precisely two weeks later the trustees elected Edward A. Cowles, then superintendent of Boston City Hospital, as Jelly's successor. This rapid-fire sequence of events has all the earmarks of a carefully prepared plan. Though Cowles's name never shows up in the records before his election, the trustees' negotiations with him surely predated Jelly's formal letter. The change of power was orchestrated so smoothly as to leave no hint what went wrong between Jelly and the board, yet something obviously did. The arrangement saved face for those faces that needed saving: Jelly agreed to serve through June, and the first assistant physician would hold the fort until December, when Cowles was scheduled to take office.

In selecting a man who had administrative experience in general hospital medicine, the trustees broke with the pattern of promoting a McLean physician or appointing someone from the network of mental institutions. Bell, though not an asylum doctor, had immersed himself in the subject during his political efforts in New Hampshire. The unorthodoxy of the trustees' choice suggests that they had special expectations of Cowles. Unfortunately, however, trustee records are deliberately obscure when it comes to motives. They reveal who was elected—though not who was considered and *not* elected, and never the critical *why*. All of that—the discussions, arguments, and compromises—is dirty laundry not to be hung out for posterity. History receives the sanitized account scrubbed, starched, and ironed into an annual report.

But some inferences can be drawn from Cowles's record. He was born in Ryegate, Vermont, in July 1837 into a family of accomplished men and women. His father, George, served for many years in the Vermont state legislature. Edward went to school in Ryegate and to college at Dartmouth. He earned his A.B. in 1859 and took his medical degree from the College of Physicians and Surgeons at Columbia in New York in 1863, in the midst of the Civil War. Dartmouth awarded him another M.D. degree the same year. Cowles next became an assistant physician at the Hartford Retreat, his singular and brief encounter with asylum medicine before McLean. After a few months he joined the U.S. Army Medical Corps and received the rank of assistant surgeon. Shortly after the Battle of Gettysburg, which occurred in July 1863, he was placed in charge of a general hospital in Harrisburg, Pennsylvania, to tend the Union wounded and ailing—an administrative trial by fire. Later he was attached to General Ulysses S. Grant's Army of the Potomac. The Civil War, like both future world wars, had a tremendous impact on medical practice and delivery systems in peacetime. Cowles's understanding of hospital organization and the role of nurses matured quickly in the field.

After the war ended, Cowles stayed with the Army, going wherever he was sent. In one assignment he spent two years as medical director of the military district of the Rio Grande, Texas, where he had to manage epidemics of yellow fever and cholera. Nobody knew anything about mosquitoes then, and Cowles had no better defenses against yellow fever than the people he was trying to help. He nearly died of it.

He left the Army with the rank of captain in 1872, went to South Boston, and became a visiting physician to the Carney Hospital there. A few months later he accepted an invitation to join the Boston City Hospital as medical superintendent. Cowles built a stunning record at Boston City Hospital, an episode in his career usually overshadowed by his even more original achievements at McLean. His Boston City Hospital successor, Dr. G. H. M. Rowe, reflected that Cowles had

> elevated it from a position quite ordinary among the hospitals of that time; under his administration, it was enlarged to twice its size when he assumed charge; new buildings were added in which many new features of hospital construction were first used, and although at that time new, they still [in 1904] remain as accepted features of good hospital construction. During his first years there, hospital gangrene, pyaemia and surgical sepsis obtained to a frightful extent. By his work in the reconstruction of the system of heating and ventilation, all blood poisoning diseases, except those due to the surgical technique of that day, disappeared. Many improvements and reorganizations based upon military lines, and suggested by his army experience, were perfected. (1)

The speed, efficiency, and excellence of the construction program at Boston City Hospital did not escape the notice of the McLean trustees intent on building a new asylum. It was probably that aspect of Cowles's accomplishments that caught the board's collective eye. And the prospect of building a new hospital from the ground up, to his own specifications, no doubt appealed to the candidate.

Cowles had done a great deal more at Boston City Hospital than oversee the expansion of facilities. He had enlisted the aid of Linda Richards, the first woman in the United States to hold a diploma as a trained nurse and superintendent of the Massachusetts General Hospital Training School for Nurses, and begun the Training School for Nurses at Boston City Hospital in 1878. In contrast with the MGH school, which was administratively independent of the MGH, Cowles designed the Boston City Hospital training program as an integral part of the hospital. This form of organization pleased that part of his mind formed in military service. He liked orderly power structures and clear chains of command, Army-style administrative pyramids with a benign father rather than a general at the top. He took the view that

> a hospital household is an organized social unit; as a family of men and women, young and middle aged, it should be under a controlling head, *in loco parentis*. The hospital is the home for those who live in it, and the lives, liberties, and happiness are largely in the hands of the controlling authority, for order must reign. It is a household organized to do busi-

> ness where the people live. The moral, ethical, and business atmosphere of the place must be calm and wholesome in its influence upon the sick and insane. . . . (2)

Though Cowles's administration of Boston City Hospital is customarily associated with the development of the nursing school, it was in his role as chief admissions officer that he made his greatest imprint on its character. Historian Morris J. Vogel contrasted the Boston City trustees' inclination to admit only the "legitimate, acutely sick, and deserving citizen" with Cowles's willingness to challenge the board with a liberal admissions practice.

> While Edward Cowles remained superintendent his humane attitude minimized the effect of the trustees on the actual operation of the hospital. His valedictory reports in 1878 and 1879 were catalogs of rules he had broken and strictures he had neglected in promiscuously opening the institution to all. Patients who could not pay had not been pauperized. He had not rejected—if they could benefit from admission—the "professional invalids, shiftless and improvident persons, frequent applicants for relief [and] victims of their own vices with alcoholism or injuries from drunken quarrels or accidents". . . . Even those suffering attacks of insanity had been welcomed, and the hospital had responded to their needs by organizing a department for diseases of the nervous system. (3)

Surely the McLean trustees had read Cowles's Boston City reports and noticed his independence of spirit; evidently it did not faze them, for they trusted him with broad authority from the moment he took office.

Cowles at 42 was a short man with a military bearing, a florid complexion, and according to a contemporary, a genial expression. He was married to the former Harriet M. Wainwright; they had no children. He was a capable, experienced executive who ran a no-nonsense operation, habits of organization acquired in the Army that had proved themselves serviceable in civilian life. He expressed his thoughts in unadorned prose. But his Boston City Hospital record showed that he was no stiff-necked, rulebook soldier. He governed with imagination, bending, breaking, or changing rules in the interest of principles. The quality that does not come through very clearly in the Boston City reports, but that revealed itself when Cowles was at McLean, was intellectual vitality of a high order. Though sometimes obstinate in his convictions, he possessed the self-confidence to admit what he did not know, but needed to know, and to find it out.

After he accepted the McLean superintendency and completed his duties at Boston City Hospital, Cowles set off on the trustees' behalf for an autumn tour of asylums in France and Britain. He had several items on his agenda. He wanted especially to see those institutions where women nurses were employed on male wards because he planned to introduce this practice at McLean, and there were no examples in the United States. He also inspected architectural features on all scales, from the general site plan down to the details of windows. Meanwhile, he reacquainted himself with asylum medicine. He returned to the United States and assumed his responsibilities in Somerville in December 1879.

Cowles's first decisions signaled that he would not await the construction of new facilities—which he judged to be in a future too remote to benefit the current patients—to start shaping the new McLean. He surveyed his domain and pronounced himself dissatisfied. Whereas Jelly had submitted to the trustees' reluctance to pour money into a physical plant slated for abandonment, Cowles insisted on replacing most of the plumbing, which he discovered to be in a perilous condition of disrepair; on renovating several rooms and wards; upgrading the ventilation; and installing new carpets and furniture. Although the trustees had already started selling off portions of the Somerville property to accumulate a building fund for the new asylum, they supported Cowles's requests by approving a hearty budget increase. One suspects that his financial demands did not come as a surprise to the board and that he had, in fact, made improvements in Somerville a precondition for accepting the McLean post.

Cowles rapidly extended the range of patient liberties initiated by Tyler. He further reduced the use of mechanical restraints. The building modifications accomplished during 1880 included the removal of ornamental gratings that acted as bars from several windows; Cowles had the sashes stopped so the windows could be opened six inches at the top and bottom. He unlocked the doors in six male wards, day and night. (Women on four or five wards had enjoyed this privilege since Tyler's administration, though only during the daytime hours.) In 1881 the door leading from the five principal male wards was fitted with an ordinary handle and left unlocked most of the day. This entailed some risk because the door opened onto an unsecured enclosure, but only two patients escaped during the first year the door was open, and one returned voluntarily. The door of the Appleton House for men, which stood on open ground, was also left unlocked during the day. The great danger, of course, was that an escaped patient would wander over the railroad tracks and get killed by a train. Cowles, aware of the hazards as well as the likelihood that such an accident might cause a public scandal, pressed on with his open-door policy, posting attendants where they could intercept endangered patients. At least one incident of this nature occurred in June 1888 when a man escaped, tried to board a moving train, and received fatal injuries (4). But fortunately for Cowles, the misadventure was construed as one more reason to quit the Somerville industrial slums rather than as an error in administrative judgment.

Cowles further liberalized the conditions of parole and the reception of friends and relatives at the asylum; he permitted short visits home and minimized the censureship of correspondence. In 1883 he ordered bars removed from more windows. That summer McLean rented a cottage by the seashore in Lynn, Massachusetts. Half a dozen women patients passed most of the season there, and weekly parties of women traveled by train to spend the afternoon taking tea or strolling on the beaches. The practice continued until McLean moved to Waverly, where the pastoral delights were sufficient unto themselves.

On the surface Cowles's relaxation of the rules governing institutional confinement appeared as the next generation of Tyler's reforms. But Tyler had loosened a few strings here and another few there, without reference to a well-articulated vision. Cowles, by contrast, measured every step deliberately against his grand design for redefining the asylum as a hospital. He spelled out this program in his annual report for 1882, and he stuck with it for the 24 years he ran McLean. It was true that McLean's founding physicians, Jackson and Warren, had used "hospital" and "asylum" interchangeably in their appeals and that the distinction between the two did not amount to much during the first two or three decades of McLean's existence, when general hospital medicine was not much to brag about. Since then, however, the general hospital had started to present itself as a more worthy model and by the 1880s was recording spectacular advances, notably in surgery. Meanwhile, asylums had floated so far away from hospitals, both in medical practice and in public perception, as to require a willful push in the direction of mainstream medicine. Cowles, a veteran of general hospitals, put his shoulder to the asylum and shoved.

One of the earliest, and surely the least expensive, measures he took was a change in vocabulary. "Once within the hospital," he wrote, "the conduct of physicians and nurses toward the patient should show that he is regarded as simply ill, as having no reason for being ashamed of his illness. Therefore, he should always be called a 'patient,' and not a 'boarder,' as is the custom in some hospitals, and has been in this one from its earliest days. The latter term implies an evasion of the fact of illness, as if it were a disgrace, and by a euphemism fosters the very feeling of which we are trying to disabuse the patients." Cowles dignified the power of names to form expectations: If I am an "inmate," a word that occasionally crept into very early McLean reports, then I must be guilty; if I am "boarder," then why am I locked up? If I am a "patient," then I must be sick.

By the same logic, Cowles banished attendants. "'Attendants' may attend the infirm and incurable; but 'nurses' attend the sick, and the experience of recovery from illness is so common that the very idea of a presence of a nurse logically carries with it the other idea, that something is being done to promote recovery, and that itself inspires hope and is curative" (5). Naturally, he objected to the term "asylum," which by his time had acquired a bad connotation, and lobbied for an institutional name change; given legal formalities and Bostonian attachment to tradition, this took longer than reeducating the habits of speech of McLean personnel. But in 1892 the McLean Asylum was rechristened the McLean Hospital.

Words, after all, are only words. A reform of language quickly loses its force if it is not accompanied by fundamental changes in the reality the words are meant to express. McLean attendants had a new label but no new skills. For decades they had acted as caretakers, companions, and watchers of the "boarders," as well as ward sweepers, dusters, dishwashers, bed makers, and window wipers—duties for which hands-on experience had always been considered an adequate teacher. When Cowles promoted attendants to nurses, he also relieved them of many household chores by employing "ward-maids to perform duties that distract the attention of nurses from more important ones," namely, active medical care of patients. He found that though many attendants handled patients with adeptness and compassion, their ignorance of principles of medicine and observation prevented them from being effective medical agents. Cowles had gained a great respect for the work of trained nurses, first in the Civil War and later at Boston City Hospital, and was determined to provide McLean with a nursing service "qualified for the task of treating a houseful of acute cases" (6). When he arrived at McLean, he introduced the attendants to some general hospital methods on the wards and set up a few classes. In 1882 he hired a proper superintendent of nurses, Mary Palmer, who had graduated from the MGH Training School and spent 12 years as an attendant and then matron at the Vermont Asylum. Together they worked with Linda Richards at Boston City Hospital to design a curriculum especially for training nurses to work with mental patients. The beginning of the McLean Training School for Nurses traditionally dates from this year, though regular classes did not start until 1883.

Previous attempts had been made to formalize the education of mental nurses both in the United States and in Europe, but McLean's attempt was the first to succeed. In Cowles's opinion the earlier efforts had been "too tentative and not sufficiently well organized.... The professional element in the work of nursing as a prospective means of livelihood was not made sufficiently important as the proper and necessary stimulus to undertake and adhere to a methodical course of study..." (7).

Cowles, who did not have a tentative or disorganized bone in his body, nevertheless ran into some early obstacles. The admirably qualified Palmer, who was supposed to introduce the training program, became ill and had to leave after two years. As Palmer's health started its decline, Cowles singled out Lucia Woodward, who had been at McLean for 15 years—six as an attendant and nine as a supervisor—and sent her to learn general medical nursing under Richards's guidance at the Boston City Hospital Training School. By the time Palmer resigned, Woodward was ready to take over her job.

The second problem proved more troublesome. The curriculum had been designed to balance education in general nursing with special instruction in the care of the mentally ill. Cowles expected trained hospital nurses to help get the general medical aspect of the program off the ground. Between 1880 and 1885, he hired nine hospital nurses to work on the female wards and train the old attendants. The plan failed miserably. The nurses complained about having to be companions to listless patients, refused to learn special skills required for nursing the mentally ill (many of which the attendants could have taught them), and generally hated the asylum atmosphere. All but one quit after a month or two. Cowles realized that teaching nurses would have to be generated principally by McLean itself, hence his logic in sending Woodward off for her course in general nursing. For these reasons, and because Cowles was proceeding with caution, the training school got off to a faltering start.

Nevertheless, the McLean Training School for Nurses graduated its first class, 15 women, in 1886. The same year the school formed a section for men and arranged for the MGH Training School to receive McLean graduates who wanted more clinical experience in general nursing. By the end of the 1880s, the training school had found solid footing. It assured McLean a source of quality nurses because some graduates naturally applied to stay on the staff. Others, as Cowles had intended, found work in other mental institutions or with private patients.

After a few years, the training school began receiving applications from people outside McLean. One of the earliest of them came from Annie Bolton, a young Quebec woman, who was attracted to Somerville by a friend's letter filled with "glowing accounts" of nursing at McLean and a desperate urge to get away from home. Bolton arrived in Boston in 1887:

> After many hours' ride, we at last reached the North Station. I gathered up my things and hurried out, fearing that I would not find my friend in that vast crowd. I found her waiting and we at once took a horse car for the Asylum, as it was then called.... After an hour's ride we arrived at

> Fitchburg Street, better known as Brick Bottom. The street swarmed with men, women and dirty children. We made our way through the crowd, crossed the railroad track and through the gate that led to the Asylum grounds.

Bolton was introduced to the superintendent of nurses early the next morning:

> After breakfast—to the library to meet Miss Woodward. I could hear the nurses shh-sh-sh. After a few minutes I heard a very determined footstep. I caught my breath, conscious only of a sharp look from piercing blue eyes and a stern mouth. She was tall and bony and reminded me of the Statue of Liberty, she was so cold. At last her face softened, her mouth relaxed and she said "Good morning. I only hope you have come here prepared to work and keep your mind on your patients and lessons. Remember, there is no *romance* in this hospital." I was given clear and concise instructions to that effect. . . . "You must put your best efforts in your work, rise to your superiors, and be loyal to the Asylum. This is no place for rattle-brained girls." (8)

(Woodward was not quite as formidable as she appeared. Nurses who worked with her over the years detected a shy woman of fragile self-esteem beneath the stony exterior. But first impressions are hard to erase.)

Bolton also recalled that during both winters of her student years Cowles sent her and two other nurses to a gymnasium in Boston to learn medical massage and gymnastics. Bolton viewed the extra education with mixed emotions; for months Woodward ordered her to give massages once a week from nine to ten in the evening, normally an off-duty time for her. But Bolton, a plucky woman, stayed on at McLean after graduation. Cowles, by contrast, was delighted with the results of massage and gymnastic exercises: "It has been surprising to see how a torpid melancholiac can have his interest aroused in the development of his biceps," he reported in 1888.

While building the training program, Cowles gently introduced more women nurses into the men's wards. "To put a man accustomed to the comforts, or even if no more than to the habits, of a domestic life, into a restricted association with men, would be to him an experience of which he probably has had no previous conception," Cowles argued. "Such a way of living would be unnatural and unattractive to most men, and to the sick man, whose mind is already disturbed, a cause of added discomfort" (9). His "experiment," as he called it, seems to have precipitated a minimum of Victorian hysteria, nothing that caused the trustees to lose any sleep. By 1887 there were three female nurses and two ward-maids deployed in five wards where men patients tended to quietness and/or advanced age. Cowles observed the new regime with satisfaction: The patients expressed their gratitude for the presence of females while the male attendants responded with more civilized, gentlemanly behavior. By 1889 he proclaimed the experiment an "established success."

Contrary to expectations in Jelly's era, McLean did not save a single penny with Cowles's arrangement. Women nurses who worked in men's wards were the highest paid of all and the only ones to earn more than a beginning male nurse, a wage scale that indicates that Cowles considered some sort of hardship pay appropriate. Moreover, the women did not replace men but were added to their numbers. A visitor in the year 1887, when McLean's patient capacity was 170, counted a total of 81 attendants and nurses, almost 1 for every 2 patients, by contrast with the 1-to-6 ratio that had obtained during the 1850s and 1860s (10).

Cowles was also reinforcing his medical staff. In 1880 the trustees authorized him to nominate two medical interns for McLean and to appoint a full-fledged apothecary in the place of the medical student who used to perform that role. The interns took over the work of clinical clerks that had previously fallen to the two assistant physicians, freeing the latter for more attention to patients and medical studies. Though provisional at the outset, the extra medical help proved so satisfactory, especially to the liberated assistant physicians, that it evolved into a permanent intern system. In 1882 the trustees approved Cowles's recommendation to invite physicians as consultants so as to form a temporary consulting staff for McLean. And in 1887 Cowles was permitted to appoint a third assistant physician, Horace M. Locke.

During Cowles's tenure the modern triad of "patient care, teaching, and research" began to emerge, and it was Cowles's aggressive development of the third element that seems to have caught the trustees off guard, though he had given them ample warning of his intentions. "It seems to me," he wrote in 1882, "that in [small, well endowed] hospitals, where the means and opportunity are liberally given, while due regard is to be had to a proper conservatism, it is a special duty to explore new paths, if any there be, beyond the beaten ways of procedure in the management of the insane. To stand still is to fail, when progress is demanded and is possible; for even negative results are valuable." His initial requests were modest: a microscope and other paraphernalia for converting a room into a laboratory and a budget for a consulting pathologist. The trustees yielded graciously. The room was fitted out and Cowles retained Dr. William W. Gannett, a Boston physician, to perform autopsies and run a systematic pathology course for the staff physicians. Cowles also began to assemble a proper medical library.

McLean "research" remained on this primitive level, albeit a wildly progressive one by comparison with other mental institutions, for five years while Cowles channeled most of his energy into the McLean Training School for Nurses. By 1887 the nursing program had acquired its own momentum and did not require so much of his attention. He asked for a leave of absence on account of his health, and the trustees granted him a one-year sabbatical. Presumably, he recovered his health promptly because during that leave he went to Johns Hopkins to study psychology with G. Stanley Hall, who was then teaching in the medical department. This is one of those line items in Cowles's professional biography that his contemporaries seldom mentioned, in some cases for selfish reasons; therefore, it often got overlooked by later generations or, if noticed, got treated in a ho-hum fashion by writers who took intellectual cross-pollination for granted. But at a time when asylum superintendents were largely ignorant of the existence of psychology, let alone its potential significance to their profession, Cowles's instincts were dazzling. He had obviously been reading something besides the *American Journal of Insanity*: He may have been pointed in Hall's direction by Henry P. Bowditch at the Harvard Medical School.

Cowles and Hall turned out to be kindred spirits and formed one of those precious friendships that survives adversities and nourishes thought. Cowles warmed to Hall's physiologically oriented psychology and his view of its application to the study of mental disorders. Hall encouraged Cowles to develop laboratory research at McLean and recommended one of his former fellows, Dr. William Noyes, as a potential candidate for the McLean staff. Noyes, at the time an assistant physician at the Bloomingdale Asylum, had graduated from the Harvard Medical School and had received training in psychology. But when Cowles proposed appointing him to McLean as a full-time pathologist, the trustees balked and advised Cowles he could have a third assistant physician or a pathologist, but not both. Cowles settled on Noyes, who arrived in 1888 with the title of "pathologist and assistant physician." (Horace Locke, the third assistant physician, filled in for absent staff members and then departed in 1889.) Cowles asked the trustees to invest $1,200 in expanding laboratory facilities for Noyes; they voted to give him $600 (11).

Cowles's excitement as McLean was poised on the brink of a systematic research program was transparent. Noyes's appointment, he wrote,

> enables us to undertake the investigations of the new questions that are now becoming so interesting and important. The lines of inquiry are in so many branches of the "new psychology" that no pretence is made beyond the purpose of beginning them. The Asylum study of these problems may include, besides pathology, "what the nervous system can do" both in health and disease, whatever is open to mechanical experiment in physical and mental phenomena of nervous action, and whatever pathological psychology may present for analysis and explanation. (12)

By 1890, Noyes's research had found a more precise focus:

> The problems that first manifestly present themselves for such inquiry are those relating to the nature and source of nervous energy, the phenomena of its expenditure and exhaustion as clinically observed in the prodromic and acute stages of ordinary insanity, and the remedial measures that best affect the arrest of exhausting processes and promote the restoration of the vigor of bodily and mental health. . . . These questions involve a study of the laws of nutrition, rest, and physical exercise, and the exact observation of the conditions attending progress toward recovery in individual cases. Such problems as these are strictly physiological and lie at the foundation of scientific psychiatry, as much as those relating to the structure and pathology of the nervous elements. . . . The complexity of all this would be discouraging at the outset, were it not so plainly to be seen that the only way to begin is to begin. . . . (13)

Cowles's plan for what he was now calling the Pathological and Psychological Department provided for a few months in Europe every year for whomever held the research position to study laboratory methods. Hall's spirit hovered benignly in the background. Cowles had been eager to develop McLean research; his encounter with Hall at Johns Hopkins had provided the gentle nudge that gave those impulses direction. Hall guided in the selection of Noyes and, with additional counsel from William James and Bowditch at Harvard Medical School, in the equipping of Noyes's laboratory for psychological experimentation.

Once Noyes settled in at McLean, Cowles arranged a weekly seminar of all the medical officers, including the interns, as a vehicle for exchanging laboratory and clinical data. Every week a staff member presented a history and review of the literature on some topic, with a summary of the current knowledge. The group discussed possibilities for further investigations. Cowles set up the seminars in a flexible format so that any pressing subject—with reference, say, to a McLean patient—might be substituted on the agenda, or interesting discussions could be carried over to the next week. In a fastidiously structured world, this was another act of administrative imagination, and it proved to be a stimulating system of study within the hospital.

Cowles did not confine his zeal for scientific investigation to McLean. He was a feisty participant in the Association of Medical Superintendents of American Institutions for the Insane—an organizational moniker that grated on his nerves. After his stint at Johns Hopkins, he brought Hall's work to the attention of the association by reviewing his publications in the *American Journal of Insanity*. When Hall—by then president of Clark University in Worcester, Massachusetts—organized the American Psychological Association, Cowles and Noyes were among the founding members. In 1891 Cowles stood before the members of the Association of Medical Superintendents of American Institutions for the Insane, who were becoming less stuffy and reactionary as new faces and inquiring minds refreshed the ranks, and insisted on the necessity for systematic research on "all subjects relating to the care and treatment of the insane." He was among the members who agitated in behalf of changing the association's name to one that would reflect a scientific orientation rather than a custodial function. When the matter came up for discussion in 1892 someone proposed "the American Psychiatric Association" but was voted down on the grounds that the name, "especially to the laymen, would be a very embarrassing one to translate" (14). The group decided instead to copy the British formula and become the American Medico-Psychological Association (AMPA).

In 1894, when AMPA was gearing up to celebrate its 50th anniversary, Cowles was instrumental in securing S. Weir Mitchell, the neurologist, as a speaker for the event. When first approached, Mitchell responded frankly that "if he spoke at all, criticism rather than compliment must predominate his remarks" and that he was therefore reluctant to accept. But AMPA membership had at long last reached that point where it was willing, even eager, to entertain outside advice and persisted with its invitation (15). And so, on May 16, Mitchell rose before his hosts and gave them the scolding he had promised:

> Once we spoke of asylums with respect; it is not so now. We, neurologists, think you have fallen behind us, and this opinion is gaining ground outside of our own ranks, and is, in part at least, your own fault.... Where, we ask, are your annual reports of scientific study, of the psychology and pathology of your patients?... What have you taught us of the 91,000 insane whom you see and treat?... You live alone, uncriticized, unquestioned, out of the healthy conflicts and honest rivalries which keep us [neurologists] up to the mark of the fullest possible competence. (16)

After he had finished his speech, the association made him an honorary member.

McLean remembers Cowles best for commanding the construction of the new hospital in Waverly. But the fact is that he accomplished an essential part of the building program, the transformation from asylum to hospital and the embryonic research program, amidst the railroad yards and slaughterhouses of Somerville. "When we build our houses," he said, "we try first to lay a firm foundation, and then to raise a good superstructure." So he laid the foundation in Somerville and raised the superstructure in Waverly. "It is simply a matter of organization," he explained (17). And organize he did. Duties, routines, and avenues of responsibility were all spelled out with unambiguous clarity. Forms were written and printed to control this and that: There were forms for itemizing laundry, forms to record temperatures in the wards three times a day, forms to paste on newspapers and magazines to regulate their circulation, forms to record the number of knives, forks, and spoons after each meal, forms to take inventory of supplies kept in the wards. (Onc startling item on the standard list of ward supplies was "grenades, hand.") Cowles presided with benevolent despotism over a platoon of cooks, nurses, physicians, laundresses, groundskeepers, firemen, seamstresses, gardeners, farmhands, ward-maids, coachmen, interns, various craftsmen, an apothecary, and the indispensable steward, who in turn managed the bureaucratic blizzard of paperwork. Altogether, McLean employees and staff numbered 169 in 1887. One imagines Cowles like one of those tough-skinned, soft-hearted officers in a Hollywood film—respected and adored by his troops.

The intern program, the Training School for Nurses, the staff seminars, the medical library, and the laboratory work in pathology and psychology all started in Somerville. Clinical charts for temperature, pulse, respiration, and urinalysis were introduced. The administrations of medicines, which were once casually entered into the records if the physician had time, were now dutifully itemized. Cowles stopped using clumsy volumes for case records, a system that had become impractical decades earlier, and started keeping individual folders so each patient's entire history could be easily reviewed. Bars were removed from windows, doors were unlocked, attendants became nurses. The boarder became a patient, "treated as a reasoning being. In other words, from the moment he enters the hospital, it should be assumed that he will understand more or less correctly all that is said or done to him" (18).

An important change in admissions practices did not originate with Cowles but nevertheless advanced his interests. In 1881 Massachusetts enacted the first voluntary admission law in the United States. The mechanism for entry to McLean consisted simply of a signature upon a form reading "I hereby request to be admitted to the McLean Asylum for care and treatment," and, less simply, of evidence that someone would cover the costs of hospitalization. Under the state law, voluntary patients could not be held against their will and had to be discharged upon their written request. The percentage of McLean patients who admitted themselves rose steadily and, by 1890, constituted about 40 percent of all admissions. Though practical problems occasionally presented themselves—most often in the form of a patient who applied for discharge against medical advice, whose friends refused to take responsibility, and who suddenly found him- or herself committed involuntarily—Cowles applauded the principle: "it is invaluable at promoting the mutual confidence which strengthens the good work of hospitals, making them truly hospitals in their helpfulness to the sick, and not forbidding to those who should early seek such aid" (19). The presence of voluntary patients was believed to raise the morale of committed patients and to make the hospital seem less like a prison. Voluntary admission also altered the medical profile of the McLean population. Whereas "mania" dominated the diagnoses among committed patients, 50 to 75 percent of the voluntary patients suffered from "melancholia."

A review of the statistics and case records from Cowles's administration of McLean in Somerville, undertaken with the advantage of a more sophisticated model of mental illness than existed in the 1890s, leads to the unhappy conclusion that the transformation from asylum to hospital meant more to the staff than it did to the patients. The program of scientific medicine provided doctors, nurses, ward-maids, and other caretakers with a sense of professional purpose such as had not existed for decades. But though Cowles's reforms may have made the experience of hospitalization more dignified for some patients, they did not appreciably alter the course of their illnesses. Cowles had nothing in his medical armamentarium to address mental disease; beneath the surface of nurses, clinical charts, and medical vocabulary, McLean still depended on moral treatment as a therapeutic program, albeit a liberalized, individual form of moral treatment. Cowles viewed moral treatment as a principle of management "calling into normal exercise the rational part of the disordered mind," but he did not suppose it altered the pathology or physiology of disease, in which, unlike Pinel, he firmly believed. Though he reported higher recovery rates than his predecessor, between 30 and 40 percent, he assigned these results to better general medical attention and better organization.

Cowles saw clearly that nothing had been accomplished for Patient Number 7160, a young woman who had graduated at the top of her high school class, performed brilliantly during her first year at Radcliffe, and then gradually retreated inside her home, like a snail within its shell, where she existed in a world of private language and fantasy for four years prior to her commitment to McLean in 1888. Seven years later she had not improved at all, and McLean persuaded her family to transfer her to Worcester State so that her place in the hospital could be occupied by a more promising case. Cowles also watched Number 7097, a 29-year-old woman also admitted in 1888, become more frequently and dangerously violent during her hospitalization. In 1891 one of the physicians recorded his impression of increasing dementia. In 1894 it was noted that Number 7097 was occasionally excited or destructive and that she rarely spoke, but she sometimes did some sewing and she spent a great deal of time outdoors; during the summer she dug holes in the dirt; one day she assaulted another patient with a chair and had to be restrained.

Even the resourceful Cowles failed to solve the problem of chronic patients. Like most of his predecessors, he stated his preference for treating acute and recent cases; and also like them he received individuals whose illness appeared hopeless. Of 102 persons admitted in 1888, 38 were reckoned to be chronic or incurable.

Cowles never had any illusions about the curability of insanity under existing treatment methods and could not, therefore, be disillusioned.

> It is probably true that the majority of the insane can be best and most practicably treated away from their homes and in hospitals and these are not yet accomplishing what has been hoped of them in curative results. Instead, however, of treating this fact in terms of reproach, it should not be forgotten that mental disease involves the disorder of an organ of a highly complex and delicate structure, and comparisons between its diseases and those of other organs of the body should not be drawn unfairly. It has its own physiological and pathological laws; and, at the best, its diseases may have to be regarded as largely incurable.

It is a grim evaluation, barely rescued by the two small words, "not yet." Cowles tendered patients the slim hope of scientific research and an active hospital regimen designed to deliver the message: "You are ill, you may get well" (20).

Trees grew taller, spring wildflowers raised their shy heads, and small animals frolicked on McLean's rolling wooded site in Waverly (now Belmont), undisturbed by rude intrusions of construction crews and their machinery, save for a spell between 1880 and 1882 when the trustees allowed the Massachusetts General Hospital to build a convalescent home on the southwest corner of the tract. A flurry of activity soon after the initial purchase in 1875 had signaled the trustees' apparent desire to move quickly. The Committee on the New Asylum retained Olmsted, the landscape designer who had advised on the site selection and who also had experience with mental institutions, to advance his ideas on development and planning of the grounds. Joseph Curtis, a civil engineer who styled himself as a "landscape engineer," was hired to prepare a topographical survey. Carl Fehmer, a German-born architect who had been living in Boston since 1879, was engaged as an architectural consultant. A letter from committee chairman Charles H. Dalton to Olmsted, dated June 27, 1875, confirmed that the trustees had already settled on a "cottage type" hospital, a building system that originated in England in the late 1850s: "I think you are aware that we do not intend following the present fashion of State Asylums, . . . but on the contrary to avoid both the structural appearance and the economical methods, which are, probably, all right in them—but to adopt to a liberal extent what may be called a domestic plan, in distinction with that of a public institution" (21).

The fashion to which Dalton referred was the so-called "Kirkbride plan," a form of asylum construction advocated by Dr. Thomas S. Kirkbride, one of the Original Thirteen, during the 1850s. It consisted of a center structure for the superintendent and other resident officers, flanked by patient wings, and it was widely adopted for at least a generation of institutional construction. Kirkbride's simple scheme made sense when he developed it: Medical staffs were tiny and building budgets, particularly for public institutions, miserly. But the drawbacks of the monolithic asylum soon revealed themselves, among them the difficulties of separating the chronic from the curable, the quiet from the excited, and the affluent from the poor and of individualizing treatment. Despite objections from some superintendents, publicly funded institutions stayed with the Kirkbride plan because it offered an economical solution to construction and staffing. Even today, the sight of huge state mental hospitals, some of which are still in use, stirs the darkest corners of the imagination and raises the images of abuse, overcrowding, neglect, and despair that the public connects with the word "asylum."

Bulfinch's McLean, with the central Barrell mansion linked to the two patient wings, though predating Kirkbride, had employed a similar logic, as had later appendages to the wings. But Wyman departed from the unified structure in 1825 with his design of the separate "lodge" for violent patients. The two Appleton houses, built in the early 1850s just as Kirkbride was marking his text for the printer, represented a further gravitation in the direction of smaller, discrete units. By the time McLean's trustees had committed themselves to moving out of Somerville, the Kirkbride plan had been widely attacked; they never considered it.

> A large class of our patients are most unfavorably affected by being brought in contact with those more insane than themselves, and *by the feeling of restraint and confinement that is inseparably connected with a large asylum building. The more closely we can approach to that of a large family living in different houses, the better result we can hope to attain.* Our purpose is to build a number of small cottages surrounding a large one that would be used for administration purposes. (22)

As Dalton said, the Kirkbride plan might be all right for state hospitals, but it would never do for McLean. A site study dated November 1875, very likely prepared by Olmsted, showed a dozen separate buildings, set about 50 feet apart with below-grade service corridor connections, and arranged more or less in a rectangle except for a centrally located kitchen. (At that point, Olmsted's connection with the development of the new McLean seems to have ended, although there was a tragic epilogue. Olmsted, the unrivaled master of American landscape design during the latter half of the nineteenth century, became mentally disabled in his old age. According to his physician, he suffered a series of brain hemorrhages. His family finally placed him at McLean, where he spent the last five years of his life within the landscape he had helped to plan. The fog that obscured his intellect occasionally lifted sufficiently for him to notice that much of his advice had been ignored. "They didn't carry out my plan, confound them," he complained [23].)

A few more sketches for the new McLean were drawn in 1876, and then the promise of imminent construction faded and expired. Nothing happened for the rest of the decade. Vague references to financial obstacles failed to explain adequately why the work came to a halt. "Financial obstacles" cover a lot of territory. A Massachusetts tax amendment passed in 1877–78 taxed the Waverly site until McLean actually occupied it. This objectionable piece of legislation ought to have spurred the trustees to get on with the job, yet they continued to wait. However, they would not have been the first clients whose dreams had exceeded their pocketbooks. The bottom-line costs of the cottage plan must have become increasingly evident during the early planning process as price-per-square-foot figures bounced back and forth between them and the architect, and questions were raised about staffing individual buildings. The building fund around 1880 was $122,076.30; by the time the buildings were erected, the first two alone cost more than twice that sum. Also, the sequence of superintendents' departures and arrivals suggests problems between Jelly and the trustees: Either Jelly did not wish to oversee the construction program or the trustees did not have confidence in his ability to do the job.

Enter Cowles, experienced builder. The principle of the cottage plan was fixed before his arrival, and he was expected to carry it out. His acceptance of the position signaled his approval of the principle. In this context his development of the "hospital idea" acquired another dimension. Cowles, a hospital man to the core, would have remodeled the character of McLean even if it had been destined to stay in Somerville (though one wonders whether he would have taken the job without the challenge of the building program; he had plenty of challenges at Boston City Hospital). But given his cast of mind, the plan to relocate the asylum and redistribute its patients in segregated quarters made hospital-style reorganization both urgent and imperative. All the time Cowles was reinforcing and training professional staff, he was mentally redeploying his medical troops in the unbuilt cottages in Waverly. Meanwhile, he was conferring with architects and redesigning floor plans and ventilating systems. Only the idea of the laboratory seems not to have been fully formed at the beginning of Cowles's tenure, but he seems to have felt it necessary to develop at least a primitive laboratory in Somerville—to institutionalize the idea of research—to assure a permanent, more expansive laboratory effort in Waverly. Altogether, Cowles's program became one of the "financial obstacles" by requiring an investment in the moribund asylum in Somerville.

Some delay in the construction program helped Cowles test and refine his administrative reforms. Meanwhile, the Bell Telephone Company began mass production of the telephone, a new device of inestimable value to the cottage plan. However, after five or six years of talk and hours bent over architectural plans, Cowles began to get impatient. He pressed the trustees to move ahead with at least one building that might be used for convalescing patients, a precursor to the halfway house. In 1885 and 1886, the trustees purchased two more parcels in Waverly, adding 68 acres to the original tract, but they did not authorize any construction. In 1888 Cowles thought the building plans sufficiently advanced to present them formally to the trustees, who listened thoughtfully but still took no action. Later in the year, Cowles informed the trustees that he had received an offer to become medical director at the new Johns Hopkins Hospital, then under construction, a disclosure he may have used to gain reassurances that the new McLean would indeed go ahead in the foreseeable future. In 1889 Cowles exhibited and explained the plans at the annual meeting of the corporation; the corporation applauded his presentation and renewed its fund-raising efforts. Another presentation to the trustees five weeks later also failed to elicit a vote to get on with building.

A small gesture in 1890 gave Cowles faint cause for hope: The trustees asked for estimates on a house for the farmer, for there was to be a farm at the new McLean just as at the old one. In 1891 they authorized the new asylum committee to confer with

Cowles about starting to build. Curtis, the "landscape engineer," drew up a detailed site study that differed from Olmsted's 1875 sketch and, since it resembles what was built, presumably based on Cowles's recommendations. Otherwise, however, 1891 passed in talk and drawing board exercises. The farmhouse disappeared into some cranny in the agenda.

The gears of construction, locked in place for more than 15 years, began to turn in 1892 and were suddenly whizzing. Early in the year, anticipating a successful resolution of negotiations to sell the entire Somerville property, the trustees at last approved Fehmer's and Page's (Fehmer had acquired a partner by now) plans for the Appleton and Belknap houses, both for women. They also announced an offer by George P. Upham to donate a third building entirely at his own expense; the Upham Building, counterpart of the old Appleton Building for men, went into construction almost immediately. The sale agreement was concluded shortly thereafter. The Boston & Maine Railroad Corporation contracted to buy the old McLean for $750,000. The trustees then voted to proceed with the construction of the two approved houses. They further requested final plans for 11 more buildings, and they bought a farmhouse and barn for $8,000.

Construction workers descended on the Waverly woodlands, trampled the flowers, and scattered the wildlife with a vengeance. By the end of 1893, two patient houses and the power station had been completed, nine more cottages were well advanced in construction, and two were on the drawing boards, leaving only a gymnasium yet to be designed. In April 1895 three patients were transferred from Somerville to Waverly: two women to the new Appleton House and one man to Upham House. On November 15, when the last Somerville occupant departed for Waverly, all the buildings in the plan had been finished except for the gymnasium, which was under construction. The old asylum stood empty and silent upon its hill above the railroad yards and slaughterhouses. The next day the trustees delivered the property to the new owners, who wasted no time in razing Bulfinch's buildings.

PART *II*

The Hospital

CHAPTER

6

McLean in Belmont

The year of the hospital's removal to Belmont, 1895, passed relatively tranquilly without either major financial crisis or large-scale military conflict; small skirmishes occurred in Cuba where native insurrectionists objected to Spain's ruthless and exploitive presence. Grover Cleveland again occupied the White House, after having relinquished it to the Republicans for four years, and was gradually losing his grip on the Democratic Party. Sears, Roebuck Company opened a mail order business. George Westinghouse built enormous power generators at Niagara Falls.

Nearly 700,000 men, women, and children lived within a three-mile radius of Boston City Hall, more than three times the population in 1850. Immigration from Ireland had long passed its peak, but more and more eastern and southern Europeans were arriving in the port. A posh residential section in Boston, the Back Bay, had been built on landfill. The trees in Olmsted's Boston park system, the splendid "Emerald Necklace" that stretched from the Public Garden to Franklin Park in Roxbury, had almost reached maturity. On a muggy summer day at low tide the Charles River, unrestrained by any dam, reeked of raw sewage, industrial wastes, and dead fish. The Massachusetts Institute of Technology held court in Back Bay; its Cambridge home was still Charles River mudflats. In downtown Boston, laborers were digging the first American subway between Park and Boylston Streets. Meanwhile, the electric streetcars which had recently supplanted horse-drawn trolleys carried passengers between the inner city and its swelling suburbs.

McLean's trustees—who so often appear in these pages as *the trustees* that one is apt to forget that they were individuals who got sick or died and came onto the board or left it—were, as always, gentlemen of the upper crust. The foundations of their family fortunes had shifted from shipping to railroads, industry, and banking. Though generous in their support of public cultural and charitable institutions, many kept the thrifty personal habits of their ancestors. Amory tells how George Wigglesworth, who came onto the MGH-McLean board in 1896, gave MGH hundreds of thousands of dollars but "never considered a pair of shoes worn out until he had had them resoled three times" (1). Whereas earlier generations of trustees had usually resided on Beacon Hill, many of the new board members lived in the more spacious Back Bay.

The trustees and other men and women of privilege figured prominently in the literary, cultivated, urbane, Harvard-educated, socially connected, intellectually enlightened, progressive, rarified Boston of popular history: the Athens of America. In more plebian Boston a woman stenographer earned around $15 per week, a dressmaker started at $12, and an "office man" at $20. A six-room apartment with steam heat at the corner of Massachusetts and Harrison Avenues was advertised at $35 a month; a "pleasant" heated room on Huntington Avenue could be let for $2.25 a week; room and board went for $20 a week or more, depending on the circumstances. Jordan Marsh sold iron beds with brass fittings for $6 and an all-wool, pleated and ruffled dress for $2.98. A dentist promised to extract all your teeth painlessly by soaking the gums in "methyl"; he charged $8 for a full set of false teeth. Murphy's, down on the docks, sold "Pure Whisky" for 10 cents a glass. Warde's Health Home in Melrose claimed that "those suffering from Nervous Prostration, Melancholia, Rheumatism and all chronic diseases can be cured at his home by magnetic movement" (2).

Newspapers, sources of information and entertainment, complemented the reporting of sober events with cultural dissertations and bizarre or gory items. Their pages told of murder trials and railroad disasters, of which (in Luther Bell's defense) there seem to have been a horrendous number. The *Boston Globe* of the day, only a few cuts above today's *National Enquirer*, was prone to running screaming headlines about such things as an "invasion" of a gang of professional safecrackers who eluded Boston's police, or about Mrs. McEachen's murder (which might have been a suicide), along with curiosities like the strange case of a wealthy Brooklyn man who passed his days in his wife's crypt (3). The newspapers also serialized essays and novels. On September 3, 1895, the *Globe* carried the continuation of Chapter XX of Scott Campbell's *Aimed at Her Honor*, beginning "She broke off abruptly as if this thought of causation had spurred to renewed life her former alarm, and, dashing away the tears which blinded her, she again fell to wildly studying Gramley's message." One hopes this man's career as a writer was mercifully short. Lovers of the language can take comfort in the knowledge that Stephen Crane's *Red Badge of Courage* was published in the same year.

Boston offered a wide variety of entertainment ranging from elevated lectures on philosophy, science, literature, or horticulture to symphony and band concerts to burlesque. On any given night there were at least 10 theatrical performances, for which the cheapest seats sold for two and a half times the price of Murphy's Pure Whisky. One might attend a naughty show at the Howard or catch Lillian Russell's latest extravaganza. In September 1895, she was playing in something billed as a "Russian Comic Opera" called "La Tzigane." A reviewer's comments capture the flavor of the evening and the times: "Something always goes wrong on Miss Russell's opening night in Boston," he wrote. "Last year in the 'The Grand Duchess' the trained ponies which were to draw her in a sleigh before the expectant audience struck at the critical movement and Miss Russell was forced to make her entrance in a very ordinary, plebian prima donna style, standing on her feet. Last evening, in a lively portion of the first act, the electric fuses burned out" (4).

Boston had beaches, parks, museums, great public holiday celebrations, and—when the wickedness of city living seemed too much to bear—railway trips to the countryside. There were sporting events appealing to every level of interest and income, from polo and yachting to prizefighting. Boston's baseball team of 1895 was not faring much better than the Red Sox of 1985. On September 12, 1895, after a 9-5 loss to New York witnessed by some 8,000 frustrated spectators, the *Globe* observed ruefully that "Boston's batting again has its ludicrous features. They swing at the ball but it always escapes."

Though it all sounds quaintly appealing, the thoughtful Daniel Patrick Moynihan once quipped that anyone who longs for the good old days doesn't know very much about them. It is easier to wax sentimental over an existence without automobiles, the Sony Walkman, nuclear weapons, and television sets than one deprived of novocaine, refrigeration, Social Security, universal suffrage, fresh green vegetables in February, penicillin, zoning laws, no-fault divorce, and Wassermann tests. The average life span was short. The infant mortality rate was 200 per 1,000, and babies who survived the first year had to run the gauntlet of the contagious diseases of childhood. Most adults and many adolescents worked long hours, often under harsh conditions, as in, say, the slaughterhouses of East Cambridge or the railroad yards of Somerville, or on the impoverished farmlands of western Massachusetts—and for meager gains. The unemployed poor huddled in squalid, vermin-infested, unheated wooden tenements if they had any housing at all. The current assumption that violence was less pervasive than it is now finds little support, especially if one counts saloon brawls or violence within families, which the constabulary tended to ignore unless it escalated to a public disturbance. Boston politicians raised corruption to an art form compared to which more recent varieties have been but second-rate imitations. Altogether, the Athens of America had a seamy side which seldom found its way into history books, a substratum of prejudice and social unjustice and a human dimension of misery, boredom, resilience, and daily courage which does not make good mythology but which is a great deal more authentic than the usual expurgated histories of the city.

If, in the fall of 1895, an innocent wayfarer had trespassed on McLean's territory in Belmont, he might have believed himself to have strayed into some curious residential development for very affluent people with excessively large families. He would have been astonished to discover that what he was looking at was, in fact, a hospital for the care and treatment of the mentally ill, because it did not resemble any asylum or hospital he had ever seen. Nor would he have mistaken it for another kind of institution such as a college; the buildings were sited too far apart and too unceremoniously with respect to one another. The initial impression, to quote one observer, was of "gentlemen's country residences" irregularly dispersed in a pastoral landscape (5).

This illusion, of course, was precisely what the designers, Cowles, and the trustees had intended by their interpretation of the domestic plan. The architects had looked to residences rather than institutions and to country estates rather than towns for their models. Whereas Olmsted's 1875 sketch, an orderly arrangement of more tightly packed buildings, had been suggestive of a village, the final scheme favored privacy and distinctiveness over a sense of community.

Though most of McLean's buildings were harmonious in scale, constructed of red pressed brick trimmed with light-colored marble, limestone, or sandstone, and shared common structural characteristics as well as similar mechanical systems, no two of them looked alike. The architectural firm of Fehmer and Page designed 7 of the original 12 structures. Shepley, Rutan, and Coolidge designed North Belknap, the service building, and the administration building, which was distinguished from all other structures by its yellow-brick exterior. Thus, instead of trying to follow garbled instructions ("you can't miss it: third building on the left after you pass the big oak tree—and the one with the Flemish gables"), the first-time visitor to McLean simply had to watch for the yellow building. Benefactor Upham's architect, William Y. Peters, was responsible for the design of the Upham Building. All the patient buildings, except Upham, plus the administration and service buildings, were connected by a below-grade tunnel-corridor system which carried steam and electric lines while allowing for the distribution of food and laundry carts. At above-grade level the tunnel walls, supplemented by freestanding brick or wooden fences, enclosed recreational yards behind the patient residences. In the eye of the beholder the internal tunnels appeared as simple garden walls. Please remember the steam lines; they are going to cause headaches!

The setting of the architecturally varied structures into the thoughtfully modified landscape reinforced the illusion of country residences. McLean grounds owed their inspiration, if not their execution, to Olmsted, who had popularized the English school of landscape design. The grounds at the old McLean, originally laid out after the continental fashion at the end of the eighteenth century, had been highly stylized geometrical dispositions of terraces, formal flowerbeds, and stately trees marching in rows. The landscapers at McLean in Belmont made a different bargain with nature. Three miles of roads curved gently in compliance with the natural contours of the site. Expanses of lawn yielded to meadow and then to the soft edges of woodland. Well-formed trees had been spared the axe so as to shade and seclude the buildings or, perhaps, to stand as noble specimens introducing texture and vertical form into a vista across an open lawn. (One of them, a stately oak, was injured by a bolt of lightening while I was writing this book; it bears its wound with dignity.) New plantings of flowering trees and shrubs added color and seasonal variation. The hand of man concealed itself carefully; the landscape seemed to have been created by Nature in a particularly benevolent mood.

Two female patients and one male patient had been transferred from Somerville to the new Appleton and Upham houses, respectively, in April 1895, along with adequate nursing and service personnel. Two months later, Cowles, who had good public relations instincts, hosted the annual meeting of the American Neurological Society and showed off his new domain. And, on October 1, about two weeks before the patients were scheduled for transfer, the trustees held an enormous reception. "The magnificent buildings of the new McLean Asylum for the insane, situated on the high hills of Belmont and Waverly, were thrown open today for the inspection of physicians and such other persons as are interested in hospitals," reported a local newspaper, in disregard of the fact that McLean had changed its name to hospital three years earlier. " . . . More than a thousand persons availed themselves of an opportunity to visit the buildings during the day, many coming from a great distance" (6).

The visitors saw comfortable patient quarters and sunny parlors opening onto wide views of the Charles River Valley, Boston Harbor, or the Blue Hills of Milton. They saw elegant reception rooms and intimate dining rooms with broad windows and open fireplaces; they saw oak paneling, finely crafted stairwells, and up-to-date lavatories, kitchens, laundries, and laboratories, as well as plumbing, heating, and ventilating systems. Superintendents condemned to running state institutions on miserly appropriations must have suffered sharp pangs of envy as they toured McLean's grand facilities. Another 2,000 visitors, largely from the general public, inspected the premises on October 2 and 3.

Well before the effects of this idyllic environment on the mental health of patients had been evaluated, it was observed to have becalmed the community of Belmont. The *Boston Evening Transcript* carried a letter from "R.B.C." of that town, on October 5, which read in part:

> The coming of the McLean Hospital to [the local inhabitants'] staid town was not entirely welcome. There was no prejudice against the class of invalids for whom it was to provide, that might have been felt in a less intelligent community. But there was a feeling that a great corporation had absorbed a large piece of territory, and that the growth of the town had consequently been arrested in that direction. But the opening of these superb buildings with their reminder that all of this comfort and elegance is provided for the alleviation of suffering has brought its lesson. . . . It is true that her ministries are largely to a class of educated people of means. But the recovery of some of these people with powers and sympathies quickened by the discipline of illness will have fruits in liberal gifts to other hospitals who minister more distinctively to the poor.

However, in the immediate present such charitable benefits accrued directly to McLean. A month before the new plant had been put to service, Mrs. Sarah Matchett offered to finance the building of a cottage to house a single patient on the grounds. The trustees accepted her proposal, and "Hope Cottage" was completed in 1896.

The great removal from Somerville to Belmont began on October 17.

> Patients had for some time heard that the move was coming soon and every day were wondering if it would happen "today," and how they would all be transferred. Some made up their minds that it would be a long procession of carriages of one kind and another winding its way through the streets of Somerville and Cambridge, and then on into the country until they finally arrived at the new hospital all together; and all along the way sidewalks would be lined with people waiting to see the curious procession pass. But when the time came, not a patient knew that anything was happening. For a number of days little groups filling two or three carriages were invited to go to ride—not at all an unusual occurrence—and the "rides" ended at Waverly. Then one day, much to their surprise, they found that they were all in the new McLean; and as for the public, they read about it in the newspapers after it was all over (7).

There are always bugs that must be worked out of new buildings, and the new McLean had its share of them. No sooner had the staff and patients settled into their quarters than they began to remark upon flaws in construction—little leaks and drafts that revealed themselves when the rain or wind came from a particular direction, doors that did not hang quite properly as the building settled, leaky faucets, windows that refused to open—minor but irritating errors which had to be corrected and which added unbudgeted expenses to the overhead. The persistent misbehavior of the steam heating system turned out not to be trivial at all. When it started to malfunction during the first year, the engineers studied the problem and recommended expensive changes, which were made. But by 1899 the iron return pipes were discovered to be almost completely corroded, and the engineers could not explain what had happened. In desperation, they recommended the substitution of brass pipes for iron, at a cost of $10,000. The price tag horrified the trustees, who turned to chemical engineers at the Massachusetts Institute of Technology. MIT's experts conducted a series of elaborate tests and found a high concentration of carbonic acid in the feed pipe drawn from the springs on the grounds. They prescribed the addition of an alkali to the water, thus saving the cost of brass pipes. Though relieved, the trustees were still vexed by all the money that had already gone into the system's maintenance along with the other unanticipated expenses of the new hospital.

If it was not one thing, it was another. A "coal famine" in 1903 added an unwelcome $13,600 to the wrong side of the ledger.

The new McLean was running the kinds of budget deficits that make conservative monetarists uneasy, and the trustees were taking Cowles to task. As time passed, his annual reports read more and more like exercises in financial justification. Just as married couples sometimes fall to squabbling over money, so did Cowles and the trustees begin to find themselves at odds over the budget.

Though both the property and the building square footage in Belmont greatly exceeded what had been available in Somerville, the new hospital had been designed for fewer patients than the old asylum, where in 1890 the average daily census had been about 174. (In fact, the number of beds at McLean had been shrinking since mid-century, an anomalous phenomenon in an era when growth was equated with progress.) McLean in Belmont had been built to accommodate 160 patients, all in private rooms and including about 20 apartments with private parlor, chamber, and bathroom. The figure of 160 had been determined during the planning process as the lowest one that at a minimum weekly rate of $20, up $5 from Somerville, would yield an income to balance operating expenses. Also, the small professional medical staff in residence at that time could comfortably manage 160 patients and offer them proper individual attention.

Admissions had been kept low during the last year at Somerville, and many chronic patients had been discharged in anticipation of the move. Approximately 120 patients finally went to Belmont, and space was therefore available to "the more strictly recent cases, as having a stronger claim." During 1896, the first full year of operation, 125 persons were admitted, of whom 80 were recent cases and 45 were thought to be chronic. The average daily census was 138. Of the patients discharged, 24 were listed as recovered. These were not exactly encouraging statistics, but Cowles nevertheless believed Belmont had a salubrious effect. "The patients are, doubtless, so influenced by the improved comforts and attractions of the new houses, within and without, as to permit greater freedom in granting the liberty of the grounds," he wrote; "the tests of self control can be sooner applied, and, while these are naturally contributing to the curative influences, the convalescing patient earlier shows self reliance and trustworthiness" (8). Furthermore, he did not have to worry about patients tripping on railroad tracks.

Predictably, some patients did not respond at all to the new surroundings. Number 5843, one of the few long-term patients who had come over from Somerville, seemed not to have the slightest idea where he was. The entry in his case record for December 31, 1895, noted that "since coming to Waverly Mr. ______ has shown no special comprehension or appreciation of his new surroundings. He has rather improved in physical condition, but not mentally. He walks about or sits silently in the ward, never speaking intelligibly and taking no interest in those about him. At times he gets excited and sings, shouts, gesticulates and dances about. Occasionally he is violent and strikes a patient or nurse." (Number 5843 developed abdominal cancer and died of peritonitis in September 1902. He was 52 years old. He had been a patient at McLean for 29 years. The diagnosis in his file read "dementia praecox," which is presently known as schizophrenia.)

During 1897 the average patient population rose to 143, admissions to 137, recoveries to 42. The ratio between recent and curable and chronic cases remained approximately constant, so it is obvious that if McLean had kept all the chronic patients, it would have been filled within three or four years with individuals who were not expected to recover. This did not happen for a couple of reasons. In an effort to avoid a backlog of patients like Number 5843, Cowles started a policy of admitting patients for observation with the understanding that McLean would treat those who could be helped and transfer those with poor prognoses to state facilities. Money could buy an exception to this policy, but that kind of money was itself exceptional. McLean's rates were even more effective in discouraging use of the hospital as a guardian. Few families could afford to pay the charges indefinitely, and even those that could might be persuaded that a patient, especially one who demonstrated no signs of improvement after several weeks' trial and who seemed insensitive to the environment, would be just as well off in a cheaper state hospital.

Thus, discounting deaths, roughly 20 percent of the patients discharged represented transfers to other facilities. Still, Cowles and the trustees recognized a moral obligation; mindful of the conflict between his ideal of a healing hospital and the needs of its constituents, Cowles wrote, much as Bell had written a half-century earlier, "It is also considered a part of the legitimate work of this hospital to receive cases of active senile insanity, and those that are otherwise so difficult to manage in their homes . . ." (9).

McLean was filled to capacity within a few years. The hospital received more applications for the admission of women patients, voluntary and involuntary, than it could accommodate. Cowles fiddled with floor plans, divided some of the capacious suites into single rooms, and by 1902 claimed adequate space for 170 patients while reporting an average daily census of 175. On days when he had 180 patients, the women's quarters became "unduly crowded." In 1900 he appealed for an additional building; undaunted by the dull response from the trustees, he persisted in his requests. He produced sheafs of figures to support his contention that a new building would pay for itself in a few years by reducing the annual deficits that currently bedeviled the budget.

The trustees did not share Cowles's interpretation of fiscal reality. They were ill disposed to go after more funds until the financial viability of the new hospital had been more thoroughly tested. Also, they were distracted by a huge building program at MGH. Cowles, tenacious as a terrier with a succulent bone, continued to worry the issue, but the trustees would have none of it. They were even less eager to build a residence for the nurses, though they could not ignore Cowles's argument that "a comfortable, restful, and attractive home for our women nurses was earned by them long ago" (10). So the women's patient quarters remained crowded, and the nurses stayed in their dormitories on the top floors of patient houses.

The grand appearance of the new McLean and public knowledge of the rate of board led people like R.B.C., author of the previously quoted letter to the *Boston Evening Transcript*, to believe its patients were "educated people of means," a notion later perpetuated by the sprouting of half a dozen individual cottages like the one Mrs. Matchett had built. According to popular gossip, McLean was filled with wealthy eccentric Boston Brahmins. The rumors did not have a very good purchase on reality. True, there were several well-to-do patients at McLean. Though the registration books at the turn of the century stopped itemizing the rate of board, the mention in the 1902 annual report of the addition of 25 private nurses billed to individual patients is suggestive. There were at least 25, perhaps as many as 50, patients representing the affluent classes and paying more than the minimum rate of $20 per week.

At the other end of the socioeconomic spectrum—though not at the bitter end of abject poverty—were a small number of people whose board had been guaranteed by some sponsor: If, for instance, a faithful household servant, in those days usually Irish, became mentally ill, a kind employer might pay for treatment or observation at McLean. The majority of the patients, however, fell between two extremes and belonged to what the *Boston Evening Transcript* characterized smugly as the "self-supporting classes." There were schoolteachers, clergymen, artisans, clerks, farmers, students, seamstresses, lawyers, physicians, and shopkeepers. McLean put a financial strain on many of these patients or their families. As in the past, the hospital admitted some promising patients at a lower rate of board and subsidized their stay.

The statistical data accompanying the annual reports of this period reflected the ferment in the field of psychiatry. The most conspicuous change involved a revolution in the language of diagnosis. The old, familiar, and reassuringly comprehensible mania and melancholy fell by the wayside in the mid-1890s. More mystifying terms took their places: dementia praecox (literally, premature or early ripening dementia), depressive maniacal insanity, involution psychosis, neurasthenia, paranoiac condition, psychopathic inferiority, and so on. The new nomenclature was based on a scheme of classification of mental disease developed by Emil Kraepelin, a German psychiatrist who had studied with Wundt. The psychiatric profession still honors Kraepelin as its "Linnaeus" because his systematic description of disease entities brought some order to the anarchic study of mental illness. Since his nosology continues to provide the substructure for classification, he may also be regarded as the granddaddy of *DSM-III*, the American Psychiatric Association's *Diagnostic and Statistical Manual of Mental Disorders* (*Third Edition*), which is to the practice of psychiatry what Webster's Dictionary is to writing.

Kraepelin's scheme differed from earlier taxonomic attempts in that he described the entire symptomatic course of a disease rather than the manifest behavior or a cluster of symptoms at a particular moment. Thus, his diagnoses carried prognostic weight, something which could not have been said of earlier diagnoses: Predictions of chronicity such as had formerly appeared in McLean's statistics had been independent of diagnosis, based on the case history and empirical guesswork. Cowles heralded Kraepelin's studies as "perhaps the most illuminating conceptions of insanity that we have yet received as explaining principles. . . . The fundamental conception is that in conformity with general pathological principles there must be an underlying pathological process for every distinct form of mental disease manifested by definite symptom-complex . . ." (11).

Human behavior being as idiosyncratic as it is even among so-called normal human beings, the diseases of the mind resisted facile, inflexible categorization as long as the underlying pathology could not be identified. Mental illnesses could not be differentiated like measles and mumps; patients in the hospital often declined to fit themselves neatly into any of Kraepelin's niches. Moreover, Kraepelin, passionate scientist that he was, proceeded to becloud the waters he had recently clarified by revising his classification in subsequent editions of his 1883 *Lehrbuch*, a process of refinement that caused consternation. The volume expanded from 384 pages in its first edition to 814 pages by 1895 and to 1,370 pages in the seventh edition. Some psychiatrists, Cowles among them, wished Kraepelin had quit earlier, because as his influence spread, less-gifted minds started to play the bewitching nomenclatural game, and descriptive psychiatry threatened to bury laboratory research in a nosological landslide. During the 1890s, however, Cowles was still more thankful than not for Kraepelin's contributions.

Kraepelin had a direct representative in Belmont in the person of August Hoch, the pathologist. Cowles had hired Hoch in 1893 to replace Noyes, who had not been happy in his laboratory and had resigned to take a position at the Massachusetts Hospital for Dipsomaniacs and Inebriates, where he could spend more time with patients. Hoch, born in Switzerland, arrived in the United States in 1887 at the age of 19. He studied medicine at the University of Pennsylvania and then with the magnetic Canadian clinician, Sir William Osler, at Johns Hopkins. Somehow Cowles heard about Hoch (probably through his friend Henry Hurd at Johns Hopkins), offered him the pathologist's post, and immediately dispatched him abroad. Hoch went to Wundt's laboratory in Leipzig and thence to Heidelberg to work with Kraepelin. Along the way he married a woman from his native Basel. Husband and wife returned to the United States, and Hoch began his work at McLean. Adolf Meyer, who first met him in 1895, recalled him "living in the village with his wife and his only child, Susie—in a genial home—and [giving] his whole enthusiasm and interest to a continuation of his psychologic and anatomic studies" (12).

Though hired as a pathologist, Hoch played an important role in clinical record keeping and diagnosis at McLean. Under his direction, and with Cowles's blessing, McLean's patient records were reclassified according to Kraepelin's scheme. Hoch led the weekly clinical conferences during which the medical staff and consultants discussed the diagnosis of a newly admitted patient. The typewritten summaries of those conversations demonstrate that, whatever the advantage of Kraepelin's classification as a conceptual tool, it was not easy to apply in clinical practice.

In May 1899, concerning the condition of a woman in her mid-twenties, Hoch concluded his remarks by saying: "If the woman was 50 we would undoubtedly call it a case of involution psychosis. We know it is a deteriorating condition and we, naturally, think of dementia praecox. Whether these cases are dementia praecox or not, we do not know; but we know they are deteriorating conditions. Prognosis: I would give an absolutely bad prognosis; she has no chance for remission." Tuttle thought the diagnosis fell somewhere between the depressive phase of depressive-maniacal excitement—which Hoch had ruled out—and dementia praecox, but admitted that he did not feel sure enough to commit himself to any diagnosis at all. Two consulting neurologists supported Hoch's opinion of dementia praecox, even more firmly than he had advanced it, along with his pessimistic prognosis. But Charles Little, the second assistant physician, startled the group by saying, "I don't wish to make a diagnosis. I feel she has something from which she will recover. She strikes me as having a fundamental condition. I think quite likely there is a fundamental depression, and it is a case of melancholia. I will not make a diagnosis." Little's intuition proved correct, at least in the short run. When the patient left the hospital a few months later, the last word in her file was "recovered"; but since her acquaintance with McLean ended then, one cannot say whether her recovery was a remission or a permanent return to health.

In the case of an 18-year-old girl committed to McLean after having suffered two previous attacks of illness and accompanied by her father's observation that "something seems to be gone with her" after recuperation from those attacks, Hoch initially suspected manic-depressive insanity but, after watching the patient, changed his opinion to "essential dementia." "Our prognosis must be bad," he concluded, ". . . her remission will be less complete, her condition become more continuous, and she will get comparatively rapidly demented." The third assistant physician, E. Stanley Abbot, agreed, as did a neurologist at the conference. Tuttle, again stuck between dementia and manic-depression, leaned toward dementia. Another conference occurred at the time of the girl's discharge 10 months later. Though the record read "recovered," the group concurred that her disease was merely in remission. Hoch now believed her to be suffering from dementia praecox. Cowles thought Hoch's diagnosis was probably right but left open the possibility that "the case may resolve itself into circular insanity," that is, manic-depressive insanity. Tuttle had shifted his stance in favor of manic-depression. Little again said he would not arrive at a diagnosis.

None of this idiomatic talk made much difference to the patients during their residence at McLean. They got worse, had remissions, or returned to permanent health regardless of the diagnosis. Different diseases did not receive different therapies except in such cases as alcoholism, where cause and effect were visibly connected. Patients were assigned to quarters on the basis of behavioral symptoms rather than medical diagnosis, the quiet with the quiet, and so on. Manic-depressives, neurasthenics, and victims of dementia praecox were all submitted to the same regimen of moral treatment with its wholesome diet, physical exercise, diversions, nursing care, and structured environment. The more recent the onset of the disease, the more likely the patient was to improve. No McLean patient was ignored, however, no matter how apparently hopeless his or her condition.

Nevertheless, diagnosis was a serious business because it affected the patient's future. A diagnosis of dementia praecox carried grave implications. Kraepelin believed that nothing could be done for these patients to prevent their progressive mental deterioration, and the empirical experience of hospital psychiatrists reinforced that view. Therefore, a diagnosis of dementia praecox at McLean might become grounds for transfer or commitment to a state hospital after another attack.

By the turn of the century, some state facilities had become so overcrowded, underfunded, and understaffed that they could not offer evenhanded management or observation. They consigned untreatable cases to the back wards and focused their few resources on trying to help the "recent and curable." A patient in the back wards could get better and no one would notice, or the change in behavior would be dismissed as medically insignificant; patients with dementia praecox were not supposed to get well. Reading through McLean's case conferences, one senses some hesitancy, particularly in Tuttle and Little, to deliver a firm diagnosis of dementia praecox because it implied abandoning hope. Psychiatrists needed hope almost as desperately as patients and their families. Manic-depressive insanity was a much more auspicious diagnosis (13).

Kraepelin assumed the existence of an underlying pathology for each disease entity. Though the identification in 1897 of pathological changes in the brain tissues of certain demented patients by Kraepelin's colleague Alois Alzheimer helped substantiate that assumption, the pathology of most mental diseases remained elusive. The question of cause was equally mystifying. "We all know how important the etiology is in the question of circumscribing diseases," Hoch told a meeting of AMPA in 1900,

> for disease entities are etiological entities. In psychiatry, however, even more than in other fields of medicine, the fact has often been overlooked

> that a noxious influence preceding the outbreak of a disease is not necessarily its cause. But all such influences should, nevertheless, be an object of our study, for though they may not represent essential causes themselves, they may point out the way to a clearer understanding of them, as they may be more or less closely connected with them. What we must, however, rigorously require of an essential cause is that it has given rise to a definite disease picture and that this same disease picture cannot be produced by anything else. . . . We cannot deny . . . that our knowledge of strictly essential causes is meager. (14)

For want of a firm grasp on either the etiology or pathology of mental diseases, Cowles had no grounds for altering the course of hospital treatment from medically oriented moral management aimed at keeping the patients in optimal physical health while actively engaging their minds. This, of course, was more or less the same system that had been used for three-quarters of a century in Somerville, transplanted to vastly superior circumstances in Belmont. The new McLean had the customary diversion of games, concerts, carriage rides, classes in drawing and painting (for women) and woodcarving (for men), and walks on the lovely grounds. The new hospital also had two gymnasiums, one for each sex; built in the English Tudor half-timbered style, they lent an antic quality to the architectural ambience. Each gym was equipped with gymnastic apparatus and had an instructor in physical training; the nurses had been instructed in massage and the administration of "medical" gymnastics. Almost half the patients regularly used the exercise and massage facilities.

The gymnasiums doubled as social and recreational centers. Cowles likened the men's facility to "a gentleman's club." The women's building contained a parlor and a small conservatory. "Such incidents as a series of progressive whist parties give a hint of the manner in which the life here is made homelike. At these parties a lady patient acted in turn as hostess having given the invitations, and made other arrangements, in due form" (15). The women's gymnasium also contained a much-publicized art room, a changing loan exhibition of paintings, prints, and photographs. (One cannot refrain from remarking that classes in drawing and painting, and exhibitions of fine art, were considered appropriate only for women; yet no doubt most of the items on display had been produced by men. What a peculiar world!)

In 1899—the same year Massachusetts Institute of Technology chemical engineers saved McLean $10,000 with their solution to the problem of the steam pipes—the hospital spent $10,000 on a hydrotherapy unit which was installed in the basement of the women's gymnasium and assigned for the use of women in the mornings and men in the afternoons. The dates may be coincidental, but the image of Cowles gleefully pouncing on the "saved" sum is irresistible: the hydrotherapy unit had been designed with the gymnasium, but not equipped until two years after the building was completed. This humane reincarnation of the punitive shower baths of the old days in Somerville included a steam room, shampooing rooms, a six- by-10-foot plunge bath which had a depth of five feet, a "combined needle and rain" shower unit, hot rooms for wrapping or "packing" patients in wet sheets, and a resting room. Though not regarded as curative, hydrotherapy helped becalm agitated patients and reduced the need for mechanical restraints to practically nothing.

Overall, the patients enjoyed a great deal more comfort and somewhat more freedom than they had in Somerville. Convalescing patients often spent weekends with their families and got discharges as soon as their mental health seemed stabilized. A number of chronically ill patients were transferred to humbler surroundings. The average duration of a stay decreased; the number of admissions rose; and McLean gave sanctuary to more people than it had at any time since Luther Bell's high watermark of the 1850s. It did not, however, presume to heal them.

In Cowles's view and in the opinion of history, the centerpiece of the new McLean was the research program. The relegation of the laboratories to the first floor and basement of the service building, which otherwise held the entertainment hall and the kitchen as well as sleeping quarters for nonmedical employees, gives a reasonably accurate idea of the position of research in the world of early twentieth-century medicine. The conditions of research at McLean's sister organization, the Massachusetts General Hospital, cannot be said to have been any better at the time. Cowles, content to have any laboratories at all, did not care where they were, only that they were staffed and busy.

The first-floor laboratories consisted of an examining room with various electrical gadgets, among them Lippmann's electrometer, the first electrocardiograph—a crude instrument with a bad habit of breaking down—and devices for measurement such as Virchow's craniometer. A microscope and photography room had up-to-date equipment, as well as a dark room. The room for physiological psychology had been outfitted with such paraphernalia as an ergograph for measuring the work capacity of the muscles, two types of kymographs for measuring blood pressure, blood counting apparatus, and several optical and auditory devices. A fourth room was equipped for pathological and physiological chemistry. For reasons of delicacy, the mortuary and autopsy room occupied the basement level. According to Hall, who advised on the outfitting of the laboratories, the total value of the equipment was in the neighborhood of $1,500.

Since the trustees withheld money for staffing the laboratories while the new hospital endured its financial difficulties, Hoch *was* the McLean research program from the time he returned from his first European sabbatical until 1900. Initially he worked in the pathology laboratory and produced studies on nerve cell changes. Cowles, who governed the direction of laboratory investigation, believed energy and exhaustion were central to the problem of mental disorders. His own research, naturally limited by his administrative duties, focused on the etiology, pathology, and clinical characteristics of neurasthenia, or nervous exhaustion (16). Hoch followed Cowles's lead and conducted ergographic investigations along similar lines as Noyes's previous studies. But in 1897, following another trip to Germany for a refresher course with Kraepelin and Franz Nissl, who was then in Kraepelin's laboratory, Hoch's research interests took a decided turn toward the clinical. He began to believe that isolated laboratory research, what would now be called "basic" research, was premature.

> Only when [clinical work] is carefully conducted are we prepared for studies in pathological anatomy or pathological chemistry; and only then will all these different studies mutually support each other and lead us in

> an aimful manner to a clear recognition of the real diseases. For these reasons also it seems to me that the general, otherwise very creditable, movement in this country towards the establishment of laboratories in insane asylums is somewhat misguided and may do a certain amount of harm. We have been severely censured for our lack of interest in scientific questions. The establishment of a laboratory may give us the feeling that we have sufficed to all scientific needs, although the observation of the patients may be as unscientific as ever. (17)

Hoch's alteration of intellectual course disconcerted Cowles, who had, after all, invested years of his life cajoling the McLean trustees to pour money into laboratories and who had always promoted dialogue between staff and laboratory physicians. As Hoch's research interests became more manifestly descriptive, both he and Cowles felt some tension. Hoch had trouble carving out time for the work he really wanted to do, while Cowles felt important laboratory studies went begging for attention. Adolf Meyer later wrote, "I well remember, as an example of the diversity of expectations from a laboratory worker of those days, a task waiting for [Hoch] on the shelves—a collection of desiccated feces to be analyzed chemically by him (the aim being to find the disease in a pure culture),* and also the beginnings of a histological workshop" (18). Meyer perhaps had that image in the back of his mind when he wrote to Cowles, in his tiny script, "Administrative and obvious matters can be governed with a general's methods of discipline, but scientific research requires too much honesty and feeling of responsibility on the part of the collaborators—much more than can be found among those who submit patiently, as the traditional assistant physicians, to the unfortunate asylum traditions governing their life" (19).

However, Meyer's later remark that Cowles "never made a complete readjustment" to Hoch's new interests "so that clinical publications were retarded" (20) distorted the truth. Cowles's annual report for 1902 contradicts that opinion by listing no fewer than four clinical publications by Hoch, along with others in progress, and only one anatomically based study. Furthermore, Cowles recognized that Hoch simply had too much work and managed to supply him with able assistance in the pathologi-

*Nothing Cowles wrote suggests him to have been so simple-minded. This is one of Meyer's slights.

cal department by hiring Dr. Emma Mooers, McLean's first woman doctor, who became curator of laboratory records and materials while undertaking pathological research; she relieved a substantial burden from Hoch, who was thus freed to pursue clinical studies—a gesture of encouragement if ever there was one.

However, it is true that Cowles's heart was really in the laboratory. He was an impatient man, falling rapidly out of love with the ideas of Kraepelin, although grateful for his basic contribution, and the fashion for descriptive psychiatry which seemed to him to be leading the profession on a hopeless detour.

> Much time has undoubtedly been wasted in the naming and classifying of these diseases not yet clearly determined. . . . For example, the view already held by some was taken that melancholia and mania were simply phases of one more general form of mental disorder. But the prevailing tendency of that time was to the attempted recognition of many new forms with new names. These and other older terms are now so far discredited, however, that a very unsettled condition prevails as to correct descriptive designations of these disorders. The conviction seems to be growing that too much attention has been given to this side of the problem. It reinforces the belief so long held here which is being presented in these statements, that the true way to study mental disorders is by analyzing them to discover their distinctive elements; this leads again to the proposition that not only structural changes in the brain must be studied, but the pathology of function of the whole body, the basis of which is general physiology. . . . The physiology of mind, with the concurrent activities of the body, thus occupies the main channel of possible progress. (21)

A psychology professor from one of the great Boston area universities, sometimes driven to justify his research program, likes to tell this story: Late one foggy night a man was walking home from a restaurant when he came upon a bum crawling on the sidewalk beneath a street lamp. "What are you doing?" the man asked. "I'm looking for my quarter," the bum replied. The man felt sorry for the bum and started to help in the search. But when nothing turned up after 10 or 15 minutes, he inquired further, "Where did you lose your quarter?" "Over there," answered the bum with a vague gesture up the street. "Then why are you looking here?" asked the man. "Because here is where the light is," the bum explained.

If this tale had been told at the turn of the century to psychiatrists at an annual meeting of AMPA, it would have gotten a good laugh, and everyone in the audience would have had a slightly different interpretation of it. As medical men, the psychiatrists now shared a belief in physiological bases for mental illnesses but held diverse views on how to go about looking for them. Those like Hoch thought disease entities needed precise definition before laboratory work could be valuable. Cowles, I think, would have said that although descriptive psychiatry might expand the circle of light under the street lamp, one was more likely to find the quarter by groping around in the dark near the place where one thought the quarter *was*.

So, in 1900, after Cowles brought chemist Otto Folin and his assistant Philip A. Shaffer from the University of Virginia to put McLean's chemistry laboratory into full-time service, he clearly transferred the weight of his enthusiasm from Hoch's work to Folin's. Folin, a retiring, industrious Swede, began a series of physiological investigations of metabolism in an effort to see whether he could establish correlations between faulty nutrition or metabolic imbalances and different forms of mental disease. He went about his work quietly and meticulously, accumulating careful analytical data and designing new experiments. For a short period during 1902, for example, he put McLean patients and colleagues on a uniform diet with precise nitrogen content and then analyzed their urine to determine whether nitrogen was eliminated in significantly different forms or quantities.

Techniques of biochemistry were crude at the time, and throughout his career Folin demonstrated great ingenuity in improving them. For instance, no less than 25 cc of blood was needed to evaluate the uric acid content of blood—among other things, the diagnostic criterion for gout. Since Folin could not go around withdrawing huge quantities of blood from patients, he pioneered techniques of chemical analysis that required only small amounts; sometimes he could test for a single element in a drop obtained from a finger prick (22). He developed a new method for determining ammonia in urine and other fluids, improved the methods for analyzing ethereal and total sulphates in urine, and refined a number of other techniques. Folin's methodological worked earned him an international reputation, and he eventually came to the attention of the Harvard Medical

School, which in 1908 made him its first professor of biological chemistry.

Ironically, while advancing the science of biochemistry, Folin's metabolic studies of mental illness proved negative and, therefore, disappointing. Reviewing his work several decades later, Cecil Drinker remarked philosophically that

> all the work Folin and his successors accomplished had to be done. It was the painful spade work which goes on long before anything grows. Cowles, . . . William James, and many others would have foretold brilliant results from Folin's work and that of his successors; but all that was gained at the time was a large knowledge of what was not true, what would not work.
>
> But in science that is part of the bag. A solid negative which stands as a fact is worth much for the future. Cowles' imagination jumped far past biochemical possibilities in 1900. . . . He was a hospital administrator, and knew biochemistry only as a belief. What he wanted this new scientific tool to do was so big he was ready to gamble heavily on it, and all he gained was a succession of hard-earned negatives. (23)

Cowles's last year as superintendent, 1903, was only Folin's third year in the McLean chemistry laboratory, so Cowles left filled with optimism. Though he lived long enough to see that his horse wasn't coming in, he never abandoned his faith in biochemistry as a key to the mysteries of mental diseases.

Cowles never put all his money on one biochemical horse. In his last annual report, he stated that "efficient research, to be of value in this field of inquiry, requires expert ability in experimental physiology and its special department of psychology" (24). Cowles had a specific expert in mind: Shepherd Ivory Franz, whom he had met at the Dartmouth Medical School where he lectured, as well as at Harvard. Franz, an instructor in physiology, had been trained in psychology, though he had little experience of abnormal psychology. Franz remembers that at Dartmouth Cowles

> brought to my attention Kraepelin's newer conceptions of the manias and melancholias, which were being looked upon as one disease, not different diseases. Dr. Cowles was attempting to define more accurately his personal views of the relationships of the excitements and depressions. He thought they were mainly fatigue situations, and he was trying to bring the variety of symptoms into relations with the newer ideas of nerve physiology. . . . Informally he asked me to outline an experimental plan whereby some of the problems might be attacked. (25)

As their casual conversations continued, Cowles became convinced that Franz belonged at McLean. Franz warned him that he had to decide soon on an offer to teach physiology of the nervous system at another university. Cowles, knowing he was in his last year at McLean, hurried to get an appointment for Franz. The trustees did not cooperate, forcing Cowles to find his own money. In what was probably McLean's first fund-raising effort specifically for research purposes, he succeeded in acquiring $1,000 and promises of additional support from the same Sarah Matchett who had donated the first private cottage. Franz arrived in Belmont in 1904, after Cowles was gone.

Cowles did not retire voluntarily. For the sake of public appearances, he made a half-hearted attempt to exit gracefully in his last annual report:

> In these reports, from year to year, some expressions have been given to the Trustees of my reliance upon their confidence and support, but the fullness of this could not be put in any words. Now there is the further acknowledgement to be made of their provision for the retirement of medical officers long in service, and my acceptance of the beneficent principle, being the first to take advantage of the new scheme now applied to me with such assurances of honorable esteem. That there must be such changes as the relinquishment of the labors of a lifetime, with one's ideals yet not quite attained, finds great consolation in the assurance that the special work of research will go on with even more completeness than has been possible heretofore. (26)

During 1903 the trustees voted mandatory retirement with pension of the McLean superintendent and his first and second assistants, as well as their counterparts at the general hospital, at the age of 64. Since 64 seemed an arbitrary figure with no immediate application to anyone except Cowles—who, after 24 years of McLean administration, radiated more mental and physical vitality than most men in their forties—some sympathetic bystanders construed the trustees' decision as a not-very-tactful way of deposing him. As usual, the trustee records offer no support to this or any other theory; they say nothing at all, except that the vote occurred. But Cowles had not expressed the slightest desire to retire.

The scuttlebutt in psychiatric circles, according to G. Stanley Hall, was that Cowles had lost "his official head because he had gone too far" in promoting McLean's research program, a version of events which may have originated with Cowles himself (27). This explanation missed the central issue: money. From the Trustees' perspective the key column of figures was the one called "Excess of Expenses over Receipts." In 1900 that figure was $35,781; in 1901, $31,891; in 1902, $25,563; and in 1903, the year of the fateful coal shortage, it came in at $46,569. Desperate to reduce the McLean deficit, the trustees held back and snipped away from the most vulnerable item, the research program, which did not have a distinct and inviolate fund. They would not advance money for Franz, and when Emma Mooers resigned from the pathology laboratory in 1903, they did not replace her. Though they accepted the ideal of scientific research, as long as it could not be shown to have any direct bearing on the welfare of the hospital's patients, it presented an inviting target for budget reduction. Pruning research raised fewer hackles than, say, terminating the gymnastics program or firing half a dozen nurses, either of which would have been abhorrent to Cowles. The trustees were not prepared to accept his solution to the financial problem, the construction of a new building for women patients, until they had assured themselves better control over the budget.

In 1903, unnerved by financial conditions in Belmont coupled with a leap in the deficit at MGH, the trustees reviewed their entire administrative structure and came up with a plan that would, in their words, "put into the hands of one department all the purchasing power of the Institution, together with such merging of the various mechanical and industrial departments as will effect the greatest economy, together with the greatest efficiency" (28). This decision put the resident physician of MGH, then Herbert B. Howard, in the role of chief executive officer of both MGH and McLean. Fiscal authority, the chief source of the hospital administrator's power, passed from Belmont to Fruit Street in Boston. This was the move that really unseated Cowles; mandatory retirement was merely a device. While the trustees pondered a great many factors while redesigning the administrative apparatus, Cowles's independence and their inability to withdraw authority that had been granted him back in the 1880s influenced their thinking. The revised structure guaranteed that no McLean head would enjoy such powers as Cowles had wielded. In the end, Cowles extracted some small satisfaction by sneaking Franz in under the wire.

On January 24, 1904, some of Cowles's friends gathered at the Union Club in Boston and surprised him with a testimonial dinner. Among the speakers were Jelly, Tuttle, G. H. M. Rowe of Boston City Hospital, Henry Hurd of Johns Hopkins, and Walter Channing, a distinguished Boston psychiatrist. As if at a wake, they recited flattering phrases about Cowles's contributions to psychiatry, emphasizing the nurses' training school and the research program; they enumerated his achievements at Boston City Hospital, as a builder of hospitals and as a leader in the psychiatric profession. Two speakers who had not compared texts referred to the "Indian summer" of his life, a gooey metaphor that must have made Cowles wince. But the superintendent of the Pennsylvania Hospital for the Insane remarked that Cowles was entering retirement "with judgment and mental powers undimmed as yet by age" and that the news "has come as a shock to all of us."

When Cowles finally rose to respond, his friends could see he had been moved by what he correctly recognized as both congratulations and condolences. He spoke frankly of "mixed feelings," "regrets," and "running the gamut of emotions."

> Thus accepting with equal mind both congratulations and sympathy, I find that my replies take spontaneous expression in such figure[s] of speech as "it is like pulling oneself up by the roots," or "leaving the plough in the furrow." There must be some lingering regrets, for the roots grow deep in such a soil, and the desire is strong to turn the furrow around that beautiful curve yonder, now so near but that has seemed so far distant for so many years. (29)

The friends presented a loving cup. The dinner would have been a ghastly event if Cowles had not been in a good mood. Fortunately, he had learned that very day that Mrs. Matchett had donated an additional $5,000 that would assure Franz at least two years in the McLean laboratories. He knew, therefore, that the chain of research would not be broken with his departure.

Cowles lived until 1919. His pension ($2,746.30) was modest compared with the salary ($4,000) and housing that had been his as superintendent. He moved to Plymouth, Massachusetts, and opened an office in Boston. He continued to teach at Harvard until 1905 and at Dartmouth until 1914. Hall, who thought the trustees had treated Cowles very shabbily, invited him to be a lecturer on mental disease at Clark. He also kept an eye on the evolution of events at McLean. So Cowles stayed busy and kept abreast of his field. Intellectually he got crankier and crankier, involved in what he admitted were "obsessing fermentations" about Kraepelin's influence on American psychiatry as he became increasingly impatient with the inherent weakness of a classification scheme that was not grounded in pathology or etiology. He fretted that "the total ignoring by the psychiatrists of the basic genetic principles of general medicine afford a large vacuum for the chaotic effects of working without any coordinating principle" (30). He wrote muddled letters to Hall that revealed his continuing struggle to clarify his own concepts of mental disease. His ideas, when they could be ferreted out of the disorder, resembled those of Meyer.

Cowles had some cause for bitterness. From the moment he left McLean, this man who had helped guide AMPA out of the backwaters of nineteenth-century alienism into a new century of scientific psychiatry, who had served as its president, who had introduced some of the first research laboratories to mental hospitals, and who had advanced the careers of Hoch and Meyer, sank into professional obscurity. Meyer held a grudge against him that went back to the turn of the century, when Cowles had advised in the organization of the New York Pathological Institute, of which Meyer later (and, later still, Hoch) became head. The details of the story are too complicated to repeat here, but Franz summed up the damage to Cowles's reputation when he explained to Hall that because of Cowles's advice, "when Meyer took up the work, . . . the way had been cleared. . . . In other words, without any wish to criticize Meyer, Cowles got the discredit for the formulation of the functions of the Pathological Institute and Meyer got the credit. The magnification of one was usually at the expense of the other, and this continued for some years" (31).

Meyer owed a great deal to Cowles, who in 1895 had recommended him for a position at the Worcester Lunatic Hospital and drawn him into the circle of influential thinkers such as Hall, James, and McLean's own Hoch. Meyer, who possessed a creative intelligence, rose to prominence in American psychiatry during the first decade of the twentieth century. He formulated a system he called "psychobiology" that attempted to resolve the mind/body dualism which had so long plagued the profession and that joined psychiatry and neurology. He proposed that "mental activity is really best understood in its full meaning as the adaptation and adjustment of the individual as a whole, in contrast to the simple activity of single organs." "We are quite sure," he stated, "that man undissected is more real and important to us than the paradox of the divided individual" (32). In his view, understanding the nature of mental disorder required thorough study of an individual's heredity, environment, and physical, social, and emotional being—the living, functioning human.

Meyer stayed at the top of the profession for years. A 1935 report on psychiatry in *Fortune* magazine referred to him as "unquestionably the No. 1 U.S. *research* psychiatrist. . . . His theory of 'psychobiology' is the guiding star of most American Psychiatrists." When addressing past history, he habitually minimized Cowles's role. Loyal friend Hall found Cowles's situation "pathetic almost to a point of tragedy, to have his pioneer work apparently forgotten . . . even by men like Meyer and Hoch, whose careers he made possible" (33). Cowles, meanwhile, regarded Meyer's work with respect. "Psychiatry is having a tremendous struggle in breaking out of bondage [to Kraepelin]," he wrote in 1914. "Perhaps Meyer is doing it" (34). He worried about scientific research, not about his place in posterity, and shrugged off Meyer's slights. He was blessed with a sense of humor that stayed with him even on his death bed.

Cowles's reputation sank even further after his death in 1919 as Freudian theory gained professional ascendance. Cowles, who had missed a chance to get a front seat on the Freudian bandwagon (he was interested in Freud, but not convinced), seldom got credit for anything beyond the development of nurses' training programs. But reputations rise and fall on the tides of fashion. Cowles's name has been resurrected by more recent generations of laboratory researchers and biochemically oriented psychiatrists. Franz, one of Cowles's loyal defenders, would not have been satisfied. "I am not one who believes in waiting to erect monuments to the dead," he wrote in 1916. "Such monuments may be instructive historically but the individual in the living state often suffers privation and dies, but would go on doing a man's work if the stimulant of approbation and appreciation were applied soon enough. . . . The application of this in Doctor Cowles' case is evident" (35).

CHAPTER

7

New Views of the Patient

During the decade after Cowles's reluctant retirement from McLean, psychiatry entered an extended restless phase when disconnected forces tugged at its theoretical and institutional assumptions from different directions. From the biomedical front, Cowles's preferred line of attack on mental diseases, there came two stunning advances. First of all, there was some progress in the understanding of syphilis, a widespread disease that caused immeasurable physical and mental misery. In 1906 a German bacteriologist, August von Wassermann, isolated the spirochete protozoon that causes syphilis and developed a method of testing for its presence. Wassermann tests of mental patients suffering general paralysis (paresis) disclosed the presence of the spirochetes, sometimes in the blood and always in the spinal fluid. In 1913, Hideyo Noguchi and Joseph W. Moore published their discovery of the spirochete in the brain and confirmed the link between syphilis and paresis.

Institutional psychiatry greeted this revelation with excitement. Victims of general paralysis occupied approximately 10 percent of the beds in mental hospitals, where they invariably deteriorated and died. For instance, of 167 patients admitted to McLean in 1909, 16—12 men and 4 women—had general paralysis. The staff could do little more than keep them as comfortable as possible and watch them die. But the identification of an essential cause contained the promise of treatment and cure in the proximate future.

A year after Noguchi and Moore revealed their findings, Joseph Goldberger established that a dietary deficiency—later pinned down as a lack of niacin—caused pellagra, a condition which produced a wide range of psychoses and accounted for a large percentage of admissions to mental institutions in the southern United States. Cause, cure, and prevention came in one neat package: Given a niacin-enriched diet amplified by niacin tablets, pellagra patients soon disappeared from hospital wards. McLean's self-supporting patients being well nourished, Goldberger's discoveries about pellagra did not make a dent in their numbers. Nevertheless, both his work and that on syphilis appeared to justify Cowles's faith in research on the physiology of mental illness. Note that neither breakthrough had come out of a psychiatric laboratory; Goldberger worked with the fledgling U.S. Public Health Service, Noguchi and Moore at the Rockefeller Institute. As Cowles persisted in complaining, Kraepelin's disciples still dominated the psychiatric picture.

Meanwhile, Meyer, Hoch, E. E. Southard, and a few other psychiatrists were pulling away from the center, and another figure appeared fuzzily at one edge of the frame: Sigmund Freud, archaeologist of the psyche. Freud had been publishing his theories since the 1890s, but they had not been well received in Europe and were slow to cross the Atlantic, where, among other problems, his terminology was difficult even for those with a reasonable command of German. Yet isolated references to Freud started to pop up here and there around 1893 or 1894, first in a speech by Morton Prince, a professor at Tufts, and then in a favorable review by Robert Edes, Harvard's professor of materia medica, and most conspicuously in William James's "Lowell lecture" of 1896 (1). But is was Massachusetts General Hospital's neurologist James J. Putnam who published the first paper in English on the clinical use of psychoanalysis in 1906 and really put Freud on the American psychiatric map.

In 1909 Putnam and G. Stanley Hall invited Freud, Carl Jung, and Sandor Ferenczi to deliver a series of lectures on psychoanalysis at the 20th-anniversary celebration of Clark University. (The Clark symposium accumulated historic significance, like a stone gathers moss, with the passage of time. Freud himself called it "the first official recognition of psychoanalysis." Also, since the occasion turned out to be his only visit to North America, the members of the audience acquired a privileged position in the pantheon of psychiatry.)

F. Lyman Wells, assistant in pathological psychology, was the only representative of McLean at Clark. Though fresh out of graduate school, he was not the least bit bashful and registered his unfavorable impression of Freud's views with Hall (2). William James, 67 years old and under the weather, trekked to Worcester "to see what Freud was like." Afterwards he wrote a friend, "I hope that Freud and his pupils will push their ideas to their utmost limits, so that we may learn what they are. They can't fail to throw light on human nature; but I confess that he made on me personally the impression of a man obsessed with fixed ideas" (3). Translations of Freud's papers began to appear shortly after the conference; the New York Psychoanalytic Society organized itself in 1911.

I shall assume that readers are reasonably familiar with Freud and take the liberty of a detour around the quicksands of psychoanalytic theory for fear of getting sucked into their rich, tantalizing, and sometimes murky depths. Crudely stated, he proposed a theory of human personality, a method of research into abnormal psychology, and a technique for curing some forms of mental illness.

There is one piece of Freud's thinking that people tended to overlook, no doubt because they were overwhelmed by the more salacious elements of his concepts: Freud, a neurologist by training, maintained a belief in the physiological bases of mental disorders. "The edifice of psychoanalytic doctrine which we have erected is in reality but a superstructure, which will have to be set on its organic foundation at some time or other," he wrote; "but this foundation is still unknown to us. . . . Psychoanalysis aims at and achieves nothing more than the discovery of the unconscious in mental life. The problems of the actual neuroses, in which the symptoms probably arise through direct toxic injury, offer no point of attack for psychoanalysis; it can supply little towards elucidation of them and must leave this task to biological and medical research" (4). Freud did not belabor this point; to have done so would have distracted from his principal argument. But in view of some of the distortions of Freudian theory, it is important to review the perimeters its originator himself drew around it.

Once Freud had been in the United States under the sponsorship of respectable individuals like Putnam and Hall and some of his papers had been translated into English, psychiatrists had a hard time ignoring him. A few—Ernest Jones, A. A. Brill, Smith Ely Jelliffe, and William A. White among them—became his protagonists. Others, like Meyer, an early reader of Freud, withheld their full enthusiasm. While Meyer acknowledged debts to Freud and Jung for their "demonstration that what is at work in the center of the stage is a complex or group of complexes consisting of insufficiently balanced experience in various ways, modified by symbolism" (5), and his own description of personality profited from Freud's elucidation of psychological dynamics, he was uncomfortable with what he saw as Freud's single-minded emphasis on sexuality and the unconscious. Hoch, who studied with Paul Bleuler and Jung in 1908 after he had left McLean, found his insights sharpened by Freud and Jung, and became one of the most articulate defenders of psychoanalysis. Shortly before World War I, papers with Freudian-inspired themes invaded the pages of professional magazines, including the *American Journal of Insanity.*

On the whole, however, institutional psychiatry received Freudian theory with contempt. The atmosphere was decidedly chilly at the 70th annual meeting of AMPA in Baltimore, Maryland, in May 1914, when Charles W. Burr, professor of mental diseases at the University of Pennsylvania, presented his critique of psychoanalysis:

> Freud's idea that mental processes are ruled by law will be accepted by many of us; indeed it is no new thing, but came into the world as soon as the idea of natural law was first thought of, and has been battled over ever since. When, however, he adds to that idea that such laws of mental action can be explained by psychological terms only, there arises in the minds of some a feeling of resistance, of antipathy; a feeling that he is getting into a very fanciful realm. Those of us who are inclined to the view that there is always a physical cause for a mental act, and a perver-

> sion of physical function whenever there is a perversion of mental acts, want proof before we accept his opinions. . . .
>
> Psychic insult is, according to Freud, the large cause of certain mental disorders. . . . [I]t is common when a boy or girl breaks to say, out of kindness, that it was the stress of over-work at school or too much practicing of music that caused the mental trouble, but everyone who has investigated the matter knows that public school work is carefully arranged so that a very ordinary boy or girl can accomplish it and that it is the weakness of the person and not the greatness of the stress which causes the breakdown. We are continually talking about the strenuousness of modern life. There is a great deal of humbug about this. . . . The normal person can and does withstand all the stress and strain of life without mental breakdown. Of course the strains and stresses I am speaking of are conscious, but the argument holds for the unconscious. Really it would seem that more progress in discovering the cause of the psychoneurosis would result from the study of heredity and human chemistry and physiology and pathology than from the fanciful interpretation of hysterics' dreams. . . .
>
> I remember an old and distinguished professor of medicine in Germany who, when some years ago I told him I had aspirations to become a neurologist and alienist, looked at me kindly and a little quizzically and then said: "Be careful, my young friend, alienists are all a little queer." The old gentleman had some justification then, but what would he think now could he be told what we are often told, that psychanalysis [*sic*] is one of the greatest contributions to therapeutic art?

Burr's scathing criticism was well mannered by comparison with the remarks of the next speaker, F. X. Dercum, who characterized Freud and his followers as a "sect" and concluded "that it should be a matter of keen humiliation and chagrin that an epoch when psychiatry is beginning to unfold a practically limitless field for actual scientific research, men should be found willing to devote themselves to a cult, to an ism, which like a salted mine returns to the investigator only that which he himself puts into it. Blind pockets from which even the semblance of light is excluded, are his portion, nothing more."

William A. White, feeling as though he had been "pretty well raked over" by the previous speakers, gathered his courage and rose in defense of Freud: "Psychoanalysis, speaking very simply, pretends to do with the human mind what we learned to do with the human body hundreds of years ago," he explained:

> We had to learn to dissect the human body to find out what it is made of, and our efforts to do that dissection of the human mind must be made in the face of just about the same kind of arguments, the same kind of prejudices that hampered the efforts to dissect the human body years

> and years ago; every scientific advance, every step forward, every opening of a new door is made the same source of the same kind of resistance.

Beyond the intellectual and emotional objections of most practitioners, Freudian theory hit the stone wall of institutional psychiatry, and practically all American psychiatrists worked out of mental hospitals. To quote Burr again:

> What sort of diseases are suitable for psychoanalytic treatment? Freud states its use is limited. The patient must have a certain degree of education and his character must be reliable. Only those who are prompted by their sufferings to seek treatment can be aided. Those who subject themselves to it by order of relatives are unfitted. Psychoses, confusional, and marked toxic depressions are unsuitable. Later it may be possible to disregard these contraindications, but not now. Persons near or over fifty are not psychically plastic enough—not educable. Youthful persons, even before puberty, make excellent subjects. Psychoanalysis should not be attempted when it is a question of rapidly removing a threatening manifestation, such as hysteric anorexia. These are Freud's statements.

Well, sort of, and taken out of context. (Freud is a bit like the Bible in that some quotation can be recruited to support almost any argument.) The qualifications listed by Burr effectively ruled out the application of psychoanalysis to mental hospital patients, who were characteristically psychotic, confused, and well into adulthood.

But Freud, in fact, imagined that some modified form of psychoanalysis might be used to treat hospitalized patients. Hoch, who took on this particular aspect of Burr's diatribe, was even more optimistic about deploying psychoanalysis as a research tool for understanding the psychoses: "[I]t must be admitted that the interpretation of dreams and of the material contained in the neuroses is difficult," he said, "and that every conscientious observer is bound to have a period of uncertainty which can be overcome only by painstaking work and the collection of a large amount of evidence. It is therefore fortunate that a careful study of the psychoses, more especially of the delusions and hallucinations in the constitutional disorders, gives any one who really desires to get at the facts, an easier and quicker way to obtain this knowledge" (6). Hoch's peers were not impressed by his reasoning.

Yet even if institutional psychiatry had been more receptive to

Freud's concepts in principle, psychoanalytic treatment and research posed a practical obstacle so fundamental that no one even mentioned it. The problem simply hung in the air as a given of institutional life. Psychoanalysis required many hours of conversation with individual patients and, therefore, a doctor-patient, or analyst-patient, ratio that in 1914 no mental hospital in the United States even approached or could imagine affording. In another decade or two, the economic resistance to psychoanalysis would prove to be much tougher than intellectual opposition.

There were no psychoanalytic fifth columnists at McLean in the pre-World War I period; the word "psychoanalysis" was barely whispered in annual reports, where it showed up now and then in small print in some item in Wells's bibliography. However, there were signs of subtle changes in the hospital's approach to patients. Statements during Tuttle's administration revealed the direct influence of Meyer and, to the extent that he helped shape Meyer's ideas, the indirect spirit of Freud. "A most hopeful tendency in psychopathology as well as in normal psychology is founded on the conception of the mind as an adaptive mechanism," Tuttle wrote in 1914. The report for 1916 read in part:

> . . . In accordance with modern trends there is an effort at more intensive study of the patient on admission, with the view of determining more minutely the adaptive mechanisms of the patient, and the type, nature, and causes of the alterations in them. The patient has been able to adapt himself to the circumstances of his life as successfully as the average up to the time of his illness. He then began to adapt himself less well. In his past life we try to find what general situations he has had to adjust himself to, what special or significant experiences or difficulties he may have had, what sort of make-up he had with which to meet them, what his methods and success in meeting and handling these difficulties have been, and what handicaps he may have had in the way of inherited endowment or tendency to disease or physical disabilities, of mental deficiencies or tendencies of the illness itself. We try to get as many details of fact as possible concerning his attitude, his general and particular behavior in immediate reaction to his situation, and his comprehension of his situation and condition. From the patient himself we try to get as full an expression as possible of his own comprehension of his present and past, near and remote situations, of himself as related to them, of his reactions to them; of his own condition, and of the causes for his failure to adapt himself well. . . . We are trying to gather data for an interpretive as well as a descriptive psychiatry.

This model of study differed substantially from the one in use at the turn of the century. In Cowles's administration the patient had been viewed as a human receptacle of disease; the object of scrutiny was the disease, not the individual in whom it happened to have set up house. Descriptive psychiatry, represented by the Kraepelin-trained Hoch in his pre-Freud–Bleuler days, focused on the symptoms of disease, including the history of former episodes of illness. Information about the healthy patient was irrelevant, and the patient was not asked about his or her understanding of the illness. Laboratory researchers looked for clues to disease in brain tissues of deceased patients, in the chemistry of blood, stools, and urine of living patients, in rates of muscular exhaustion, and in physiological phenomena. This was a rigid medical model of psychological illness. Gallstones were a disease; manic-depressive illness was a disease. People were hosts. Such a crude translation of their perspective would no doubt have offended Cowles and his staff. "But we *care* for these patients," they would have countered, while pointing to ample evidence of their caring and kindness. Indeed, they did care. But they made a sharp intellectual distinction between patient and pathology.

The model, essentially Meyer's, that began to come into focus at McLean during Tuttle's administration united disease and patient, enlisted the patient as an observer of his or her own symptoms, and wove the illness into the fabric of an entire life. Psychobiology, like Freudian psychology, enlarged the definition of evidence so as to draw in data that had previously been considered biographical rather than medical.

The problem of essential cause tended to get obscured in the density of detail. Meyer hypothesized both somatic and psychological causes of mental illness, with emphasis on the latter; his critics complained that he did not establish comprehensible connections between the two and that his concepts were muddled. The statement in McLean's annual report, cited earlier, was also unclear in this respect, suggesting a mix of physiological and psychological causes: There is "illness" on the one hand, and the patient's "failure to adapt" on the other. The formulation squared with Meyer's view "that to try to explain a hysterical fit or a delusion system out of hypothetical cell alterations which we cannot reach or prove is at the present stage of histophysiology a gratuitous performance. To realize that such a reaction is a *faulty response or substitution of an insufficient or protective or evasive or mutilated attempt at adjustment* opens ways of inquiry in the direction of modifiable determining factors" (7). For all their difficulties and ambiguities, the complex images of the patient proposed by Meyer, Freud, and their followers intuitively appealed to those psychiatrists who were trying to help living, breathing, feeling, reacting, social human beings and who felt let down by the strict medical approach.

Another more severe model of man emerged from the psychology laboratories at Johns Hopkins in 1913. John B. Watson, elaborating Pavlov's studies of conditioned reflex, published an article called "Psychology as the Behaviorist Views It" and fathered a school of psychology based on the premise that behavior and personality resulted from training or conditioning rather than heredity. His theories implied methods for predicting and controlling human behavior. Watson and Meyer were colleagues, the latter having moved from the New York Pathological Institute in 1908 to direct a new psychiatric clinic and teach psychiatry at Johns Hopkins. He and Watson exchanged views, collaborated briefly in a psychology course for medical students, and then returned to their separate intellectual paths, but not before Watson had influenced the thinking of the eclectic Meyer.

While the psychiatric profession was embroiled in debates about psychoanalysis, psychobiology, nature, and nurture, the lay public started to make noises about the quality of psychiatric care. With the appearance in 1908 of Clifford Beers's book, *A Mind that Found Itself*, the noise became impossible to ignore. Beers had been a mental patient and passed more than three years in different institutions, moving from one to another as his family groped for help and, later, ran out of money. His book is a powerfully written account of the shortcomings of mental hospitals and the insensitive, sometimes brutal, treatment of patients. It aroused the public as deeply as Dorothea Dix's descriptions of the mentally ill chained in jail cells had shocked people during the mid-nineteenth century. Since Beers had been shrewd enough to line up professional endorsements before publication, his book also made an impression in psychiatric circles. Meyer, who seems to have been everywhere during this period, wrote a favorable notice in the popular *North American Review* and put the profession on alert.

While preparing his manuscript, Beers imagined *A Mind that Found Itself* as a vehicle for launching a reform movement to improve mental institutions and for educating the public about mental illness. When he solicited advice about the form such an organization might usefully assume, Meyer proposed a society for mental hygiene that shifted the focus from institutional reform to showing people "better ways of healthy living, prevention of trouble, and efficient handling of what is not prevented" (8). In 1909, a coalition of 12 lay and professional people—Beers, Meyer, Hoch, and William James among them—established the National Committee for Mental Hygiene, which took as its goals the prevention of mental illness, higher standards of care, promotion of research on mental disorders, and the gathering of more accurate, systematic information. The committee's work started slowly for want of funds, but the organization gained momentum during the war and evolved into a public information and political instrument of some consequence.

The establishment of psychopathic wards in general hospitals and later as adjuncts of state mental hospitals, though initially independent of the proddings of the National Committee for Mental Hygiene, represented an effort to create an institutional framework for preventive psychiatric intervention. The Boston Psychopathic Hospital, set up by the State Board of Insanity as a department of Boston State Hospital and opened in 1912, was designed to "receive all classes of mental patients for first care, examination and observation, and provide short, intensive treatment for incipient, acute and curable insanity" (9).

Directorship of the Boston Psychopathic Hospital was placed in the hands of neuropathologist Elmer Ernest Southard, a man whom Meyer described as possessing "an unusual intellectual endowment, going far beyond what made him the champion chess player he was. He had a very outgoing, bubbling temperament, and a great talent—to use his own word—as impresario, and as collaborator" (10). Southard naturally inclined toward research in neuropathology, but as a student of James, he was acquainted with Freudian theory and interested in dynamic psychology; accordingly, the research program at Boston Psychopathic Hospital was broad ranging, lively, and exciting. Southard inspired many a budding psychiatrist, including Karl Menninger.

Boston Psychopathic Hospital did not provide long-term care. Patients admitted for treatment were discharged home if they improved and transferred to other institutions if they did not; this screening role resembled the "observation" system Cowles had started at McLean a decade earlier. Boston Psychopathic Hospital accepted children as patients and operated an outpatient department to give free consultation and medical treatment to aid in home care of mental patients. It also developed a superb social service department, guided by Mary Jarrett, to facilitate early discharge and aftercare of patients and to help in filling out case histories by assembling information on domestic and work environments, family background, and other biographical data pertinent to a patient's file. Altogether, Boston Psychopathic Hospital quickly overtook and outran McLean to become the most progressive mental hospital in the Commonwealth. This sprint to the forefront was due largely to Southard's iridescent leadership; however, one notes that he enjoyed a great advantage in not having to bear the burden of chronic patients (11).

The discoveries concerning syphilis and pellagra, the gathering influence of the theories of Freud, Meyer, Jung, and others, the founding of the mental hygiene movement, and the establishment of psychopathic hospitals and various outpatient clinics all occurred within 10 years after Cowles left McLean, between 1904 and World War I. Within that decade, the relatively unified image that American psychiatry had presented for half a century began to decompose into fragments. As the frail agreements about cause, identity, and treatment of mental illness fell apart, psychiatry diversified. Decades of argument ensued. Some of it was petty bickering; most of it was stimulating. Age-old questions resubmitted themselves for answering. What is insanity? Who is insane? What kinds of problems should psychiatrists work on? In what order and by what methods? How should insanity be treated? The questions were now set in the context of accumulated experiential data, increasingly elaborate physiological and psychological models of humans, and more powerful research instruments and methodologies. They were being asked during the same decade when Albert Einstein published his theory of relativity and Pablo Picasso introduced *Les Demoiselles d'Avignon*, a canvas generally conceded to be the first cubist painting. That decade challenged cherished perceptions of the way the universe worked, of progress, and of human perfectibility and set off a chain reaction of interrogation.

Although psychiatrists did not come up with hard solutions to the stubborn problems of cause and treatment of mental illness, the nature of their questions and their speculations about the role of environment and emotions in the development of mental disorders slowly altered the configuration of psychiatric practice. The definition of the psychiatric patient was liberalized. Southard, for example, described the "essential function" of the Boston Psychopathic Hospital as "caring for the non-insane," meaning people at risk of becoming insane if they did not get professional help (12). Freud treated benign neurotics: "A young officer, home on short leave of absence, asked me to treat his mother-in-law, who was living in the happiest surroundings and yet was embittering her own and her family's lives by a nonsensical idea. I found her a well-preserved lady, fifty-three years of age, of a friendly, simple disposition who . . . [suffered from] a *delusion of jealousy*."

Since such patients were not candidates for institutions like McLean or state hospitals, new forms of practice responded to their needs. By 1920 the Massachusetts state mental hospital system operated 33 outpatient clinics. At the same time, a few psychiatrists began treating patients in their offices. Both trends seemed to be fulfilling Walter Channing's turn-of-the-century prophecy that there was a big field for psychiatrists outside the hospital.

A very gradual change also occurred in the quality of encounter between psychiatrist and patient. Psychiatrists actually began to pay attention to what mentally ill people told them. (Freud scolded: "Physicians pay so little attention to neurotics and listen so carelessly to what they say it has become impossible for them to perceive anything in the patients' communications" [13].) Psychiatrists practicing for nearly a century according to the principles of moral treatment had acquired the habit of ignoring the conversations of the mentally ill. The aim had been to deflect the patient's attention from "diseased thoughts" to healthy reflection; the last thing an old-fashioned alienist wanted to discuss with a patient was why he thought he was Napoleon. Freud and Meyer urged psychiatrists to attend carefully to what the patient said, to ask questions, and to listen to the eloquent silences. Freud refined listening and questioning into an exacting art and therapeutic method. In Meyer's scheme, information gleaned from the patient supplied pieces to the puzzle of total personality, of disease as one facet of that personality, and of adaptive behavior and where it might have run off the track. Whatever the motives, and precious few psychiatrists practiced psychoanalysis before World War I, psychiatrists were spending more time with patients.

Cowles's departure and the new administrative structure achieved what the trustees wanted at McLean: an interval of prosperous dullness. Executive power rested officially in the hands of Herbert B. Howard, resident physician and administrator of the general hospital, a man distinguished by his muscular physique and an obstinate belief that electricity would prove to be the preferred energy source for automobiles. He bought an electric runabout for MGH and, "in order to have enough power he placed in it a double set of wet batteries. This placed the driver high in the air. The vehicle was steered by a tiller, had a short wheel base, and was very heavy. The tires were solid and smooth." Howard's secretary, a novice driver, was at the helm of this contraption one day out at McLean when he got confused by the tiller and drove the car up a hill. Luckily, both he and Howard were thrown clear of the heavy batteries when it overturned (14).

Howard's empire was in Boston, and though he visited the Belmont colony at regular intervals, he spent little time there. He watched over budget items and the physical plant but did not meddle in staff issues or medical policies. When he left MGH in 1908 to oversee the building and development of the new Peter Bent Brigham Hospital—for he was, like Cowles, an expert in hospital planning and construction—he was succeeded by

Frederic A. Washburn, who handled McLean administration in a similar fashion. Whether by personal preference or trustee design, the MGH-based executive officer made little difference to McLean. He served principally as a symbolic brake on costly ambitions of the McLean superintendent, should he have any. The real power lay with the trustees, who controlled McLean's purse strings.

George T. Tuttle ran the day-to-day McLean operation within these constraints. He was a graduate of Dartmouth College and the Harvard Medical School. As mentioned earlier, Cowles had known him as a 29-year-old intern at Boston City Hospital and welcomed him in Somerville in 1879. He had spent 25 years as Cowles's chief lieutenant and then been promoted to his rank. Nothing exposes the hypocrisy of the trustees' retirement "policy" as applied to Cowles better than this excerpt from Washburn's history of MGH: "In 1903 Dr. Cowles reached the age limit for active duty and was succeeded by Dr. George T. Tuttle. Dr. Tuttle was born in Northwood, New Hampshire, in 1850. . . . He was Assistant Physician at the McLean Hospital, 1879 to 1904, and Medical Superintendent, 1904–1919." Maybe Washburn never learned arithmetic. Tuttle served until the age of 69!

Tuttle spent 40 years as a McLean physician and left behind few traces of himself. He was short. He liked wine jelly. His health was frail, and he guarded it carefully by living as quietly as it was possible for a man in his position to manage. His father had died when Tuttle was a young man and left him as effective head of a sprawling family. He took this responsibility very seriously and helped numerous siblings and step-siblings throughout their lives. His stepmother spent her last years in his residence at McLean, where she died in 1913. The next year Tuttle, then age 64, surprised his staff by marrying a Dorchester woman, Celeste Weed Albright.

This self-effacing, orderly man made practically no imprint on the character of McLean, let alone on the broader field of American psychiatry. The assistant physicians respected his clinical abilities, and the nurses like him. He produced very little in the way of professional literature: an article about the colony of mental patients at Gheel, Holland, which he had visited in 1889

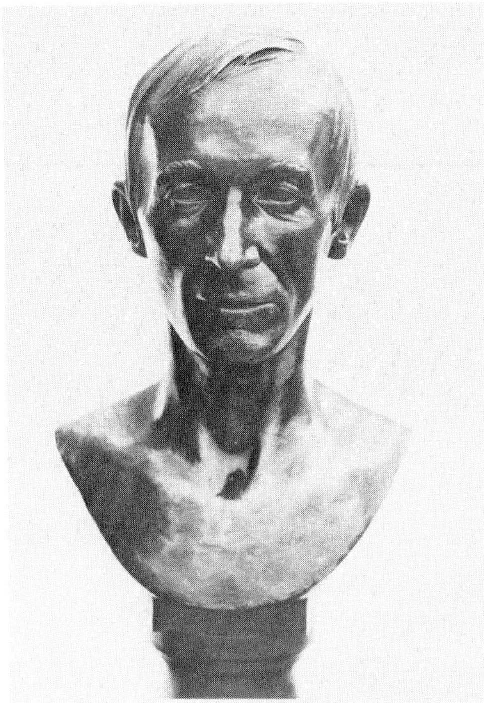

Photo courtesy McLean Hospital

Bust of Rufus Wyman, M.D., from a death mask by T.B., 1897.

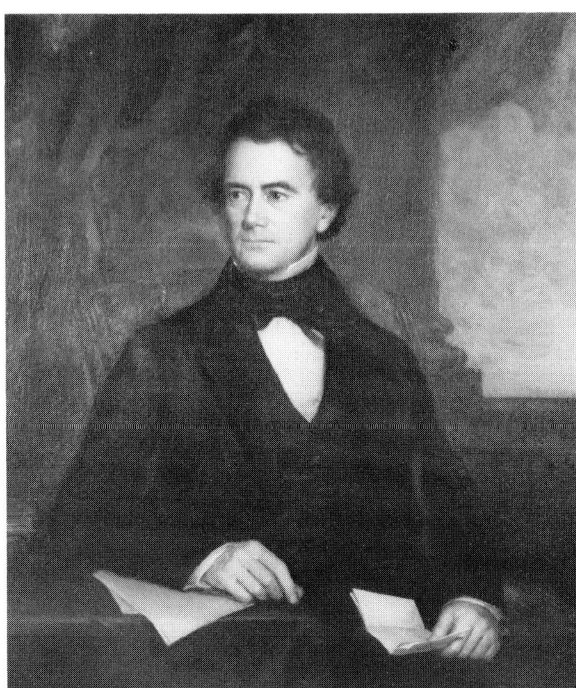

Photo courtesy Chuck Kidd Photography

Portrait of Luther Bell, M.D., portrait by Moses Wight, 1857.

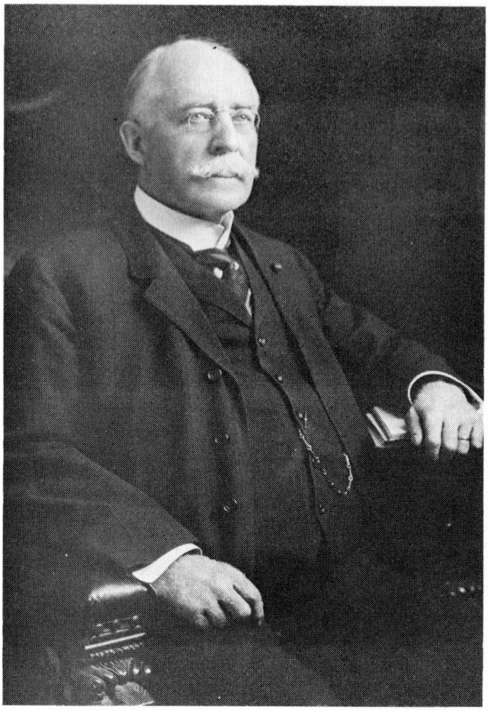

Photo courtesy McLean Hospital

Portrait of Edward Cowles, M.D., by Wilbur Dean Hamilton, 1913.

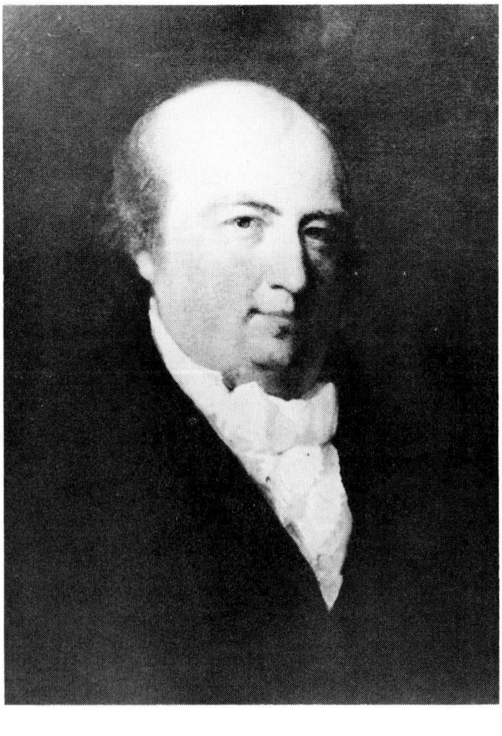

Photo courtesy McLean Hospital

Portrait of John McLean, by Gilbert Stuart, 1824.

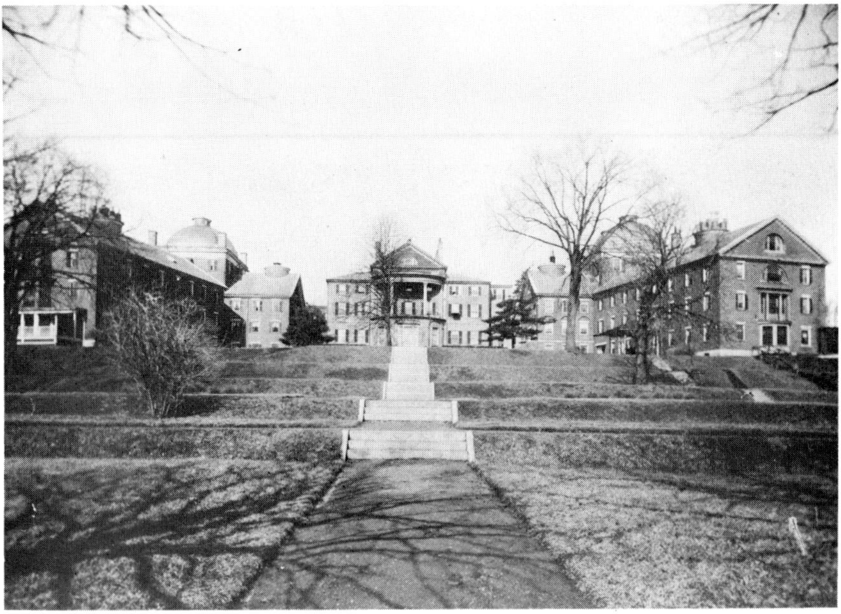

Photo courtesy McLean Hospital

Rear View of the McLean Asylum ca. 1890. The buildings are (l-r): Women's East, Women's Belknap, Administration Building (original Barrell mansion), Men's North, and Men's East.

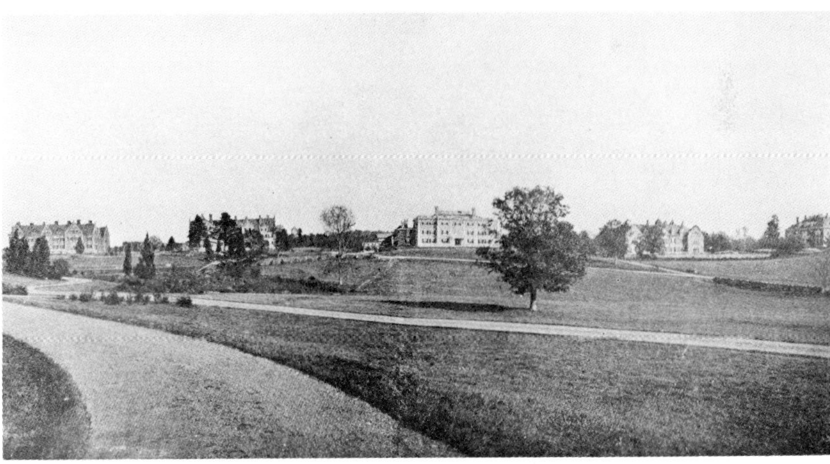

Photo courtesy McLean Hospital

Panoramic view of McLean Hospital, ca. 1910.

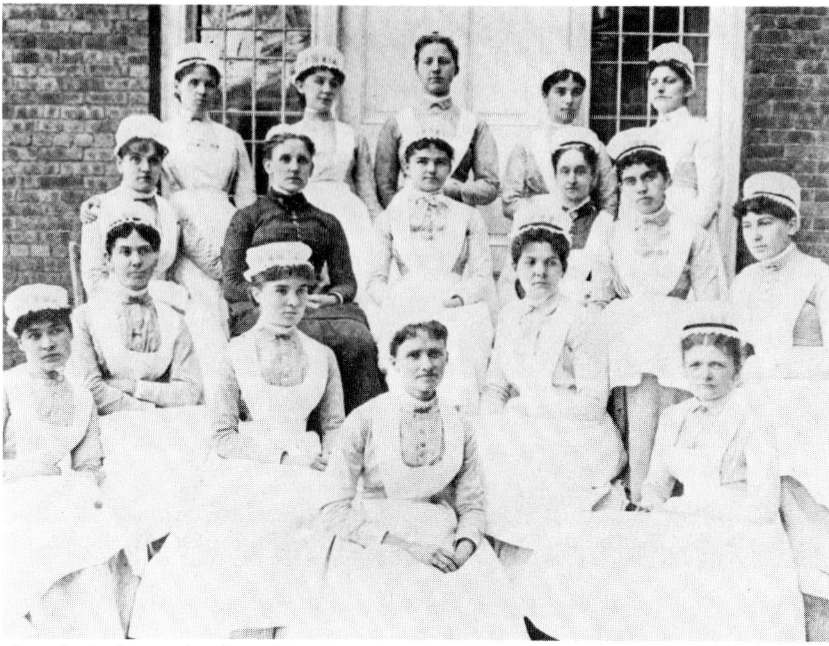

Photo courtesy McLean Hospital

America's first trained psychiatric nurses, graduation day, McLean Asylum, 1886.

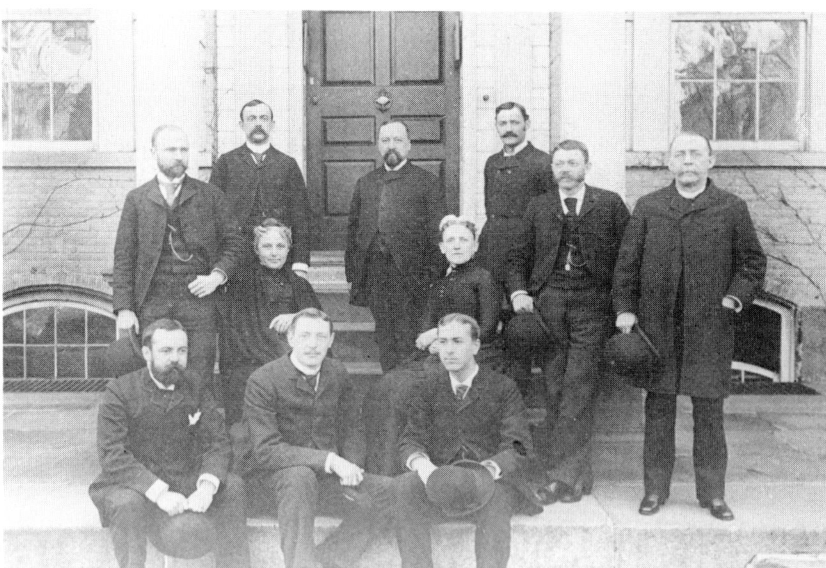

Photo courtesy McLean Hospital

Asylum professional staff, 1891. Back row (standing l-r): Dr. Locke, Dr. Babcock, Mr. Willis, Mr. Bradbury, Dr. Tuttle (First Assistant Physician), Dr. Cowles (Superintendent); middle row (l-r): Miss Gilbert and Miss Woodward (Superintendent of the McLean Hospital Training School for Nurses); front row (l-r): Dr. Noyes (Pathologist), Dr. Huddleston, and Dr. Fuller.

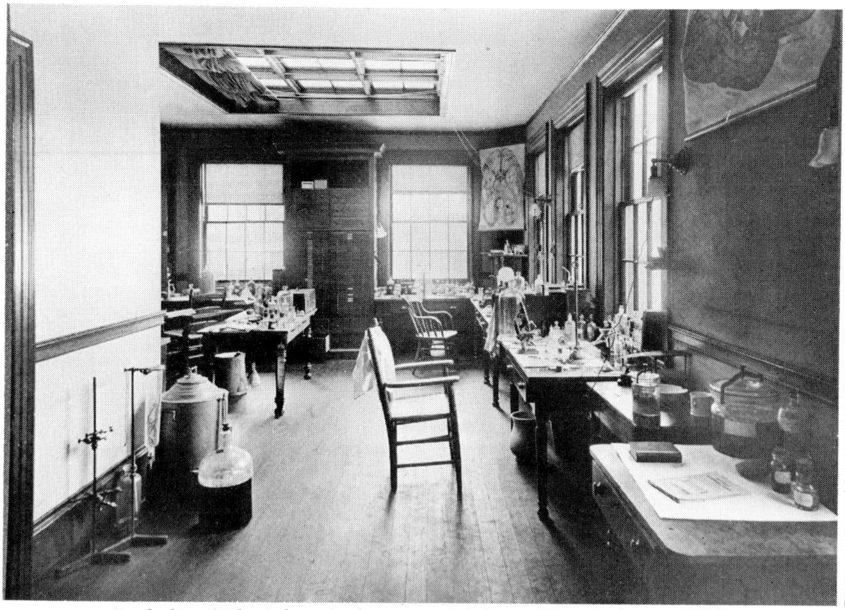

Photo courtesy McLean Hospital

Pathology/Physiology Laboratory, McLean Hospital, ca. 1905.

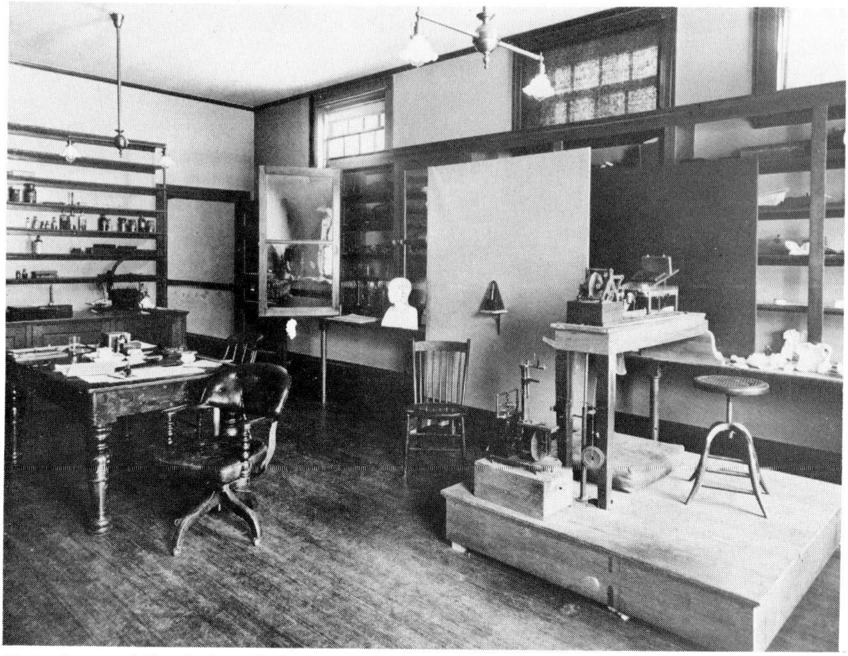

Photo courtesy McLean Hospital

Experimental Psychology Laboratory, McLean Hospital, ca. 1907-1910; Apparatus: a perimeter or campimeter, a Hipp chronoscope, a phrenology bust showing the areas of the skull corresponding to the various faculties of the brain according to Gall and Spurzheim, a metronome, a Kymograph, an Erograph, and a Rheostat.

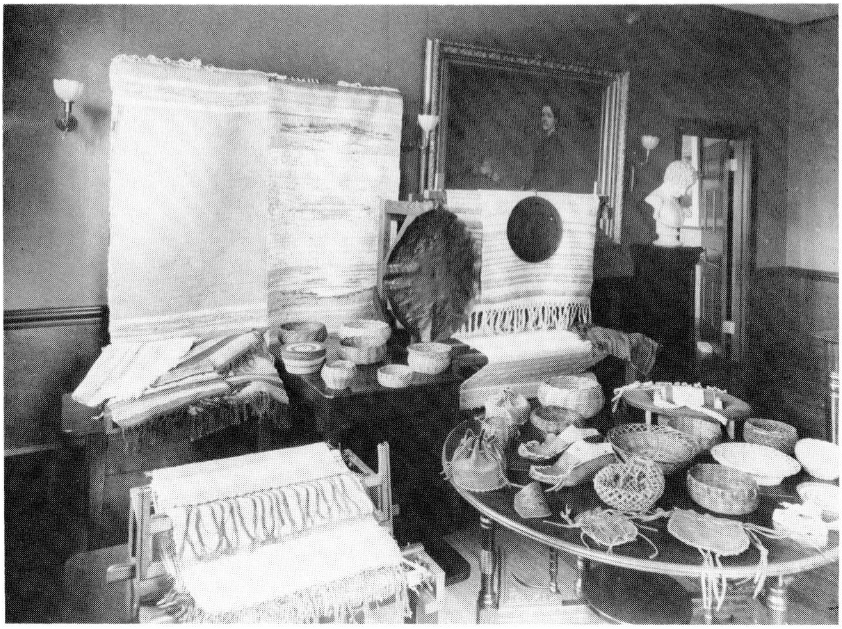

Photo courtesy McLean Hospital

Women's Occupational Therapy, Women's Gymnasium, ca. 1910.

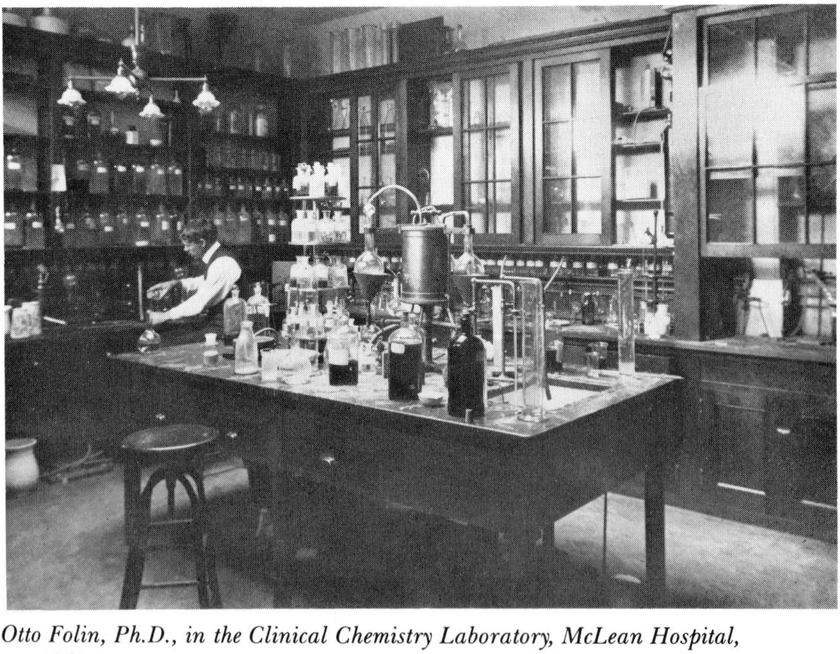

Photo courtesy McLean Hospital

Otto Folin, Ph.D., in the Clinical Chemistry Laboratory, McLean Hospital, ca. 1905.

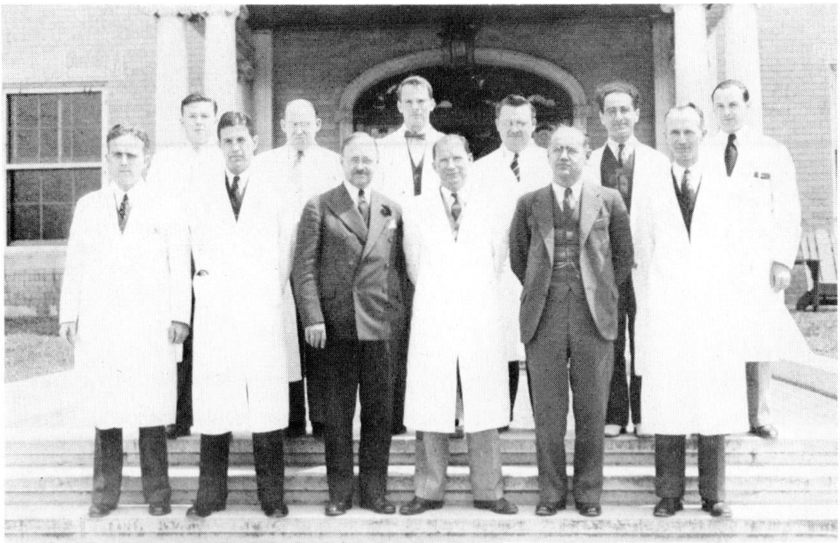

Photo courtesy McLean Hospital

Professional staff, ca. 1938; back row (l-r): Dr. Varney, Dr. Tompkins, Dr. Peltz, Dr. Semrad, Dr. Weiss, Dr. Sulzbach; front row (l-r): Dr. Howard, Dr. Young, Dr. Wood (Director), Dr. Tillotson (Psychiatrist-in-Chief), Dr. Whitehorn (Director of the Laboratories), and Dr. Chittick.

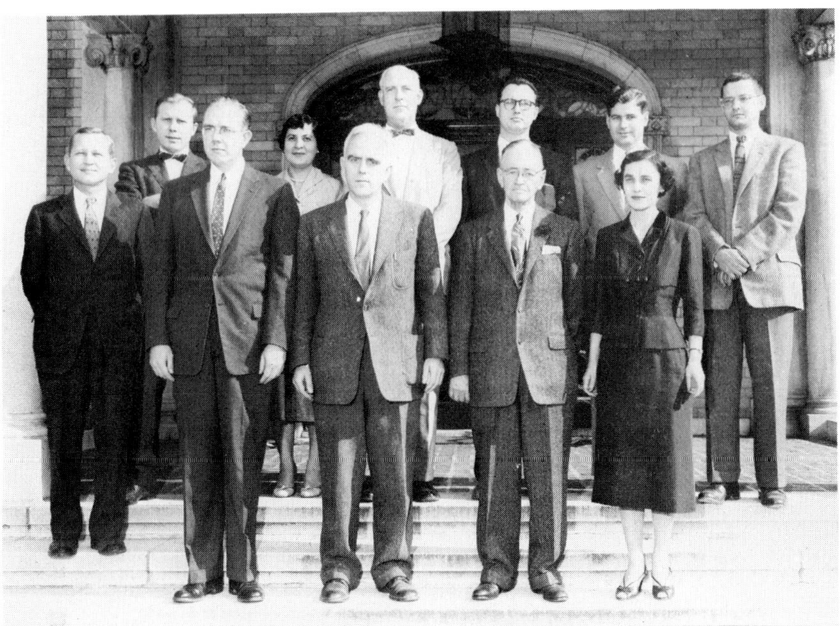

Photo courtesy Ralph H. Hutchins, Jr., Photographer

Clinical professional staff, 1955-1956; back row (l-r): Dr. Haycox, Dr. de Marneffe, Dr. (Pierce) Stiver, Dr. Sharpe, Dr. Walter, Dr. Cain, Dr. Clark; front row (l-r): Dr. Stanton (Director/Psychiatrist-in-Chief), Dr. Howard, Dr. Wood (Director, Emeritus), and Dr. Lorenz.

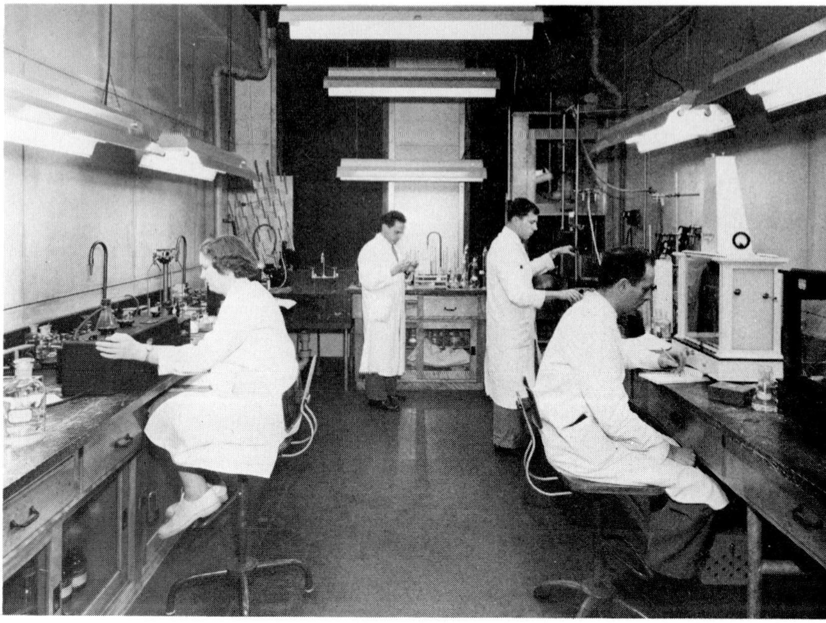

Photo courtesy McLean Hospital

Dr. Helen Hess, Dr. Folch-Pi, Dr. Francis LeBaron, and Dr. James Meath in the Constant Temperature Room, Biological Research Laboratory, November 11, 1952.

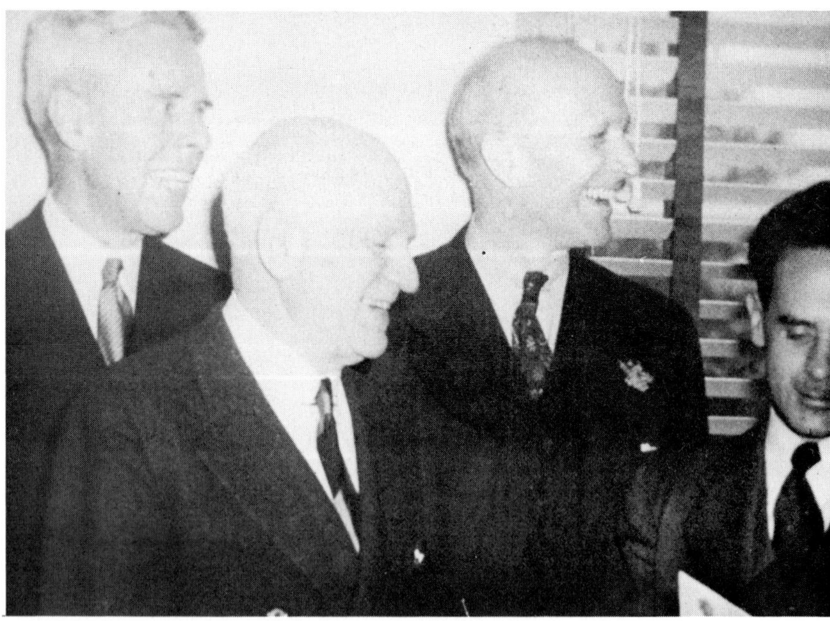

Photo courtesy McLean Hospital

Dr. D.D. Van Slyke, Mr. Francis C. Gray (Chairman, Board of Trustees), Dr. W. Penfield, and Dr. Jordi Folch-Pi (Director of Scientific Research) at the dedication of the Biological Research Laboratory, May 17, 1946.

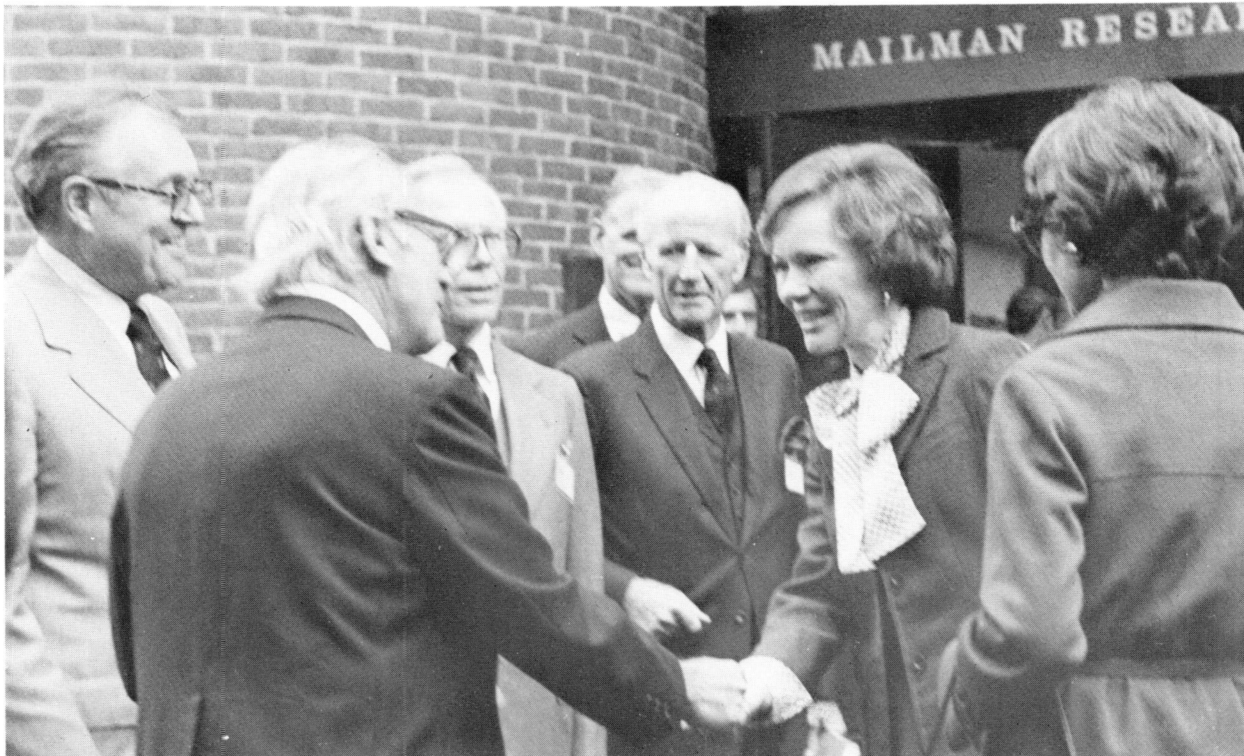

Photo courtesy Hutchins Photography, Inc.

Dr. Kety (Director, Laboratories for Psychiatric Research), shaking hands with Mrs. Carter, Dr. Frazier (Psychiatrist-in-Chief), Dr. de Marneffe (General Director), Mr. Lawrence (Chairman, Board of Trustees), Mr. Putnam in background (Chairman, McLean Hospital Committee), Dedication of the Mailman Research Center, October 3, 1977.

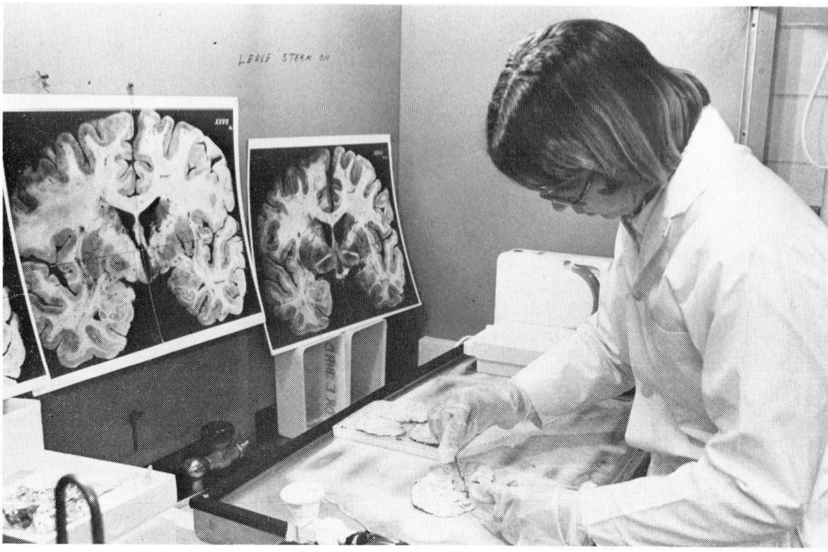

Photo courtesy McLean Hospital

McLean Hospital establishes one of only two brain-tissue banks in the United States, 1978.

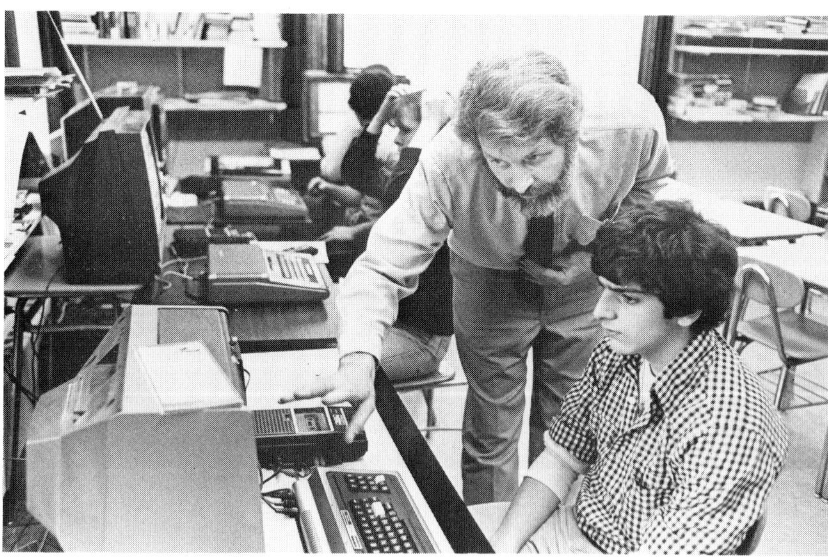

Photo courtesy McLean Hospital

Computer training at Arlington School. [To protect patients' privacy, only hospital staff and friends are recognizable in photographs.]

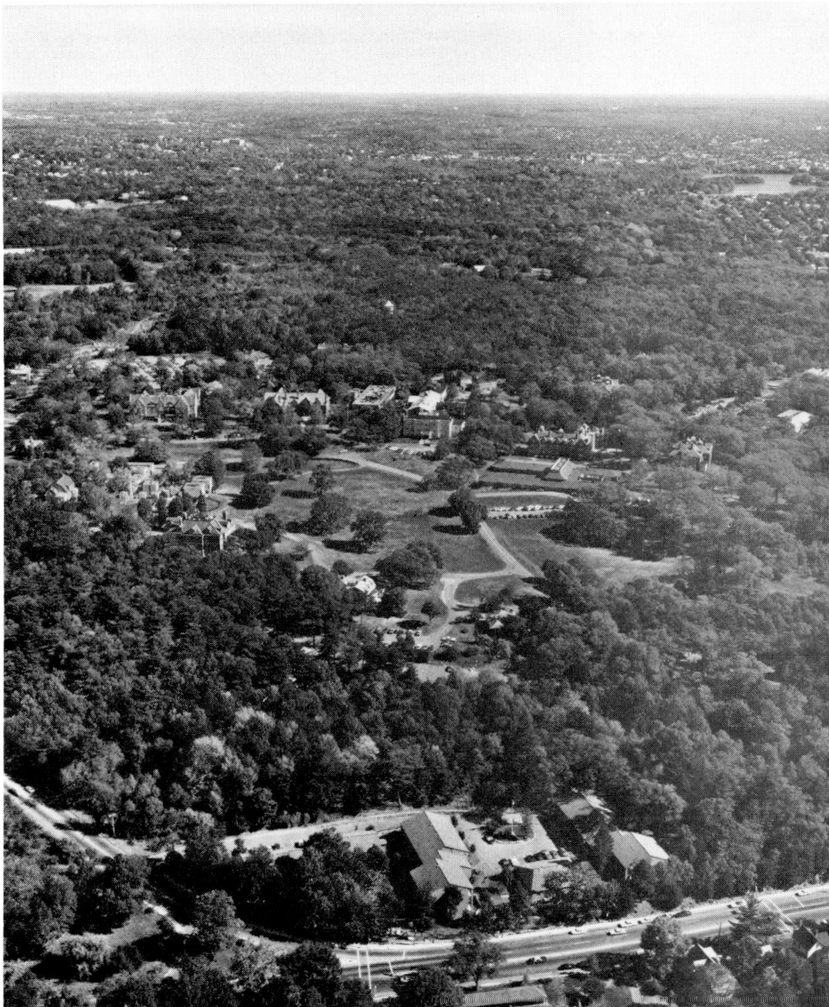
Photo courtesy Aerial Photos International, Inc.

Aerial view of McLean Hospital, 1981.

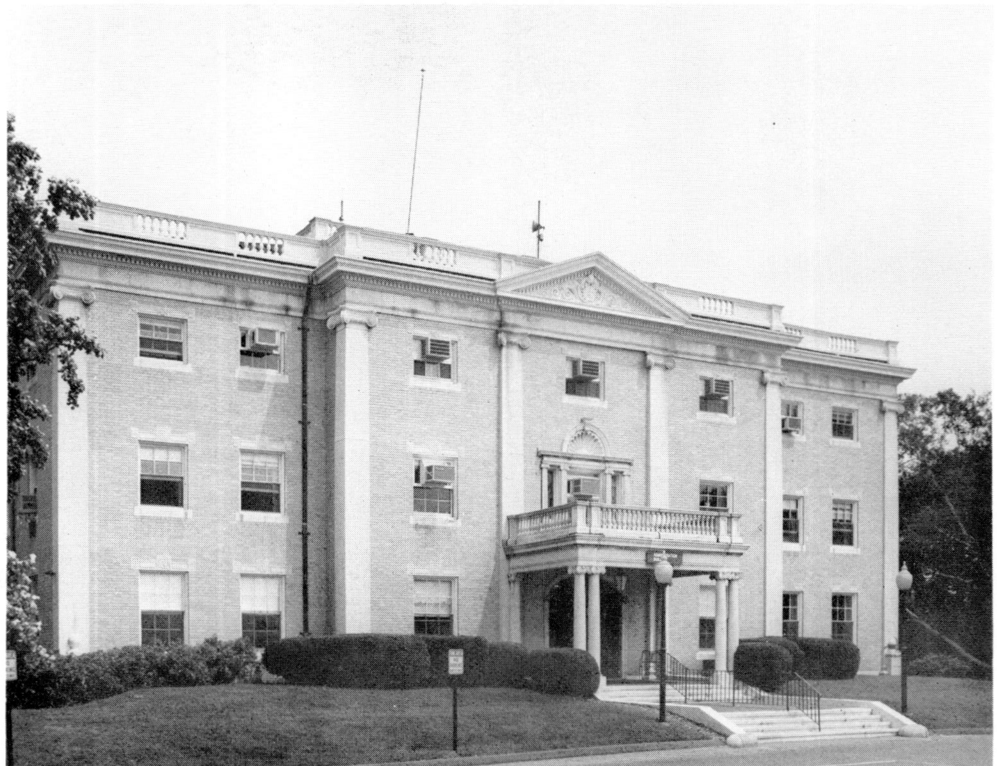

Photo courtesy Chuck Kidd Photography

Administration Building, McLean Hospital.

when Cowles sent him on a trip to Europe; another, as chairman of the AMPA committee on nursing education, with curriculum recommendations; and a few workmanlike research papers. His annual reports reveal the pens of others: The sections on scientific work were set in quotation marks and probably written by the laboratory staff.

After Cowles retired from the Harvard Medical School in 1905, Tuttle was appointed in his place as clinical instructor in psychiatry and conducted rounds at McLean until 1912. But when the Boston Psychopathic Hospital established itself in the medical school's back yard, the scene of clinical education in psychiatry migrated there, leaving Tuttle and McLean estranged from academia. Tuttle was not bitter. He had foreseen the shift all the time he was supporting the creation of the Boston Psychopathic Hospital. Tuttle did not deliver rousing speeches at annual meetings of AMPA or provocative talks at the Boston Society of Neurology and Psychiatry. Perhaps having spent 25 years in Cowles's shadow, he could not quite tolerate the light of day.

Abbot, who had seen the team of Tuttle and Cowles for a decade, observed that "one cannot write of Dr. Tuttle without reference to Dr. Cowles and his work. At the end of their 25 years together the latter wrote with feeling of his own work that through all those years 'Dr. Tuttle has borne a large and worthy share.' Dr. Cowles, with his comprehensive, far-seeing visions, needed the matter-of-fact, practical judgment which Dr. Tuttle contributed. Dr. Cowles had imagination, initiative, energy, ambition; he saw needs and possibilities, not only in the hospital but in the whole field of psychiatry, in a large way. Dr. Tuttle saw what could be done practically, at the time and under the conditions, and how it could be done; he also saw what could not be done, and why." If this is not the stuff one wants engraved on tombstones, Abbot also recalled Tuttle as "uniformly courteous, gentle and gentlemanly. To his patients, especially, this trait, together with his consideration, his sympathetic understanding, his straightforward and utter integrity, his sound judgment, and his quiet ways, gave a feeling of confidence and security that were immeasurable in their distorted world or troubled lives" (15).

Tuttle's modesty of ambition, perhaps a product of his ability to see what could not be done, delighted the trustees. The budget finally began to behave itself during his administration. The horrifying $46,569 of excessive operating costs during Cowles's last year, 1903, plummeted to a mere $7,468 in 1904. A greater turnover in male patients helped on the income side of the ledger, while the cost of supplies was substantially reduced either by efficient management or the trustees' stern orders. Interestingly enough, Tuttle's remark on the financial turnaround carried forth Cowles's banner of scientific research: "The improvement in the financial condition has settled, temporarily at least, the question of a continuance of the work of the laboratory, which has been maintained for so many years at a serious tax on the hospital resources." However, it will be seen that as time went on, such "continuance" became more and more tentative.

The first year of Tuttle's leadership was no fluke, and the budget stabilized despite such extraordinary expenses as a $7,000 war, in 1906, against an infestation of gypsy moths, who avenged themselves by redeploying their forces in greater and more costly numbers in 1907. In 1906 the hospital built a small place of worship, the Samuel Eliot Memorial Chapel, and Codman House, the facility for women patients for which Cowles had argued years earlier. The latter, a red-brick structure more frankly institutional in character than the original McLean architecture, brought the hospital capacity up to 220. Greater capacity increased the income, just as Cowles had predicted. By 1911, when the average daily census equaled the number of beds, receipts finally exceeded operating costs, even though the staff had been augmented to accommodate the larger number of patients.

There was a great deal of fluctuation in the professional ranks during the prewar decade. August Hoch left for the Bloomingdale Hospital in 1905, and the pathologist's post passed to Frederick H. Packard. Shepherd Ivory Franz accepted an offer from Washington to become psychologist at the Government Hospital for the Insane (St. Elizabeth's); when Tuttle asked him to nominate a successor for the psychological laboratory at McLean, he suggested F. Lyman Wells, who arrived in 1907. Wells himself resigned to work in New York in 1910 but came back the next year. Folin went over to Harvard Medical School in 1908, and though he continued to be listed as a consultant, the place of a full-time chemist was open. It went to Charles C. Erdmann, a German who had come to Boston via Canada. He had no advanced training in chemistry and did little more than routine analyses, but he was a genial fellow, well liked by his colleagues. He kept a boat in Boston Harbor and often invited them for a sail. Early in 1914 he went to Germany, joined the German army, and was never heard from again, leaving McLean staff members to imagine, during the war, that he might have been a spy.

With all this coming and going, the presence of E. Stanley Abbot provided some continuity; having come in Cowles's time, he had a longer term than any physician except Tuttle and was a source of spiritual leadership. He and Packard traded places in 1909; Packard became the first assistant physician, and Abbot became the pathologist and effective head of laboratory research. The venerable superintendent of nurses, Lucia Woodward, who had been connected with McLean since 1864, retired from active service in 1912, and was succeeded by Jennie McIntosh. (Woodward left the hospital and shared an apartment with a friend, but advanced age eventually compromised her independence. When she was 84 the trustees invited her to live on the grounds as a guest of McLean. She accepted and passed the last years of her life among old friends. She died in 1934, at the age of 91.)

There was also plenty of turnover within the lower echelons of the medical staff. Earl D. Bond, a fresh Harvard Medical School graduate who had chosen psychiatric training over an internship in general medicine, arrived at McLean as a junior assistant physician in 1908. Within a few months, he had been catapulted to the rank of second assistant physician in charge of male patients, because two junior and the former second assistant physician had all departed. Bond accepted his new duties with great presence of mind, "eager, confident, sure that I was in the right place at the right time." Many years after he had left McLean and become a prominent psychiatrist and educator in Philadelphia, Bond reminisced about his four years at Belmont. His unpublished manuscript paints a picture of an agreeable life. He recalled the quiet, rural atmosphere of the landscape, with its tennis courts and a "rough and ready golf course." At first, when he was still a bachelor, Bond lived in the administration building.

> There were two long tables in the staff dining room which were presided over by the first and second physicians and to which came the psychologist, the superintendent of nurses and her assistant, the dietician and her assistant, the pharmacist, the librarian, the chief clerk, the steward and all the physicians except Dr. Tuttle who had his own house nearby. The two groups were cheerful and friendly, and after dinner on good days were accustomed to adjourn to the front steps to watch the sun go down.

Bond's promotion carried a salary increase, and he married his sweetheart in 1909. That year the trustees acted on Tuttle's urging and acquired a small parcel of land with a wood frame house a few minutes' walk to the buildings for men patients. Bond and his bride moved in.

Bond worked hard. He visited all the male patients, anywhere between 90 and 100 of them, every day. There was no room for psychotherapy in that schedule! On Wednesdays and Saturdays he, Packard, and Tuttle made a grand tour of the hospital, "visiting every patient and having a walking discussion about what should be done in each case." Bond visited Packard's female patients every other Sunday, and when Bond went on vacation Packard returned the obligation in kind. The clinical conferences initiated by Hoch had been institutionalized on a weekly basis, with visiting neurologists frequently in attendance. Tuttle, commenting on the conferences in an annual report, noted that "the cases of disagreement [in diagnosis] show that there are differences in point of view or in fundamental concepts among the members of this staff as well as in the psychiatric world at large, and indicate the great need for further investigations" (16)—an invigorating, if not a comfortable, professional climate. Bond also lectured on the subject of hygiene to first-year students in the Training School for Nurses. As an aspiring academician, he managed to produce two papers on his own and a third in collaboration with Abbot. He did all of this while holding down first base on McLean's baseball team, which was composed principally of male nurses.

Contrary to what one might suppose given McLean's distance

from Boston and the difficulties of transportation, Bond emphasized that he felt neither socially nor intellectually isolated in Belmont. In part because he had studied there, he had easy access to professors at the Harvard Medical School. He regularly attended meetings of the Boston Society of Neurology and Psychiatry, traveling by McLean's horse and carriage, which "took us slowly but comfortably to the Society meetings in Boston at the Boylston Library in Fenway." In 1911 Bond arranged to work in E. E. Southard's laboratory and spent every afternoon there for a month. "I insisted on this," he wrote, "because Southard was the embodiment of the idea of Research for the whole state of Massachusetts" and, by implication, because McLean's own diminished research program did not satisfy Bond's curiosity.

"As I look back upon McLean Hospital after many years and after knowing other hospitals," Bond reflected,

> I see it as a microcosm holding all kinds of psychotic patients in pure culture. They were not contaminated by "wonder drugs," tranquilizers, psychoanalysis and shock treatments. They were in the care of a splendid group of nurses—a rarity then and a rarity now. And they were under the influence of therapeutic forces well described by the founder[s] of the American Psychiatric Association in the eighteen-forties.
>
> The first force was space. Each patient at McLean had a room. There was no overcrowding which makes treatment difficult. The second was classification and the third promotion. Patients deeply depressed or confused or overactive were placed where they could be protected and where they assumed no responsibility. As they improved they were moved up through five wards to the convalescent building with less protection and the assumption of much responsibility for themselves until they (hopefully) were promoted to their homes.
>
> A fourth force was occupation therapy and lectures, recitals, library service, recreation.
>
> A fifth force was the removal of a patient from his home complications—from the place where his unusual conduct created consternation in the people he loved most. In the hospital his unusual behavior was met by understanding and tolerance.
>
> A sixth force would now be called psychotherapy. It was then called "meeting patients as equals and companions," accepting suggestions from them.

Thus did Bond describe moral treatment, vintage 1910.

Bond carried memories of McLean patients with him throughout the remainder of his long, productive life.

> A man with one of the most honored names in Boston was admitted to my service because his family found that he had lost his memory. He had been made guardian for many widows and orphans. It turned out that he had lost all the properties entrusted to him. A reconstruction of events brought out what must have happened. He would open a deposit box, take out the stocks and bonds and stuff them into his pockets and go to his office. There he would find his pockets uncomfortably full and empty them into the waste basket and the maid would put them in the trashcan. At the hospital he could not remember where he was; sometimes he thought he was at home, sometimes in his office, for he did not realize any change in his environment. He died of a large brain hemorrhage in a month.

Bond remembered one woman who suffered general paralysis and believed she had a gold baby, and a paranoid man who thought fire whistles were blown every time he entered a city. "One day I went with him to a baseball game in Boston. As we passed through Cambridge the fire whistles sounded. Neither of us mentioned this fact." A woman who saw him taking notes while she was talking said, "I am supposed to be crazy, but if you think what I say is worth writing down, you are crazier than I am." He never forgot the morning when "a nurse telephoned me to view a miracle. A widow who had been depressed, tormented, moaning for thirteen years had gone to bed as sick as usual and had awakened cheerful, calm and clear." Such are the inexplicable changes that bedevil the lives of psychiatrists.

Bond noticed another phenomenon: during the four years he spent at McLean, not one single properly qualified physician applied for a position on the staff. This fact, he realized, reflected on the lowly status of psychiatry within the hierarchy of medicine rather than on McLean's reputation. It also suggests how much courage and conviction the choice of a career in psychiatry required.

Bond grew restless in his fourth year at McLean. Tuttle's retirement was presumably imminent; he would reach the magic age of 64 in 1914, and Packard appeared destined to succeed him. Though Bond had not objected to working alongside Packard, he did not want to work under him for reasons he was too polite to enumerate. Therefore, when Southard recommended Bond for the position of pathologist at Danvers State Hospital, he accepted. He left McLean in 1912 (17). Tuttle, who did not have to live by the same rules as Cowles, remained in place until 1919.

Bond observed correctly that psychiatric patients, like people in general, are much more interesting as individuals than in groups. Nevertheless, it is instructive to review McLean's statistical data from time to time for an overview of the population. In 1909, five years into Tuttle's administration and during Bond's stretch as second assistant physician, McLean admitted 167 patients: 85 women and 82 men. More than 50 percent of these people came to the hospital voluntarily. One hundred and eleven of them had never been mental patients before. Some 70 percent came from Massachusetts, most often from the greater Boston area. Most had been born in the United States, though there were 10 Canadians, two women who had been born in Ireland, one Austrian, one Italian, one Russian, one Scot, one Spaniard, and one Swede—not exactly a melting pot, but there was at least some diversity. (The State Board of Insanity required statistics concerning the nativity and parentage of mental patients. State mental hospitals had a large foreign-born population, and one school of public opinion used such data to argue for tough immigration policies on the grounds that foreign nations were dumping their madmen and idiots on American shores.)

The list of occupations ranged from manual labor to capitalists, proving that mental illness distributed itself democratically. Among women could be found one bookkeeper, one librarian, one maid, two nurses, three each of stenographers, students, and teachers, 14 without any occupation at all, and 24 housewives—numbers that reflected accurately the positions that middle- and upper-class women held in Boston society shortly before World War I. The men, by contrast, represented 27 job categories, including dentist, carpenter, farmer, florist, laborer, manager, manufacturer, physician, steamship captain, druggist, lawyer, merchant (7), clerk (6), and salesman (5). There were more married than single patients among both men and women, though widows outnumbered widowers by 11 to two. There were no divorced patients.

The two youngest patients, a boy and a girl, were teenagers older than age 15. One new admission was over 80 years old. In between the two extremes, the curve of ages rose more or less regularly, peaked in the 40- to 50-year range, and then declined, resulting in a mean age for all patients of 44.42. Manic-depressive disease was by far the most common diagnosis, accounting for 75 cases admitted, broken down on the charts as manic-depressive depression (49), manic-depressive excitement (22), and manic-depressive mixed phase (4). Depression at this time at McLean was classified as one pole of the bipolar syndrome; no patients were listed under "involution melancholia," for example. A total of 16 patients suffered general paralysis; 17 had either arteriosclerotic dementia or "senile insanity"; eight were thought to have dementia praecox. There were also seven alcoholics, a morphine addict, an epileptic, and a scattering of other patients with individual diagnoses or unknown illnesses.

The statistics relevant to etiology fudged the issue of essential cause by listing "exciting" and "predisposing" causes. Of the 111 patients first admitted to any hospital, 31 had histories indicative of hereditary tendencies toward disease. "Worry" was the chief exciting cause, followed by "unknown," "overwork," and syphilis, in that order. Notes on a case conference concerning a 33-year-old woman illustrate a variety of opinions about the sources of mental illness. In this instance all five physicians agreed on the diagnosis: psychoneurosis. But the consensus dissolved on the subject of cause. Three conferees were impressed by the patient's family history, a ghastly one comprising a mother who had suffered "nervous depression," two insane first cousins, and an alcoholic brother. Another psychiatrist raised the issue of worry. Tuttle summed up his views with "she has been spoiled and it is a matter of inheritance, too much money and nothing to do."

Of 137 individuals discharged from McLean during 1909, 27 were listed as recovered; 22 as "capable of self-support," a new and refreshingly realistic category; 31 as "improved" but, by implication, incapable of self-support; and 25, mostly transfers, as not improved. An additional 32 patients had died, among them 14 victims of general paralysis and two of suicide. A reader of the annual report pondering the fact that the sum total of patients under treatment during the year was 384, of which only 49 (12.7 percent) returned to the world apparently recovered or at least able to resume their ordinary activities, would not have felt much encouraged about the treatment of mental disease. Wyman's and Bell's statistics had been far more promising; Tuttle's, however, were more accurate.

The case records in this period differed from those of the Cowles era principally by the inclusion of detailed histories pieced together by careful interviews with the patient, family, and close friends. The files revealed an intensified probing in an effort to understand what was going on within the patient, both physiologically and psychologically. Proper documentation started with a thorough medical history of the patient and all relevant branches of the family tree. There was a body of social, economic, and psychological data—much of it anecdotal—with emphasis on events immediately preceding the onset of illness. Franz, and later Wells, put some of the patients through batteries of psychological tests, measuring psychomotor activity, fatigue, and intellectual functioning. The 1909 annual report mentions free-association tests, and some records note that the patient had been given the "cowboy" test. This exercise, one of several designed to assess levels of aggression, presented the patient with an imaginary scene of two cowboys facing each other; the patient was asked to demonstrate what he or she thought would most likely happen next by choosing from a selection of pictures showing one cowboy shooting the other, one cowboy punching the other, and both cowboys riding their horses in a race (18). Some records also mention the "gilded boy" test, which I have not been able to identify. (Maybe the latter had something to do with the woman's delusion of a gold baby, mentioned by Bond.) The administration of such tests was entered into the patient's file but usually not the results, because psychological testing was viewed as experimental research without clinical significance. It was also at this time that McLean began to try to follow up discharged patients and record the course of their conditions.

Although conversations between psychiatrist and patient would not be considered psychotherapy—and certainly not psychoanalysis—by later standards, they were often recorded in some detail. The folder assigned to Number 9808, a 36-year-old stenographer admitted in early March 1908 and diagnosed with manic-depressive insanity, mixed phase, carried this entry for March 16:

> When seen this morning the patient was found lying in bed; she appeared very unhappy. When asked why she hadn't slept last night she said, "I couldn't, that's all. I was thinking of staying here forever." (Were you afraid?) "Yes." (Afraid of what?) "Afraid of the people out on the hall—the patients." (Are you worrying about anything?) "Yes." (At this point the patient begins to cry a little) "About staying here." When asked if she didn't feel hopeful of getting well and going home she said, "I won't get well any sooner than the other people around here, and the people here never get well and that's why they're brought here."

Dialogue of this nature had not previously been considered worth putting on record, and the reading of several random cases circa World War I does not reveal any discernible pattern to the conversations in frequency, in whether they got committed to paper, or in the questions posed by the psychiatrists; so it is not clear what significance was attached to them. But they do show that McLean staff members were beginning to take the utterances of patients seriously. Incidentally, Number 9808 gradually improved. By the fall she felt quite contented, and her disposition was noted as "sunny." She went home on Christmas Day, recovered.

Though information about the patients was piling up, the changes in treatment since the Cowles era were imperceptible. There were the three tennis courts and the nine-hole golf course of Bond's fond memories. A set of Swedish Zander machines for mechanotherapy was installed near the baths in the women's gymnasium. The privilege of enjoying works of art was extended to men. The stage in the recreation hall was adapted for amateur theatrical productions. Manual occupations, banished from McLean for almost half a century in deference to the social classes of the patients, were revised with success; men tinkered at woodcarving and cabinetmaking in a well-equipped carpenter's shop, and a handicraft teacher was hired to teach women basket weaving, leather work, lace making, weaving, and pottery. But on any given day no more than one-third of the patients were considered well enough to engage in occupational and recreational activities.

As for McLean's research program, it was on the decline, as

Bond's defection to Southard's laboratory suggested. After Cowles's departure the energy started to drain out of research, and Tuttle lacked the persuasive powers, if not the desire, to prevent the leak. Erdmann, the German who took Folin's place, had none of his predecessor's imagination or talent. When he failed to return from Germany, the trustees did not appoint another biochemist.

The pathologists, Packard and then Abbot, were frankly overwhelmed with routine duties of autopsies and record keeping, leaving little time for original research. Tuttle's repeated supplications for a junior assistant in the pathology lab achieved nothing. Packard did not distinguish himself as a pathologist. Abbot, a talented man, was a fine observer who undertook searches for hereditary data in the case records and wrote some thoughtful papers. But he was spread thin, moving from routine lab work to record keeping to clinical conferences to interviews with patients to lecturing in the nursing school to administrative tasks. He enlisted in the armed services in 1917 and did not return to McLean after the war. The trustees let the pathologist's post remain vacant until 1920. The whittling away at the research program did not please Tuttle. Faithful to Cowles's vision, he ended his annual reports year after year with a plea for a $200,000 endowment to support laboratory work. Nothing came of it. Meanwhile, since the number of patients had increased and the number of assistant physicians had not, staff members hired for laboratory positions were impressed into part-time clinical service. When the war came along and the manpower shortage became severe, research was practically impossible.

The most interesting studies at McLean during Tuttle's tenure issued from the psychology laboratory represented first by Shepherd Ivory Franz and later by F. Lyman Wells. Franz was one of the earliest trained psychologists to conduct his research in a mental hospital laboratory. "There had been some sporadic attempts in this country to take psychology out of the clinics, and to introduce the facts of abnormal psychology to psychologists, but they were abortive, . . ." he later recalled.

> That psychiatry and other medical topics had developed and were being

> thought of anatomically (and only partly physiologically) was almost self-evident, and it was also self-evident that the psychologists of that date had not taken much account of the facts of abnormal states accompanying mental disease. My position was unique. To some, both psychologists and psychiatrists, it was an invitation for attack, and to others a warning to defend themselves. Psychiatrists considered me to be a psychologist, lacking the general medical knowledge and experience for psychiatry. Some psychologists said I was not a psychologist. Obviously, I tended to occupy a "No Man's Land," with whatever advantages that position conferred. (19)

Franz viewed his experience at McLean as a clinical apprenticeship and had a productive three years. He started by honoring his bargain with the departed Cowles and embarked on fatigue studies. Simultaneously he pursued a line of research he had pioneered when he was an assistant in physiology at the Harvard Medical School, the "training-destruction" method of brain research. He conceived the notion that one could train animals to perform particular movements or respond to specific stimuli and then remove selected parts of the brain and test for the presence or absence of the acquired response as a means of disclosing relations between parts of the brain and behavior. At McLean, Franz continued such experiments with laboratory animals and translated insights achieved in the laboratory into work with patients suffering well-defined psychological deficits associated with brain damage, such as stroke victims. His patient work with a man who had lost his speech ability after a stroke resulted in a classic study, "The Reeducation of an Aphasic."

In his last year at McLean, Franz worked with Hoch on analyses of the defects in memory and attention in senile and presenile patients. But Hoch left, and Franz accepted a position in Washington that involved him in the creation of a psychology laboratory at the Government Hospital for the Insane and promised resources well beyond anything McLean was offering. Tuttle somehow managed to convince the trustees that another psychologist should be engaged; they agreed, possibly impressed by what Franz had done. Franz suggested Wells, who had just earned his Ph.D. at Columbia. The conditions of research at McLean were deteriorating, and Wells had a worse time of it than Franz. "About half the time of the head of the department of pathological psychology has been devoted to the clinical examination of cases," Tuttle grumbled in 1909. In fact there was no department of pathological psychology; there was just the overworked Wells.

Unlike Franz, who had been physiologically oriented, Wells was a "brass instrument" psychologist interested in the technology of mental testing and in developing measures of intellectual efficiency. He produced useful criticisms of the psychological instrumentation then in common use, as well as interesting fatigue and free-association studies. Taken as a body, his work aimed at refining methods of psychological observation so as to arrive at a better understanding of the mental equipment that patients in different diagnostic categories brought to bear on their situations.

Though brash enough to have criticized Freud during the Clark conference, Wells did not slam the door of his mind on dynamic psychology. Though some aspects of psychoanalysis did not quite live up to his methodological standards, as the years went by he found himself more and more drawn to Freud's concepts. In 1919 he presented a paper at the American Psychopathological Association in which he explored possible links between experimental psychology and psychoanalytic theory. The influence of Freud shows clearly in this charming paragraph, published in 1913:

> We certainly know that the mental organism is not a close-knit, well-disciplined absolute monarchy, whose every member responds fatally [sic—faithfully?] to direction from the highest levels; rather it is a loosely gathered democracy, often with most liberal notions of State Rights. Seldom, indeed, is it altogether united on single questions of policy. The majority of the *Ichcomplex* may be able to enforce its decrees only with difficulty against a riotous minority; which, if it be a sufficiently well organized complex, may split off and set up a local government of its own; or even seize the reins of the central authority, and carry on according to its own schizophrenic inclinations. (20)

Wells left McLean in 1921 to take charge of the psychological laboratory at Boston Psychopathic Hospital and later to teach at the Harvard Medical School and the Department of Hygiene. He also held prominent offices in professional associations. He lived until 1964 and, near the end of his life, achieved the questionable distinction of being the last person alive immortalized in the by-then famous photograph of the prominent people at the Clark conference.

In 1914 a Medford woman who suffered from manic-depressive illness and who had been a McLean patient in 1903 recognized symptoms of a renewed attack and asked permission to use McLean's hydrotherapy facilities. She came in for baths for several days in hopes of holding back the tide of her rising excitement. Unfortunately she could feel the effort failing, and she committed herself to the hospital. What makes this woman historically remarkable is that she appears to have been McLean's first outpatient, the seed of an idea that did not germinate for several decades. Though sympathetic to the ideal of prevention represented by the mental hygiene movement and Boston Psychopathic Hospital, Tuttle and the trustees held fast to the image of McLean as an institution treating patients who required hospitalization. The concept of outpatients had not existed when McLean was planned, and the design had never been intended to accommodate such traffic. The bringing of not-so-sick patients—the "non-insane," as Southard called them—into proximity with the very sick was considered by professionals to be a bad idea for both groups. McLean could make an exception for the Medford woman precisely because she had been a patient herself and would not be surprised by the behavior of other patients.

The Massachusetts General Hospital, by contrast, was set up for medical outpatients, and in 1912 its General Executive Committee pondered the establishment of a psychiatric clinic along the lines of the Boston Psychopathic Hospital. Southard attended one of these meetings; Tuttle attended another. A consensus emerged that MGH should not operate an outpatient service without being prepared to provide beds for observation or immediate treatment as it did for other clinics in the Out Patient Department. However, the committee made a minimum gesture of recommending the appointment to the Neurological Service of a staff member to examine walk-in patients with mental disease. Upon Putnam's recommendation, MGH acquired psychoanalyst Louville Eugene Emerson, a psychologist whose methods stirred dark suspicions among the resident MGH medical establishment. He was assigned an inconspicuous cubbyhole underneath the stairs of the Bulfinch Building. (Emerson became a nonperson in Washburn's official history of the era. His name appears only on the staff list in the back of the book, even though he was MGH's first psychiatric appointment and the first card-carrying psychoanalyst anywhere in the MGH-McLean system!)

However, mentally disordered people arrived in increasing numbers at the MGH outpatient department, having been misdirected there by various social and charitable agencies, and the issue of establishing a proper psychiatric clinic came up again in 1916. E. Wyllys Taylor, Putnam's successor as head of MGH Neurology and, like Putnam, broad-minded on the subject of psychiatry, apologized that his department was not equipped to handle mental patients. He recommended that the hospital adopt a firm policy of not receiving any psychiatric cases and so notify the agencies. Tuttle, however, countered that he could operate a modest clinic if the trustees would give him an assistant. He described a service geared toward prevention and screening rather than treatment of acute cases; patients requiring hospitalization would not be admitted but sent elsewhere, thus eliminating the need for beds.

Tuttle's proposal seemed financially viable, as well as more humane than slamming the door on deeply distressed, possibly suicidal people ("Sorry, buddy, we don't do that here") and chucking them back into the streets. The General Executive Committee therefore voted to establish a "clinic for mental diseases" independent of MGH Neurology to be managed by McLean physicians. Abbot threw himself into planning the clinic. It operated for some months, but folded in 1917 when both MGH and McLean developed manpower problems because the United States had entered World War I.

The war, of course, put a strain on everybody. At McLean there was a sudden shortage of personnel without any compensating shortage of patients. Half the medical staff—including Abbot and Wells, most of the male nurses, and some of the women—rushed off to enlist. Tuttle fell back on untrained attendants to fill in the gaps. Junior physicians were impossible to find. In 1918 an epidemic of influenza hit hard: The hospital recorded 56 cases, resulting in the deaths of one female patient and one male nurse. But the pragmatic Tuttle carried the hospital through a shorthanded 18 months with minimal interruptions of services to its patients.

The war's effects on American psychiatry spread well beyond some transient inconveniences in the management of mental hospitals. With Europe at war, transatlantic communications were disrupted well before the United States involved itself. The long-standing dialogue between American and German researchers broke down altogether. Having spent a generation building upon foreign models, American psychiatry was forced to look for authority within its own ranks. The near-isolation provided an upward thrust to the rising professional stars of individuals such as Meyer and Southard.

As the United States began to mobilize, the surgeon general's office created a division of neurology and psychiatry and assigned the National Committee for Mental Hygiene the task of organization. Thomas W. Salmon, the committee's director of special studies, hastened to England to evaluate the psychiatric consequences of war within the British armed forces. He returned home with shocking statistics: A psychiatric disability rate of 4 per 1,000 among British troops; 20 percent of British soldiers receiving pensions suffering from war-related neuroses; "shell shock" occurring at epidemic levels. Based on Salmon's report, the surgeon general's office drew up comprehensive plans for screening recruits at induction centers, caring for and/or treating mentally disabled troops in the field, and setting up treatment facilities in the United States for those too ill to return to the trenches. Psychiatrists assigned to field divisions had the unenviable task of

> preserving, or restoring for military duty, as many as possible of the officers and enlisted men who may be brought to their attention.... This is particularly true in the case of the functional nervous disorders loosely grouped under the term 'shell shock' but more properly designated as war neuroses. Psychiatrists detailed to this duty have a unique opportunity of limiting the amount of ineffectiveness from this cause and of returning to the line many men who would become chronic nervous invalids if sent to the base. (21)

World War I was the first time the federal government and

psychiatry were involved with one another on a grand scale, and the profession demonstrated its effectiveness outside the mental hospital. Furthermore, general medicine, which had looked askance at psychiatry for decades, came to regard it with a little more respect. Physicians who had scant experience of mental illness in civilian life saw hysterical, dazed, and disoriented soldiers filing into field hospitals; the physicians' scalpels, medicines, and locker-room speeches accomplished nothing. Psychiatrists, however, sometimes seemed to help these desperate men. Though not entirely persuaded that psychiatry qualified as genuine medicine, physicians and surgeons began to take whatever the psychiatrists did a little more seriously.

Finally, the phenomenon of shell shock and the sad spectacle of homecoming troops suffering severe mental illnesses apparently brought on by war experiences alarmed the public and gave tremendous impetus to the mental hygiene movement. The incidence of war neuroses also added power to the theories of those psychiatrists who believed that psychological insult could cause the brain to malfunction.

CHAPTER

8

Between Wars

The unassuming Tuttle belonged to a different breed of McLean superintendents than those predecessors who had stamped the institution with their identities, who by force of character shaped the place. Think of Wyman, Bell, and Cowles, who together accounted for 76 years of leadership during a century of operation, from 1818 to 1918. So potent were their presences that the history of McLean during their respective tenures must weave in and out of their private lives and concepts. They were superstars! The rest of the cast—the changing assistant physicians, apothecaries, stewards, nurses, attendants—were all bit players. Hoch, perhaps, was the first supporting actor assigned a substantial role. (Just to drive the metaphor into the ground, the trustees were the producers.) This special breed of authority outlived its natural function and, according to some Darwinian law of institutional evolution, passed quietly into extinction. Never in its second century would McLean be so clearly the work of individuals, though one person with imagination and energy could always make a mark on it.

In his last annual report in 1918, Tuttle finally objected to the administrative structure that placed the MGH resident physician over the McLean superintendent with respect to the conduct of business, a condition which had obtained throughout his term in office. Though he had accepted this humbling posture for several years, he did not think his successor ought to submit to it. Meanwhile, the fact that Frederic Washburn, the resident physician, was in Europe commanding U.S. Base Hospital No. 6 rather than in Massachusetts paying weekly visitations to McLean offered a political opportunity for attacking the system of governance without embarrassing an individual. Tuttle complained about crossed signals which generated confusion and ill will among employees who could not be sure where their orders were coming from. There were also, he said, a number of economic inefficiencies. The trustees accepted his argument, returned executive authority to the McLean superintendent, and left the MGH resident physician to mind his own store.

Under these circumstances, McLean leadership passed to Frederick H. Packard, the first assistant physician and, previously, the pathologist. A Harvard Medical School graduate who had also studied at the University of Munich in 1907–08, Packard had been at McLean since 1902; he was 44 years old when he became superintendent in April 1919. Though a lackluster researcher and, in Earl Bond's view, not a particularly inspiring clinician, he demonstrated a flair for administration. He had a clear picture of the institution in his charge and good instincts about which responsibilities could be delegated and which could not.

Packard inherited a pile of administrative problems. Some, like money wasted on food and fuel procurement, went back to the two-headed organizational beast recently slain. Packard, aided by a steward and a purveyor who kept close watch on market conditions, distribution and use within the hospital, storage, and so forth, brought these expenses—which accounted for more than half the operating budget—under control and ended 1919 with a handsome surplus. However, the war had created more stubborn and serious problems for McLean, beginning with a nursing shortage. Everyone had expected this shortage to end when the war was over, but that was not happening. While more than four and a half million able-bodied men served in the armed forces during the war, many women had been hired to take their places in industry. Employers discovered with surprise that women could perform many of the jobs formerly held by men; furthermore, women worked for lower wages than their male counterparts. Even so, those wages compared favorably with nurses' salaries. When the war ended, many employers chose to stick with female labor, and the women stayed. Accordingly, discharged servicemen found a tight job market, and those whose jobs had been held open gratefully slipped back into their old slots. Male nurses returned to the McLean staff, and an unusual number of men applied to the nurses' training school. But many women failed to rejoin the staff, and women's applications to the training program dropped sharply.

Packard derived little comfort from the knowledge that both mental and general hospitals throughout the country, including MGH, confronted the same problem. McLean was committed to quality nursing care. The amateur attendants who filled in for trained nurses represented a throwback to the nineteenth-century asylum era. "No one cares to take up nursing any more," Packard noted in alarm in a letter to his old colleague Abbot; "the patients are mostly cared for by attendants of poor quality" (1). Like other hospital administrators, Packard recognized a need to make nursing more competitive with the other forms of labor that had opened up to women. As an initial gesture, he renewed the plea, advanced first by Cowles and repeated year after year by Tuttle, for a nurses' residence. The trustees submitted to the pressure created by the scarcity and agreed to build. Though precious months were frittered away revising the plans and waiting for a predicted drop in the costs of building material and labor that failed to occur on schedule, Higginson House was completed by May 1924.

Meanwhile, however, to add to the problems, Superintendent of Nurses Jennie McIntosh resigned in 1921, and Packard looked for a replacement. Though he offered a good salary, months passed before any qualified candidate responded to his overture; when one did she was an older woman, "elderly," Packard said, who could not be counted on for long. She was succeeded in 1924 by R. Helen Cleland, who also served a short, four-year term. Nevertheless, during the 1920s the training school curriculum was upgraded to conform to the standards of the Massachusetts Board of Registration of Nurses. These measures, the improved housing conditions, and a gradual return to prewar patterns of domestic and industrial life outside the hospital helped McLean replenish its supply of women students and staff nurses.

The staff over which Packard presided was badly decimated in other areas. There were neither junior assistant physicians nor a pathologist. The inadequacy of medical manpower, coming as it did on top of the nursing shortage, seriously strained the clinical personnel. A number of medical procedures had been integrated into the McLean routine: urinalyses of every newly admitted patient and of others when indicated, blood and Wassermann tests, and intravenous administration of diarsenol to patients who had a positive Wassermann reaction. (Diarsenol was one of the arsenic compounds then being used to treat syphilis. Unfortunately, it was seldom helpful in advanced cases of general paresis.) During most of 1919 all these tests, plus history taking, daily visits to patients, case conferences, nursing school instruction, and numerous other tasks fell to four full-fledged physicians—one of whom was Packard, who concentrated on administration—aided by three fourth-year medical students who could only work full time during the summer months. There was no time for psychotherapy in that schedule. It scarcely had room for perfunctory small talk. The keeping of case records lapsed into disarray. Research, already severely weakened during Tuttle's administration, ground nearly to a halt. Wells was the only staff member who enjoyed that luxury. George Bartlett, the dentist who had been added to the staff, tended strictly to teeth.

Given the rapid developments in the field of psychiatry, this was an intolerable situation for an institution of the caliber of McLean. Packard identified the problems and pursued solutions to them aggressively. His first annual report, though carefully worded so as not to alarm McLean's constituency, depicts an institution on the edge of crisis: It is operating at full capacity, even turning down applications for want of space. Simultaneously, however, it is suffering a nursing shortage which threatens to get worse rather than better, and the medical staff can barely keep abreast of essential services. The acquisition of a new assistant physician by the end of November improves the standards of record keeping, but the psychiatrists are still overloaded. The situation with regard to research is disastrous. Packard writes:

> The traditions of the institution accustom it to leadership in scientific work. For some time past, especially as a result of war conditions with attendant depletion of the scientific staff, this position has not been wholly maintained. The productivity of these departments is lessened at a time when scientific work and spirit are of heightened import and more insistently required by professional and enlightened public judgment. Resumption of scientific work in at least its former scope must be contemplated if the institution is to sustain the prestige won in other years by the extensive contributions of its laboratories to scientific progress. (2)

This little bit of understatement—"not wholly maintained" indeed!—slipped by those readers who did not study the staff list and who did not, therefore, notice that there was no chemist, no pathologist, and no physiologist. But it is interesting to see Packard arguing the case for research and identifying it with institutional reputation.

Packard lived under a dim but lucky star. Ten years earlier Tuttle's urging for more research and a nurses' residence had produced nothing; ten years later the American economy would collapse into the Great Depression. But Packard's administration coincided with a buoyant national economy and rising public expectations, so the trustees responded. That is not to say, however, that the trustees wrote Packard a blank check; while approving the recreation of old, and the creation of new, professional slots, they assigned low salaries to those positions. Most of the problems Packard had in hiring and keeping staff involved dissatisfaction with the rates of pay, and much of his official correspondence recorded his efforts to get better salaries for his people.

In this somewhat ambiguous atmosphere, McLean began the most ambitious program of staff building thus far in its 100-year history. Packard had an easier job plugging the laboratory gaps than beefing up his clinical staff. He immediately appointed James G. Plant as clinical assistant and pathologist. Though he left McLean in 1922 for a job in mental hygiene, the subsequent vacancy in pathology was due to Packard's inability to locate a qualified candidate at the given salary rather than to the trustees' unwillingness to appoint one. Otto Folin, who had been based at Harvard Medical School since 1908, returned full time to McLean in 1920. One of his gifted pupils, John C. Whitehorn, followed in his wake in 1921 and became assistant in pathological chemistry thanks to a fellowship made available by one of the trustees. The legendary Walter B. Cannon, who for years made the study of physiology a rivetting experience for Harvard medical students, went to McLean; Clarence J. Campbell was appointed to assist him. After Wells resigned for a more lucrative position at the Boston Psychopathic Hospital, psychologist Helge Lundholm promptly filled the post in pathological psychology.

Thus by the end of 1921 Packard had gathered the largest research team yet to grace McLean. He was not, however, entirely satisfied because he recognized the frailty of the enterprise. In response to a query from Meyer, who had his own problems trying to solidify research down in Baltimore, Packard observed that

> since my connection with the Hospital . . . , there has never been any definite appropriation set aside for scientific work on the whole. From time to time it has been customary to get permission to spend money for this or that assistant or for this or that laboratory purpose. . . . For some years Dr. Tuttle and myself have tried to stimulate interest in acquiring a fund of two hundred thousand dollars, the income of which should of necessity be devoted to scientific work, so that regardless of the financial condition of the Hospital and the whims of the Trustees, money would be available. So far we have not been very successful, but have a nucleus of fifty-five hundred dollars. (3)

Sarah Matchett's 1904 gift of $5,000 accounted for most of this fund; Packard had raised only $500 more by the time he wrote this letter. His subsequent efforts were not much more fruitful, producing only another $2,500 during the 1920s. Endowed research remained a mirage in the financial desert.

On the clinical side Packard had trouble recruiting and keeping people. "It is practically impossible to obtain physicians," he wrote Abbot in despair (4). McLean paid such poor salaries that student assistants would not stay on as juniors because they got better offers elsewhere. Indeed, the staff situation deteriorated to such an extent that Abbot consented to return to McLean at the end of 1922 and fill in as the temporary first assistant physician. Throughout the Roaring Twenties the clinical staff remained in a state of flux, with physicians arriving and departing like trains at a railroad station. Of the clinical physicians listed in 1922, only one, Kenneth J. Tillotson, was still at McLean in 1930, and he too had nearly slipped away. McLean's archives hold the copy of a letter dated May 11, 1922, from Packard to Earl Bond, who by that time had risen to the post of director of psychiatry at the Pennsylvania Hospital. In it Packard wrote:

> Dr. Tillotson has been at this Hospital since last July. He is a very likable man of a hypo-manic makeup, enthusiastic, and active. He is still young and his judgment is not very mature. [Then, as now, psychiatrists sometimes fell back on their jargon when commenting on colleagues; it is safer to understand these terms as character descriptions than as diagnoses.] I have liked him very much and hoped he would remain longer at the Hospital. The necessity of earning more money than any position which I have to offer him affords has made him feel obliged to look elsewhere. If you are able to obtain his services I feel sure you will like him.

But Packard contrived to keep Tillotson by promoting him from junior to assistant physician and paying him extra for assuming the record-keeping functions of the pathologist who had decamped.

Though there was no continuity of staff to speak of, there was a gradual, steady increase in numbers of physicians who worked at McLean in clinical positions. Whereas the 1922 staff chart showed only four men, in addition to Packard, who spent most of his time grappling with administrative matters, the 1930 roster showed eight, plus two more listed as "research fellows." The names are recorded in annual reports. It is not the intent of this book to itemize the details of the staff traffic, only to remark on its volume.

Packard left office in 1929. He was said to be ill, but the circumstances of his departure are mysterious, especially since he stayed on the books as superintendent emeritus until the end of his life in 1958. Though one inevitably gets curious about such details, they are fugitive, so one gives them up because they do not advance McLean's story. Upon his departure, the trustees designated Tillotson of the "enthusiastic and active" nature as acting medical superintendent. He had risen rapidly through the ranks, his abilities enhanced by the fact that he stayed put while the rest of the ranks kept changing. In 1930 he became the official medical superintendent.

Tillotson was at the time a young whippersnapper of 32, bursting with energy and ideas and interests reaching out into various corners of psychiatry—an "eclectic fellow," said one of his colleagues appreciatively. Tillotson's own words cheerfully confirmed this view. In 1932 he told the Boston Society of Neurology and Psychiatry that "on our hospital staff we have attempted to get personnel with a wide range of experience and diversification of opinion. We have the organicists and the functionalists, biochemists and psychologists, the Kraepelinians and the Freudians, as well as the adherents of Bleuler, Meyer and others. It is necessary that all these opinions should be carefully considered and judiciously applied to meet the individual patient's needs" (5).

"Tilly," as he was known among McLean patients, ran McLean single-handed for a couple of years. But even the ebullient soul has its limits, and the multiplying obligations of administration encroached upon his energies. In 1932 the trustees, who had again been studying the administrative apparatus, came to Tillotson's rescue by moving him sideways into the position of psychiatrist-in-chief in charge of clinical affairs and importing W. Franklin Wood as director with executive responsibilities. Wood came to McLean directly from MGH, where he had been responsible for opening the Baker Memorial, the hospital's new wing for patients of "moderate means" (the affluent and the indigent already being provided for). Prior to that, he had had extensive administrative experience, including some in mental hospitals. The titles at McLean were somewhat misleading in that they did not express the division of responsibilities. "Executive director" and "clinical director" might have described their respective roles more accurately. However, since Wood had power over the budget and direct access to the trustees, had the two men disagreed seriously, Wood's opinion would have outweighed Tillotson's.

Luckily the pair worked compatibly. Wood was a capable manager who ran the hospital business with only one committee to help him. He did all the hiring and firing and ran interference with the trustees as well as professional, state, and local authorities. He signed the paychecks, determined the salaries, and oversaw the running of the farm, powerhouse, garage, grounds, repairs, pharmacy, and nursing school by meeting daily with people from those departments and by virtue of his regulation of the budget, which in turn was controlled by the trustees. He knew most of the patients by name and read the nurses' night reports regularly. Though he left Tillotson to run clinical affairs, Wood paid close attention to the general character of the treatment, watching what was going on in the psychiatric and nursing services and holding daily conferences regarding patients and what difficulties there might be. Wood, his family, and their Dalmatians occupied the superintendent's residence on the grounds.

Wood and Tillotson, the latter happier in this secondary, clinically directed role, piloted McLean through the Depression and World War II. During the period between wars under discussion in this chapter, the Depression might seem to have been a particularly troublesome time for the institution, but in fact it was not all that bad. The patient census remained high. In 1932 the hospital responded to economic conditions by reducing salaries instead of laying off staff, and in 1934 the weekly rates charged to patients were lowered for the first and only time in McLean's history. There were small budget deficits in 1933 and 1934. However, some of the staffing problems that had nagged Packard during the 1920s solved themselves during the Depression. The rate of turnover among nurses declined almost to zero. As national unemployment figures careened upwards, people with jobs held on to them and accepted cuts in pay philosophically, comforted by the lower price levels that to some extent compensated for lost wages. The professional staff also became more stable and even continued its modest growth.

Packard, an able enough executive, cannot be said to have enriched the field of psychiatry. It is not clear what theories of mental illness he subscribed to. On occasion he expressed strong sentiments on the subject of mental deficits and heredity:

> The persistence of a nation or race depends mostly on the preservation of the mentality of the race and the disintegration of past civilizations has been due to the increase of mental defectives. There are indications that

> our own civilization, like those of the past, will go to pieces unless something is done to maintain the mental efficiency of the people and to curtail the propagation of the mentally defective. (6)

Though he used the term "mentally defective" rather than "insane" or "ill," one would like to know where he drew the line. A letter advising a former patient, who had been discharged two or three years earlier and maintained mental health ever since, that there was no reason why he should not marry proves that Packard observed distinctions. It is likely that very few of McLean's patients would have fit his definition of "defective." Nevertheless, his statement put him perilously close to the views of eugenicists, who had successfully championed the passage of sterilization bills in several state legislatures. Under these laws, between 1907 and 1940 more than 18,000 patients in state mental hospitals were surgically sterilized, over half of them in California. Massachusetts never legalized the procedure.

Packard's eugenicist leanings are relevant only as they permit insight into theories of the time and, to a lesser extent, into the man's thinking. (His convictions about the collapse of former civilizations are not easily supported by historical evidence.) In practice these ideas did not affect the way McLean was operated. Packard did not impose them on the staff and, on the whole, left clinical matters in the hands of senior assistant physicians while allowing laboratory researchers to pursue their own inclinations. Whitehorn, for example, who quickly demonstrated himself a worthy successor to Folin in biochemistry, prized the freedom he found at McLean and realized that very few institutions would have permitted him to do whatever he wanted. Packard respected his work and the clinicians valued his participation in staff conferences. When Whitehorn announced he had received another invitation, Packard negotiated housing and an increase in salary for him. Whitehorn stayed at McLean until 1938.

Without any strong navigational directives from on high, clinical practice at McLean followed the course of mainstream institutional psychiatry a length or two behind the avant-garde. There was a strong undercurrent of the ordinary common sense that had long been part of the institutional tradition. When, for instance, clinical conferences got bogged down in nosological dispute, Packard was apt to recite stories about bright young psychiatrists he had come across in other places trying to apply Kraepelin diagnoses out of the book with the startling results that their dementia praecox patients very often got well. There was room within this pragmatic approach for the concepts of psychoanalysis which insinuated themselves principally via new staff members who had been excited by Freud's theories. Psychoanalysis made its first official appearance in the 1924 annual report, where Packard sketched McLean's clinical policies:

> In the treatment of mental and nervous cases those things which tend to put the patient in the best possible physical condition continue to be of prime importance. Psychoanalytic and psychotherapeutic measures have their places and are important. The administration of drugs or medicines for specific mental treatment is at the present time disappointing and plays a small part.

In 1925 Packard reported that "a special attempt has been made to make use of psychoanalytic and psychotherapeutic measures as far as applicable and practical in each individual case." He stated in 1928 that "a special attempt has been made to find out what, if anything, in the Freudian methods is practical of application in the psychoses."

The last item coincided with the addition of psychologist George E. Gardner to the McLean staff. Gardner had come at the invitation of Lundholm, whom he met during his second year of graduate work at Harvard. Lundholm, apparently laying the groundwork for his own departure, was impressed by Gardner's grasp of psychological testing methods and thought his talents would serve McLean well. But Gardner had other things on his mind. "I went to McLean," he recalled,

> and at that time there were two physicians on the male side, two physicians on the female side, a pathologist, Dr. Whitehorn, and a superintendent whom we never saw, luckily. By this time, I had become thoroughly convinced that the Freudian theory was the only concept that could be applied to the psychoses, as I saw them, and to the neuroses, as I knew them from a distance. Being a frustrated teacher, I began to give seminars at McLean to the staff and what were called residents. These were held in the evening and I can still remember making large charts of the Freudian structures.
>
> I didn't meet with much success and enthusiasm. Most people were organically oriented and wished to remain that way, with the exception

> of John Whitehorn. I did earn a new name, however. I was immediately dubbed "Sigmund." (7)

Gardner did not feel beleaguered for long. Ives Hendrick, a psychoanalytically minded psychiatrist, came on staff as "assistant physician and psychoanalyst" in 1930 and began his own research into the applications of psychoanalysis among McLean's patients. M. Ralph Kaufman came the next year to serve as clinical director during 1931 and 1932. His influence shows up in the 1931 annual report, where it is written that

> during the past year, we have been reorganizing with the idea of improving our clinical approach to the patients. The attitude that is being stressed most at the present time is that of a therapeutic approach. This involves a thorough knowledge of the patient's early development, personality and character trends. Emphasis is being placed upon the family interrelationship.... To carry further our own psychotherapeutic approach, emphasis has been placed upon the personal relationship between the patient and the physician. An endeavor is made to see the patient as often as possible for an intensive discussion of the patient's problems.

Although the administrative restructuring that made Wood executive director and Tillotson psychiatrist-in-chief ended Kaufman's career as clinical director, he returned to the hospital again in the late 1930s as a research fellow studying suicide.

In 1934 it was noted that three patients had been treated by "orthodox" psychoanalysis. By 1938 McLean listed Hewitt Varney, Paul Howard, Elvin Semrad, and Eleanor Pavenstedt as staff members who, if not analysts, were practicing dynamic psychotherapy. Tillotson, whose approach was more or less in Meyer's psychobiological tradition, had by that time been through a brief period of analytic training in Europe.

Howard, who had been attracted to McLean by having observed Whitehorn on rounds at MGH, joined the staff in 1938. He remarked that although the actual practice of "orthodox" psychoanalysis had been limited to a very few patients, the analytic movement acted as a positive, humanizing force.

> The dynamic approach in psychotherapy made the patient seem more meaningfully alive. In many conferences, observation, diagnosis, and prognosis were still machine-like, and deteriorated patients looked like cases of irreversible brain disease. It was most discouraging to work with

> them, except where there was an occasional spontaneous recovery. Once the analysts brought in a dynamic developmental psychology and pathology, the hospital staff could feel that they were dealing with people who were still human. (8)

In tandem with the evolution toward dynamic psychotherapy, there occurred an apparent change in the makeup of McLean's patient population. According to the published statistics, in 1930 all but one of the first admissions were suffering from psychoses; the exception was a problem drinker whose mental functions were not so severely deteriorated as to qualify him as psychotic. But seven years later, Tillotson reported that 52, or nearly 20 percent of all patients admitted, were "not insane" and furthermore that "a careful review of the diagnoses reveals that approximately fifty percent of the patients admitted during the past year were non-psychotic or suffering from some form of neurosis or psychoneurosis." He explained this phenomenon in the context of

> an important trend in medicine as well as in psychiatry. This gives evidence of a desire on the part of patients who are in need of psychiatric care and hospitalization to seek such medical or psychiatric attention early and under conditions best suited to give them such treatment uninhibited by traditional prejudice and the erroneous impressions that a hospital giving care and treatment to the major psychoses or mentally ill patients can not give proper care and treatment as well as afford suitable accommodations for the non-psychotic or sane patients. Furthermore, it tends to disprove the idea that McLean Hospital is adapted only to the needs of the major psychotic patient. (9)

Tillotson's words invite closer inspection because "neuroses" was a new word in the McLean diagnostic lexicon. Psychoses were gross impairments of the processes of memory, thought, language, perception, and orientation, of known organic origin (such as in general paresis or stroke) or unknown etiology (such as schizophrenia); neuroses covered all other kinds of mental disturbances. Psychoses corresponded approximately to the legal conception of insanity. People afflicted by neuroses were, as Tillotson observed, sane. Since the difference between the psychotic and the neurotic was principally one of degree of disturbance, psychiatrists pronounced judgment based on symptomatic evidence that could not be measured objectively. Though some cases were clearly one or the other, there was a great mushy area in the middle, and one psychiatrist's psychotic might be another's neurotic.

To those who held with Freud that the neuroses could be treated by standard psychoanalysis but the psychoses could not, the distinction was not trivial. The greater the psychiatrist's faith in the healing powers of psychotherapy, the more inclined he or she was to arrive at a diagnosis of neurotic in a marginal situation. It is extremely likely that many of the patients classified as neurotic in 1937 would have been admitted to McLean as psychotics in 1927 and that the statistics said more about changing psychiatric concepts than they did about significant alterations in the patient population. Though McLean had a country-club reputation—due in part to its gracious external appearance and in part to the jolly section of the annual reports wherein were catalogued upper-class recreational opportunities—the patient were not self-indulgent, affluent suburbanites who checked in to talk about themselves and play a few rounds of golf.

The 1937 annual report did not carry the usual statistical tables. But the 1939 statistics listing the diagnoses of first admissions during the year supports the speculation that old afflictions had been shifted to new categories and were being thought about in new ways. Under "psycho-neuroses" one finds "manic type," "depressive type," and "mixed type," the manic-depressive diseases of yesteryear, as well as something called "reactive depression," which earlier in the century would have been classified as "manic-depression, depressed type" and earlier still would have been simply "melancholia."

Well-worn habits of thought die hard, however. A 51-year-old woman, admitted to McLean during the summer of 1938 having become progressively indecisive, agitated, irritable, and depressed since the suicide of her husband, believed herself responsible for the death or disgrace of her family; she thought she would never get well and should be put out of the way. She had no previous history of mental illness. She was classified as manic-depressive, depressed and agitated type, and considered psychotic in one research study. Moreover, the same 1939 annual report that lists manic-depressive disorders as psychoneuroses in one place shows them as psychoses in another. Fortunately for the patients, given the level of attention at McLean and the desire of the staff to help anyone whose behavior hinted that she or he might respond to any form of therapy—psycho, hydro, occupational, or otherwise—the fine points of taxonomy made no more difference to the patients during the 1930s than they had at the turn of the century.

Memories of patients and staff help reconstruct life within the hospital during the Depression years. One patient, Frank W. Kimball, wrote a small, quiet article on his experiences of more than a decade at McLean. His account was published, but the excerpts which follow are taken from the original manuscript, now in the McLean archives, because they are more spontaneous than the edited version and because they mention specific members of the McLean staff by name. Kimball, suffering from what he chose to call a "tired mind," came to McLean in December 1931 from the Channing Sanitarium in Wellesley, Massachusetts, where he had been a patient since July 1927. His record at Channing showed him to be

> retarded in speech and motion. Shaky. Self-accusatory. Afraid of arrest for imagined misuse of family funds. Suspicious of nurses, believing them to be spies. (I myself recall often shushing visitors in my room for fear of the nurse outside the door, who I thought was there to snoop.) I thought I was going to be hauled to court in New Bedford—why New Bedford, I can't imagine now!—on a charge of rendering a false income tax statement. Complained of food tasting queer. Thin (got down to 115 lbs. . . . normal 135). Thought my firm had failed, and that the family property was involved.

Though Kimball made some gains at Channing, his wife thought the richer therapeutic opportunities—occupational recreational, hydro—at McLean would speed his recovery and had him transferred to Belmont. "In my new surroundings I remained indifferent and unresponsive—slow to enter into the various activities provided," Kimball wrote.

> Gym work was an awful bore. I must have sorely tried Mac's [Angus J. MacDonald, instructor in physical training] patience with my less than half-hearted daily dozens, my dull efforts at hand-ball, table-tennis, bowling, badminton, etc., etc. The weekly movies in the entertainment hall made little appeal. Guess I was never known to admit that I enjoyed them, or those outside I went to occasionally. The automobile rides I

> could not enjoy, either. Always as we returned I would see from afar that hated yellow brick Administration building on the hill looming up as the symbol of my hopeless captivity and utter isolation.
>
> By this time I had settled well down into my "mute" status. My "good mornings" and other greetings were only perfunctory responses to the approaches of others. And I can't recall cracking a smile the whole long, long time I was a patient in either hospital.
>
> This life of semi-automatic activity, in a chronic mood of indifference, and blue fog of futility, continued from 1931, outwardly varied, as it had been in Channing, by excursions to the outside world. . . .
>
> All through my illness I had done more or less in the way of occupational therapy—woodcraft, leather work, cane and reed-weaving. Doubtless this kept alive my bent in these directions, and I found a growing liking for such handicraft. This reached a stage in McLean when I was really turning out a good deal of work; caning chairs, building garden chairs, making towel racks. . . . Mr. [Daniel] Joy, the [director of occupational therapy] at McLean, and I got along well. His patience, skill, and understanding did more for me than I realized. Dan [was] a philosopher, too, and I know I must have absorbed much good sound psychical nourishment along with a certain skill. . . .
>
> Lest it seem strange that I could do all this, . . . yet still be unfit to leave the hospital, let me explain. My demeanor was spiritless, and my conversation and social qualities minus quantities. After all, I was only partly alive—surely in no shape to return to normal living.

Mr. Kimball will continue his story later on in this chapter. At the moment, however, his description of his stay at McLean invites some comment. One notes first that his narrative is peopled by occupational therapists, physiotherapists, librarians, and nurses, not by psychiatrists. Doctors make their appearances only at some moment of critical decision; they dart weightlessly in and out of Kimball's frame of reference, but they do not anchor his time at McLean. It is the others with whom Kimball passes the long hours of his confinement who provide the ballast of continuity, human contact, and encouragement. Every employee who saw patients regularly automatically became a potential therapist.

Many patients remembered Harry Oteri, who spent 50 years as McLean's barber and became a friend to countless men whom he shaved and groomed with a soft touch while responding to their conversation with well-sharpened human skills. Kimball's perception of the relative significance of individuals in his care corresponded to the distribution of personnel in the hospital. Not surprisingly, then, he never mentions either Tillotson or

Wood, having seen little of the former and nearly nothing of the latter. He writes of "*the* doctors" but "*my* nurse."

One observes further how persistently the therapists worked with Kimball, forcing his reluctant, diminished hulk into activity. Left to himself, he would have vegetated in his room, mind and body wasting for want of exercise. Paul Howard recalled one of the more severe forms of intervention that Kimball apparently did not experience at McLean (though in view of his weight loss, may have at Channing): "A small but persistent feature of nursing and medical care until the biological treatments came in was the fact that about 4% of the patients refused to eat and had to be tube fed. The resident on twice daily rounds would tube feed about six women and one man. . . . after the preparation of the feeding by and with the assistance of the nursing staff." The formula for regular "meals" resembled a rich nonalcoholic eggnog; this was supplemented once a day with eight ounces of orange juice laced with two teaspoons of cod liver oil. "Tube feeding was a slightly dramatic but routine procedure and not very uncomfortable as expertly practiced. Without it the people refusing food would have starved" (10).

Kimball's first-person account pricks the "country club" balloon. Readers interested in a more genuine country club environment might enjoy comparing his descriptions of McLean with some accounts published in the April 1935 edition of *Fortune* magazine. Here one finds Craig House in New York State, a private, luxurious, and expensive establishment catering to mildly depressed patients: "You get plenty of personal service. There are several employees to every patient—almost a hundred nurses, a score of men working on the grounds, six doctors, dozens of cooks, waitresses, chauffeurs, etc. Each of the fifty odd patients has his own nurse, who eats with him at a table for two, who plays golf or pool or cards with him, who takes him to the movies in Beacon or driving in one of the eight Cadillac limousines maintained for the patients. Shopping trips into New York, fifty miles down the river, are frequent." Or, in Massachusetts, there was Austen Riggs at Stockbridge, "more like an extremely pleasant country club" than a sanitarium, which treated "the milder types of neurotics who wander freely about the town and form the chief support of the local golf and tennis club. . . . The average stay there is four to six weeks, but so enjoyable is the life there that three out of every four patients return for short visits every six months or so for several years after their discharge." McLean's pastoral landscape, golf course, and tennis courts might have fooled the *Fortune* reporter for a while, but if he did his research properly and spent some time on the wards, he would have soon discovered that McLean was no country club.

"Patients and their families were personally treated," Howard remembered,

> especially by the nursing service. They did not have the freedoms of the present patients since the hospital had to exert a greater degree of protection than later became necessary. For one thing, lacking more modern treatments for depression and other disturbances, patients needed more cautionary care against suicide and violent behavior. Freedom of the grounds and to visit was not often thought wise. The presence of staff constituted the principal form of care. Physical restraint and seclusion were used as little as possible, although necessarily more than later; and chemical restraint or sedation was used rarely—not massively as in some hospitals. (11)

Howard's recollections of McLean in the late 1930s include a curious piece of information: Male nurses and attendants served on the men's wards, female nurses and attendants on the women's (shades of the asylum in Somerville). There had been reason to suppose that Cowles had ended segregation of the sexes, at least with respect to employing female nurses on men's wards, some chapters ago and that such Puritan practices belonged to the past. This obviously was not the case, though I was not able to discover when or why McLean regressed to the old ways. (Speculation: Perhaps this was a by-product of the shortage of female nurses after World War I.)

So strict were the rules of segregation, Howard recalled, that once when a male patient collapsed outside the gymnasium and a female nurse happened to be nearby, she made no move toward the patient but stood by while a male nurse was fetched to attend to him. The separation of patients according to sex was also more rigid than it had during most of Cowles's tenure; men and women met only weekly at chapel and monthly at dances. A remark in the 1936 annual report to the effect that two halls for convalescent and mildly ill patients were being left unlocked during the day makes a similarly curious impression upon those who recall Cowles's open-door policy amidst the railroad yards in Somerville.

Doctors, like nurses, patients, and therapists, were assigned either to the men's or the women's wards. Patients were assigned to a specific physician upon admission, and the physician visited all his (or, occasionally, her) patients on ward rounds twice a day, during daytime hours and at night. Thus, a resident psychiatrist might be responsible for 25 or 30 patients at a time and become acquainted with others on the wards during rounds and in clinical conferences. Wood seldom made rounds; Tillotson showed up irregularly. The staff psychiatrists apportioned their time with patients according to their educated hunches about who might benefit from some form of psychotherapy. In practice, that meant 5 or 10 minutes a day with some patients, up to a half an hour with others, for there was no rule that psychiatrists must distribute their minutes equally. Kaufman and Hendrick singled out a few patients for psychoanalytic treatment. Recently admitted patients with acute illnesses were more likely to receive substantial psychotherapeutic attention than the presumed chronic or demented for whom there was scant hope of improvement.

Whitehorn, though based in the laboratory, could nevertheless often be found on the wards where the patients nicknamed him "Dr. Mosquito" because he went around drawing blood. But Whitehorn was an exquisitely sensitive man, not some automaton wielding a hypodermic needle, and he talked with the people he pricked. Early in his McLean career, he undertook biochemical studies of schizophrenic patients. Quite apart from his laboratory findings, he discovered that many of these patients apparently benefited from his attention, and he evolved an effective technique of engaging and drawing out these most inaccessible of mental patients. "Schizophrenic patients, as I see them," he wrote, "have a special position in regard to the power and influence of other persons. They are sensitive, resentful, baffled, boxed-in or withdrawn from ordinary participation in life. They respond to prescriptive pressures by further withdrawal and resentment; they respond to mere permissiveness by inertia, that is, by not having any response" (12). Whitehorn found that schizophrenics often responded to active, friendly, and firm problem-solving methods based on the physician's understanding of their individual strengths and weaknesses, as well as of how they viewed their respective situations. He similarly noticed that certain types of people had negative effects on schizophrenic patients. One of his McLean colleagues, a brisk character, actually alarmed them, and Whitehorn commented that he could always tell which patients were schizophrenic by observing who shrank when Dr. ____ passed through the wards.

Whitehorn's career in psychiatry resembled August Hoch's in its gravitation from the laboratory to the clinic. Initially surprised when his colleagues called his conversations with patients "psychotherapy," Whitehorn spent more and more time on the wards as time passed, though he never gave up his laboratory work entirely. During 1937 he could be found delivering one course of lectures at MGH not, as one might have expected, on biochemistry, but on psychotherapeutic management; another course at Simmons College School of Social Work on the "Elements of Human Nature"; and a third on the same subject to graduate students at Radcliffe College. Thus, the director of laboratories came to be the most powerful model for young clinicians on the McLean staff during the 1920s and 1930s. His rare combination of courtesy, intelligence, and insight made a profound impression, particularly on Paul Howard and Elvin Semrad.

Howard volunteered a list of McLean psychiatrists from the 1930s who later moved out of McLean and on to prominent performances elsewhere, beginning with Whitehorn, who eventually inherited Adolf Meyer's positions at Johns Hopkins and Phipps, and became president of the American Psychiatric Association. Hendrick and Kaufman both acquired national reputations as psychoanalysts. Semrad became director of psychotherapy at the Massachusetts Mental Health Center, the new name for Southard's old Boston Psychopathic Hospital. David Young became a hospital superintendent in North Carolina, as well as the state's chief mental health official. A parallel list could be drawn from the nursing staff. "I mention the later careers of some of these people," Howard explained, "to show that the clinical staff was one of ability and that they worked hard according to the information of the times." Unfortunately, however, despite all the improvements in the quality of encounter between doctor and patient, despite all the hours in the laboratory or in psychological testing, rapid effective treatment for serious mental illness remained maddeningly evasive.

Along with his duties at McLean, Tillotson played an important role in reactivating the psychiatric clinic at MGH. As mentioned in the last chapter, the hospital's earlier effort to provide services for mentally disturbed patients had withered during the personnel shortage of World War I. The clinic had reopened in 1919, but the General Executive Committee and the trustees judged the circumstances unsatisfactory and quickly closed it again. Psychiatric patients who presented themselves in the Out Patient Department during the 1920s were directed to the Neurology Department, which, lacking appropriate staff or facilities to care for them, usually referred them to other institutions. However, since there was no neon sign outside MGH to advertise the fact that it did not treat mental illness, psychiatric patients kept arriving. Moreover, some of the medical and surgical staff had become alert to psychiatric problems among patients on their own wards. By the end of the 1920s, the subject of psychiatry was back on the MGH agenda.

When Tillotson became McLean superintendent in 1930, he was simultaneously appointed to MGH as "psychiatrist at the general hospital," under the aegis of the Neurology Department. Charged with reviving the old Psychiatric Clinic, he updated some of the concepts and, in accordance with the timely buzzwords, called it the Mental Hygiene Clinic. The development of the MGH clinic explains the otherwise mysterious appearance of psychiatric social workers on the McLean staff roster. Their efforts were, in fact, concentrated in Boston, and though Tillotson claimed they were "devoting much time in a very helpful manner to the problems in connections with patients at McLean," they vanished as unexpectedly as they appeared.

The Mental Hygiene Clinic was staffed with McLean psychiatrists and psychiatrically interested MGH neurologists, including Emerson, the psychologist-psychoanalyst who was listed on the MGH staff until his death in 1939. Within a year, the clinic had more patients than had been anticipated, and sessions scheduled for the morning usually spilled over into the afternoon hours. MGH still had no beds for psychiatric patients, but plans were quietly afoot for developing inpatient capabilities.

The impulse to develop a full-scale psychiatric service got two big shots in the arm in 1933. First, the trustees hired Nathaniel W. Faxon to succeed Washburn as director; Faxon came from the Strong Memorial Hospital in Rochester, New York, which had its own rudimentary psychiatric service, and he ardently supported the program at MGH. Second, and more powerfully, the medical sciences division of the Rockefeller Foundation under Alan Gregg gave the Harvard Medical School (along with a few others) a grant to upgrade psychiatric education with the objective of bringing psychiatry closer to medicine. Since McLean, Boston Psychopathic Hospital, or any other hospital devoted solely to mental illness represented a century of institutional isolation from mainstream medicine, MGH, one of Harvard's principal teaching hospitals, became the clinical beneficiary of the Rockefeller money.

In what proved to be an inspired administrative decision, Stanley Cobb, who was the Bullard professor of neuropathology at Harvard and chief of the Neurology Service at Boston City Hospital, was selected to head the new Psychiatric Service at MGH. Though Tillotson retained a title of psychiatrist there, from that time forward the history of the MGH service belongs to Cobb and his successors (and the psychiatric social workers dropped off the McLean roll). However, given the corporate relationship between McLean and MGH, the development of a distinct psychiatric element in Boston precipitated some fallout in Belmont.

The effects were largely positive as long as Cobb ran the MGH service. He built a strong department, put psychiatry on the map, and was influential within MGH. His biographer, Benjamin V. White, noted that Cobb was particularly good in establishing the importance of liaison psychiatry in the minds of key members of the medical staff. White quoted one of Cobb's colleagues, Derek Denny-Brown, who remarked that "Stanley had to use very simple language. He couldn't talk to Howard Means, Walter Bauer, or Oliver Cope [important MGH doctors] about libido, id, or pre-oedipal situations. Instead he had to point out the effect of 'worry' in aggravating arthritis or peptic ulcer" (13).

Gradually, through Cobb's efforts, psychiatry gained some legitimacy at MGH, though to this day there remain physicians and surgeons there and elsewhere who treat psychiatry as an illegitimate offspring of medicine. But to the extent that the MGH Psychiatric Service improved the image of psychiatry, McLean profited.

On a practical level, McLean and the MGH Psychiatric Service enjoyed a close cooperative relationship. Tillotson, Whitehorn, and others were involved in clinical and teaching aspects of the MGH service. David Young of McLean consulted with the MGH Gastrointestinal Clinic because Chester Jones, chief of the Gastrointestinal Service, was much interested in the psychological components of gastrointestinal illness. McLean's psychiatric residents assisted in the clinic. Exposure to different kinds of mental patients than those usually admitted to McLean, to a general medical setting, and to the provocative questions and insights of doctors in other specialties, as well as students, expanded the experiential world of McLean psychiatrists.

The flow of traffic moved in both directions. People like Cobb, neurologist James B. Ayer, and neurosurgeon William Jason Mixter joined McLean's consulting staff and increased the stock of resources that could be brought to bear on McLean's patients. Furthermore, Cobb and his program attracted students and staff. Both Paul Howard and Francis de Marneffe, who later figured prominently in McLean's history, served as assistant residents on Cobb's service, the former in 1936 and the latter in 1952; a number of people from Cobb's staff at one time or another formed some connection with McLean. Eventually, this invigorating spirit of cross-fertilization would erode, but during the 1930s and 1940s it had a wholesome influence on McLean's development.

The author—apparently Dwight MacDonald, though there is no byline—of the 1935 *Fortune* article on "nervous breakdowns" and mental hospitals cited earlier in this chapter explored a half dozen institutions, talked with numerous psychiatrists, and arrived at this conclusion:

> The modern mental hospital treats the patient usually with kindness, sometimes with intelligence. It gives him chairs to cane (occupational therapy), it squirts water at him to tone up his system (hydrotherapy), it listens sympathetically to his troubles and tries to advise him (psychotherapy), it stimulates him to swing Indian clubs (physiotherapy). All this is very nice and usually very helpful, but when the impressive Greek names are stripped away, the whole trick boils down to very little. About all the sanitarium can do is to create around the patient an artificial environment that will be congenial enough for him to make a satisfactory adjustment to it. Once the strain of maladjustment is relieved, his neurosis or psychosis has a better chance of curing itself. Creating such a favoring atmosphere is a matter of human insight rather than medical skill. Pleasant chintz curtains may be more effective than all the Greek therapies put together.

The writer further correctly identified the roots of this form of treatment in Pinel and Tuke. Though this description trivialized what went on in mental hospitals such as McLean, where patients were gravely ill and medical intervention was often essential to manage the somatic disorders that accompanied mental disease, and oversimplified concepts of dynamic psychotherapy, it was nevertheless essentially correct. For all the years of experience, the mountains of information, the research, and the learned discourse, the standard therapy was still moral treatment, a mere stone's throw beyond Rufus Wyman's practice in the early nineteenth century. Perhaps this blunt reality revealed less about a supposed "failure" of psychiatric medicine to come up with cures for mental diseases than it did about the solidity of the humane premises of moral treatment.

Nineteen thirty-seven, the 119th year that McLean had been receiving patients and the sixth year of patient Frank Kimball's residence, may also be said to have been the last year during which moral treatment was the exclusive therapy at McLean. Kimball dated the beginning of his long climb out of depression from that year, pinning it on his involvement in a new activity: "I had been reading pretty steadily from the first: newspapers, magazines, a random selection of books. In 1937 Miss Reed, the new librarian, started the Hospital bi-monthly magazine, the *McLean Gazette*. Somehow she got the idea that I could write something for the book column of the magazine, and the book (of all books) she picked out for me was by no means light reading. It was *Middletown in Transition.*" (Kimball's three-sentence review of this classic study is a lesson in succinctness and ought to be required reading for contributors to the *New York Review of Books.*) Thus began Kimball's career as McLean's book reviewer and his excruciatingly slow return to health.

Though inventive in the elaboration of moral treatment, as Kimball's story indicates, and liberal in attitudes towards dynamic psychotherapy, McLean was constitutionally wary of medical remedies for illnesses that manifested themselves psychologically. Ever since Rufus Wyman denounced bleeding and purging, the institution held back from treating psychological symptoms of doubtful origin by biological intervention. McLean was accordingly conservative in the prescription of sedatives, about which little was known except that they got results, which were widely used in state hospitals. McLean favored becalming excited patients by packing them in wet sheets or putting them in continuous baths, more expensive, labor-intensive options from a managerial perspective; but sedatives made the patients groggy and unresponsive to psychotherapy and the other activities designed to engage and exercise their attention.

This cautious approach to biological remedies, which was generally shared by other hospitals of McLean's class and character, was grounded in the humane traditions upon which the institution was founded. The ability to act on those convictions—to treat severely ill, sometimes dangerous, patients with gentleness—was a luxury. State hospitals, understaffed and under financial pressures from their legislatures, depend on sedatives and restraints to control excited patients; some resorted to desperate therapies. But McLean patients were spared the indignities and physical pain of such off-the-wall treatments as the wholesale extraction of teeth, tonsils, appendices, and lower intestines, or the irrigation of sinuses and intestinal tracts according to a focal infection theory of mental illness that enjoyed popularity during the 1920s. Nor were McLean's schizophrenics or syphilitics given malaria, typhoid, or rat bite injections so as to induce fevers.

Thus, when reports on insulin and Metrazol "shock" began turning up in the professional literature in the early 1930s, McLean's psychiatrists followed them closely but apprehensively. Insulin treatment had developed from a serendipitous observation by a Viennese physician, Manfred Sakel, in the latter 1920s. He noticed psychological changes in diabetic drug addicts whom he had been treating with insulin; an overdose of insulin producing a hypoglycemic coma seemed to alleviate the addict's withdrawal psychoses. Sakel conceived the notion of using insulin to produce comas in psychotic patients, particularly schizophrenics. He refined his procedures between 1933 and 1935 and reported encouraging results. Insulin therapy was introduced into the United States in 1936 at the Worcester State Hospital. Inflated claims concerning its effectiveness proliferated and seeped into the lay press, raising hopes that a cure for schizophrenia had been discovered. Metrazol shock treatment, by contrast, was based on Hungarian Ladislas von Meduna's fallacious theory that epilepsy and schizophrenia were biologically antagonistic diseases and, therefore, could not coexist. von Meduna extended this logic and proposed treating schizophrenia by inducing epileptic-like fits by injecting pentylenetetrazole, a powerful camphor-like drug capable of producing convulsions and more commonly known by its trade name, Metrazol. Like insulin therapy, Metrazol quickly gained enthusiastic support among institutional psychiatrists frustrated by a backlog of chronically ill patients.

That was not true, however, at McLean, where the custom of wariness prevailed. In the 1937 annual report Tillotson wrote:

> One could not properly conclude a report on the clinical and research work of a modern psychiatric hospital without some comment on the Insulin Shock or Hypoglycemic Shock treatment of the psychoses, especially in the schizophrenias. This treatment has been carefully studied by the writer and its application closely followed both in this country and abroad from its early inception. Until recently it has not seemed sufficiently well established to justify its use as a valid therapeutic method. Owing to the demand for its use by professional colleagues as well as by the relatives of patients, we are contemplating its application in a few selected cases.

Tillotson's statement implied that McLean must bend with public opinion in order to guard its reputation as a "modern" hospital, but he certainly did not sound happy with the necessity.

> The use of "metrazol" in the treatment of the schizophrenias, [he continued] appears to the writer to be in about the same scientific category

> as the Insulin Therapy. That remissions have been obtained in psychotic patients by the applications of both forms of therapy seems definitely established, but the statements that patients suffering from the various forms of schizophrenia have been permanently cured by these methods seems [sic] untenable.

The pressure to try the new methods did not relent, and McLean bowed to it. In 1938, Sakel, on tour of the United States to demonstrate the techniques of both therapies, personally supervised the treatment of a few chronic schizophrenics at McLean. The long-term results, as Tillotson had thought, were disappointing. However, some of the short-term changes were so impressive as to compel the staff to revise some of their thinking about schizophrenia: "The fact that following Insulin and Metrazol shock treatments the patients showed some marked improvements in their social behavior and in their ability to respond to their environment suggested to some of us some changes in our concepts of the deterioration in the 43% of chronic schizophrenics who remain on for continued care in mental hospitals . . ." (14). The response to Metrazol and insulin seemed to demonstrate that the concept of deterioration, with its implication of irreversibility, was a false one and that the mental status of chronic schizophrenics might, in fact, be improved.

McLean acted immediately on this revised view and began to work intensively with its chronic schizophrenics by submitting them to an activation-motivation treatment regimen called "total push" which had been developed by psychiatrist Abraham Myerson of the Harvard and Tufts medical schools. Myerson joined the consulting staff at McLean and helped Tillotson organize the program which began in November 1938 with a group of 11 patients. They responded so well that another 21 patients were put into the program before the end of the year. "This therapy," Tillotson explained,

> is based on the principles of activating, retraining, and re-educating the inactive, apathetic, dilapidated and deteriorated patients by an active push program of physiotherapy, exercise, games, and occupational and diversional therapy. Ultraviolet, vitamins and special diets are essential. . . . We have found it possible to restore a large percentage to a better social status from whence a program of re-education and psychotherapy

> can be instituted. Already this promises to produce in the chronic schizophrenic patients some degree of social recovery. (15)

By the end of 1939, 67 McLean patients, about half of them chronic schizophrenics and another half who had been hospitalized two years or less, had been propelled through total push, and only five of them were judged to have shown no improvement whatsoever. Those few selected for Metrazol or insulin therapy were also followed up with total push. "Perhaps part of the ineffectiveness of the administration of insulin and metrazol has arisen from the inability to follow up the results with an active program designed to reintegrate the patient gradually, when the patient has reached a point at which reintegration is possible," Tillotson hypothesized (16).

Though pleased with what the program seemed to be accomplishing, its proponents were nevertheless cautious in their appraisal. "It is not . . . assumed, claimed or believed that this is a cure for schizophrenia," Myerson wrote,

> the contrary being the assumption made. The experiment thus far shows, however, (1) that the deterioration of the chronic schizophrenic, by which we mean individuals who have been mentally sick in hospitals anywhere from 6 to 20 years, who have never shown any tendency to remission or improvement, who have gradually taken on the aspect of what is called deterioration, is not altogether a natural or an entirely necessary product of the disease; (2) that it can be wiped off at least in part by effort and the patients restored to a more human and active appearance. What the future will show for this method as to its relationship to cure is for the future to determine. (17)

Total push produced sociological changes at McLean. It activated the nursing staff by diverting a good deal of their energies away from passive observation of the symptoms of mental illness or writing thank-you notes for patients and towards encouragement of healthier pursuits. It also provided a new rationale for occupational and recreational therapy.

Overall, insulin and Metrazol shock therapy accomplished more for McLean's schizophrenic patients by stimulating total push than they did by producing comas and convulsions. Though few of the chronic patients achieved a condition of health that suited them for discharge into a complicated, unstructured, uncaring world, for some life within the hospital, along with contacts with family or friends, improved substantially. The principles, if not the practice, of total push remained integral to McLean philosophy long after its somewhat intimidating name had fallen by the wayside. Meanwhile, the use of insulin and Metrazol shock subsided. Both procedures were to some degree dangerous, and Metrazol in particular had extremely unpleasant side effects. Searching for a safer alternative method of altering the internal environment, McLean tried hypothermia, a bone-chilling procedure in which the sedated and anesthetized patient was placed between blankets through which a refrigerant at a temperature of 32° F or less was circulating. In this manner the body temperature was lowered by 10 to 20° F. By 1940, however, hypothermia, along with insulin, yielded to yet another new procedure called electroconvulsive shock therapy, or ECT.

The notion that electric shock might benefit mental patients went back at least to the eighteenth century, when Benjamin Franklin and a Viennese court physician, Jan Ingenhousz, urged such treatments for the epileptic and insane (18). It was introduced in the twentieth century by two Italian physicians in 1937 as an alternative to Metrazol, over which it soon demonstrated considerable advantages including diminished risk of injury. Note, however, that the danger of fractures resulting from the violent muscle contractions during convulsions was a very real one during the early years of ECT, before muscle relaxants and anesthesia were integrated into the treatment.

ECT, like Metrazol and insulin, was originally intended for the treatment of schizophrenia and, like the drugs, produced equivocal results. It achieved some brief remissions, was helpful in calming excited episodes of illness, but resulted in no long-term recoveries. However, it was soon demonstrated to be effective in some cases of severe depression. Which brings us back to patient Frank Kimball, in 1942 still plugging away at his book reviews for the *McLean Gazette,* feeling a little more interested in life, but still unfit for the world. Even though he was over 70, the doctors decided he was a candidate for ECT.

> This was begun in late 1942, the course of treatment extending over nearly three months, with intervals of discontinuance. I don't recall the

> start of this at all, in fact my memory is quite blurred except for a dim recollection of trips in bathrobe and pajamas by wheelchair to the treatment room, where in the presence of my nurse, the chief psychiatrist, and the physician in the control room, the treatment took place. There was no discomfort, except for slight nausea at the first. I would get the very mild shock about 10:30 a.m., be carried back to my room, and the first thing I knew I was waking up in bed around noon, feeling very much refreshed.

By mid-February 1943, Kimball acted on a doctor's suggestion, went over to the administration building, and placed a telephone call to his wife in Dedham—the first time he had called home since 1927. His wife was so astonished that she did not recognize his voice. Kimball was discharged in March after a total of 15 years in mental hospitals. He returned to his home and to vigorous life as a trustee of Boston University and a mental health activist.

Despite such spectacular outcomes, ECT entailed risks and produced some undesirable side effects, such as the memory lapses Kimball mentioned (but which were explained to him and did not bother him at all), and the indications for its use were not clearcut. Moreover, while ECT obviously did work in some instances, no one understood why. So McLean was characteristically cautious about prescribing it—on occasion a bit too cautious. Howard remembered a physician suffering from depression who committed himself to McLean for treatment. The psychiatrists, always particularly conservative with patients who were doctors, decided against ECT for him. After months of psychotherapy, the patient, who had heard about ECT, took himself off to another hospital, received shock treatments, and was back in his office a few weeks later.

A more aggressive form of biological intervention was introduced in 1939 when Mixter, the MGH neurosurgeon who consulted at McLean, performed prefrontal lobotomies on two patients "suffering chronic and prolonged psychoses, characterized by agitated types of depression and diagnosed as involutional melancholia" (19). The procedure, pioneered in 1935 by the Portuguese neurologist Egas Moniz, consisted of a relatively simple surgical technique, severing of connecting fibers in the prefrontal areas from the rest of the brain. Moniz's patients were psychotic patients whose patterns of violent behavior appeared greatly reduced after surgery. American psychiatry imported the procedure and extended its application to other forms of mental disorders manifest, for example, in anxiety or insomnia. Though there were some comments about loss of "sparkle" and "spontaneity," lobotomy was widely reported to achieve immediate symptomatic relief. Tillotson wrote that both McLean patients had "made remarkable recoveries from their psychotic symptoms."

Cutting into the brain, no matter how routine the mechanics of the procedure, is under any circumstances a radical, irreversible form of treatment. It was not undertaken lightly at McLean, and some staff members did not like it. Others, however, recommended it for certain desperate patients, suffering chronic and progressive illnesses that had not responded to any other therapy. Sometimes, though indeed relieved of agonizing psychoses and able to return home, the lobotomized patient seemed to have lost his or her soul as well—that sparkle mentioned by others.

Insulin, Metrazol, ECT, and psychosurgery, all introduced to McLean in the two years between 1938 and 1940, were drastic biological treatments marking the first genuine departure from the psychological therapies based on moral treatment. They announced a new era in psychiatry. They were crude therapies, often unpleasant and frightening for patients; yet, since they held some hope for recovery, they were less unpleasant and frightening than the diseases from which those patients suffered.

Many of the horror stories the public eventually heard about ECT and lobotomy came out of institutions where such therapies were wantonly prescribed and inexpertly administered. McLean patients had the advantages of excellent, ample medical, psychiatric, and nursing staff and a foundation of psychological therapies. Some patients benefited from the new procedures. ECT, the most demonstrably beneficial and widely used of the treatments, shortened the course of many severe depressions, like Kimball's, and patients who might have wasted years in the hospital, possibly the balance of a lifetime, were discharged within months. For some others, though remaining institutionalized, the days held fewer demons.

CHAPTER

9

Dog Days

Once McLean has been placed under the historical microscope, the researcher tends to get absorbed in its small world: the fates of patients, the frustrations of psychiatrists, administrative tangles, and the inevitable politics of institutional existence. But McLean, like any other hospital, exists only in the context of a universe which touches it here and there along its edges and sometimes changes the shape of events within. So from time to time the historian must raise her head from the microscopic lens, adjust her vision, and look beyond the rolling landscape, the golf course, the stone chapel, and the other amenities that made McLean soothing to the eye.

The world into which patient Frank Kimball had been discharged in 1942 was gripped in battle, a war that exceeded World War I in geographic dimensions and human atrocities if not in numbers of military casualties. The supply of superlatives available for describing the horrors of World War II was exhausted long ago, and though there is evidence that a younger generation of Americans understands them only dimly, it is not the purpose of this book to describe them. (The Polish Nobel Prize–winning poet Czeslaw Milosz, on tour of the United States in 1985, discovered to his astonishment that some college students in his audiences thought World War II had been a nineteenth-century event.)

Around 1938 a few politically alert psychiatrists foresaw the entrance of the United States into the war and tried to set up contingency plans. Their efforts failed, and the country proved woefully unprepared for the psychiatric necessities of wartime. Such lessons, both negative and positive, as might have been learned from World War I seem to have melted from the collective memory. The federal government had spent nearly a billion dollars between 1923 and 1940 for the care, treatment, and housing of psychiatrically disabled World War I veterans, and three out of every five beds in veterans' hospitals were occupied by mental patients. Yet preparations of psychiatric services on the eve of World War II were hodgepodge at best. In 1940, for example, the Army had only 25 medical officers assigned to psychiatry. An epidemic of historical amnesia swept over the bureaucrats and institutions that ought to have been dealing with the psychiatric aspects of military service.

The American Psychiatric Association (APA) was as much to blame for this dismal state of affairs as any other group. As Albert Deutsch wrote in 1944:

> It must be said, in truth, that the steps taken by the Association to give leadership and direction to the psychiatric aspects of military mobilization were at first marked by hesitation and uncertainty of purpose. While other professional bodies quickly and firmly assumed leadership in their special fields in the national war program, the American Psychiatric Association seemed content to offer its services to the appropriate authorities and patiently await to be called. It displayed a remarkable tolerance toward inaction, unconscionable delay, and occasional fumbling on the part of the officials responsible for utilizing pyschiatric skills and procedures. (1)

One problem was a severe shortage of psychiatrically trained physicians. At the time of Pearl Harbor, there were fewer than 3,500 psychiatrists in the United States. A substantial number of them were unavailable for the military effort because they were needed to staff state institutions, veterans' hospitals, psychopathic clinics, and other facilities. Thus, the first task of military psychiatry—namely, the selection of mentally fit draftees—often fell to doctors who had little or no psychiatric background.

According to the guidelines during the early draft period, physicians had between two and three minutes to do a psychiatric evaluation—a safety net so poorly woven that a whale could have slipped through the screening process. By the time more thorough testing procedures were put in place, much of the damage had already been done: Thousands of young men psychologically ill suited for combat duty had already been drafted. Many of them became psychiatric casualties. This time around the prevailing form of mental illness was called "combat fatigue" instead of "shell shock."

If the story of the 6th General Hospital, organized by MGH, as chronicled in Nathaniel Faxon's volume of *History of the Massachusetts General Hospital* is any indication, general medicine did not do much for the psychiatric cause. Having heard about Freud, physicians and surgeons were suspicious of psychiatrists, perhaps even more so than they had been during World War I. So, when Faxon retells the formation of the 6th General Hospital, he does not record the name of a single psychiatrist. Yet he mentions, with a strange mixture of surprise and boredom, that at its first location in Casablanca, more than 22 percent of the patients admitted to the military hospital were neuropsychiatric casualties, contrasted with only 16 percent who had been wounded in battle (2). Nevertheless, the heroics belong to the surgeons who excised shrapnel and the physicians who rescued victims of epidemic diseases. Psychiatrists and psychiatric nurses are invisible in his history.

By late 1943, the psychiatric services to the military improved. Selection processes became more sophisticated, mental hygiene programs helped prepare recruits for combat stress, and field hospitals were set up for better psychiatric management than they had been during the earlier phases of the war. Meanwhile, experiences in the field gave psychiatrists an opportunity to validate long-held hypotheses concerning the relationships between psychological stress and physiological disease. For instance, the incidence of peptic ulcers among soldiers, a much higher rate than occurred in the civilian population, confirmed the psychological components of that condition and advanced the concepts of psychosomatic medicine. The Navy, which had a more enlightened attitude towards psychiatry than other branches of the armed services, used psychiatrists to review court martial proceedings and help distinguish psychologically damaged individuals from ordinary troublemakers.

Though it is true that the profession dragged its feet at the beginning of the war, it is surely the nature of modern war to inflict psychological damage, and one may well wonder just who *is* mentally fit for combat duty. One should not be astonished that an average man—a carpenter, bank clerk, or lawyer who negotiates daily life with reasonable skill and feels happy or despondent according to his fights with his girlfriend, sense of financial security, or satisfaction on the job—could pass a well-constructed psychiatric evaluation test and still go to pieces after spending weeks on some godforsaken island in the Pacific, with bombs exploding all around him and watching his buddies die. One is more surprised by the men and women who came through such experiences psychologically intact than by those who sustained deep wounds. Some of those wounds healed over well; others didn't. About one-third of all wounded were estimated to be psychiatric casualties, and mental patients clogged the wards of veterans' hospitals for years to come.

World War II, like World War I, threw a new generation of problems in the field of psychiatry into bold relief. It was with the war still in progress, in May 1944, that the American Psychiatric Association convened to celebrate the 100th anniversary of its founding. Perhaps feeling frustrated by the difficulties of the past few years, or perhaps acting on an impulse to revive a tradition set back in 1894 when they invited neurologist S. Weir Mitchell to give them a tongue lashing, the Centenary Committee called on Alan Gregg, director for the medical sciences of the Rockefeller Foundation, as their keynote speaker. (The chairman of that committee, incidentally, was McLean's old friend, Earl Bond.)

Gregg responded graciously. He did not flog his audience quite as mercilessly as Mitchell had 50 years earlier, and he showed more sensitivity to the peculiar difficulties of the psychiatric profession. "No other speciality of medicine has had a history so strange, nor a relation to human thought so intimate as psychiatry," he observed. "The three most powerful traditions or historical heritages of psychiatry are still, as they have been from time immemorial, the horror which mental disease inspires, the power and subtlety with which psychiatric symptoms influence human relations, and the tendency of man to think of spirit as not only separable but already separate from body. These are the inherent, the inveterate, the inevitable handicaps of psychiatry."

Gregg proceeded into his diagnosis of current professional ailments. "My own formulations of your major limitations would be this: you are badly recruited, you are isolated from medicine, you are over-burdened, and you are too inarticulate and long-suffering to secure redress from the public of some of the handicaps from which you and your patients suffer." He criticized both the quantity and quality of medical students who entered psychiatry, singling out only Karl Menninger for devoting time and energy in recruiting better candidates by actively courting students. (This remark slighted Stanley Cobb, who had done an able job of recruiting, aided by funds from the Rockefeller Foundation. Perhaps because Cobb lacked the promotional instincts of Menninger, he slipped easily out of mind.)

When Gregg got to the subject of the isolation of psychiatry from medicine, his criticism became quite harsh. "Most psychiatrists are so ill-trained in medicine that they cannot command the respect which would welcome them as collaborators on the wards of the general hospital. The young men entering the state hospital services in all but a very few instances are assigned to work on their wards on the assumption that, though untrained and unsupervised, they will be competent. Such a procedure would disgrace even a very quiet surgical service." Gregg further criticized the profession's ignorance of other disciplines pertinent to its efforts, such as psychology, cultural anthropology, metaphysics, genetics, and even the history of knowledge. Above all, he emphasized the necessity for an infusion of the exact sciences into the ranks of psychiatry to conduct investigations of those phenomena which could be measured, quantified, and fractionated and perhaps could yield clues to the etiology of mental illness (3).

Comparing Mitchell's 1894 text with that of Gregg in 1944 reveals differences in tone and delivery, but not much in substance. Except for the development of psychoanalytic theory and various forms of dynamic psychotherapy, to which Gregg gave due credit, one has the feeling that psychiatry had been standing in place, shifting uneasily from one foot (biological) to the other (psychological) for 50 years. Back in the nineteenth century, Mitchell's address had caused a lot of dissatisfied grumbling in the audience. When Gregg ended his speech, the room erupted with applause.

World War II was more devastating to McLean than its predecessor because there was more to be devastated in 1942 than there had been in 1917. Within months after Pearl Harbor, nursing and other personnel shortages became so acute that Director Wood shut down three private cottages and two small wards. The average daily census, which had stood at 209 in 1941, dropped to 199 in 1942 and to 181 in 1944, when Proctor House for men had to be closed. The admissions rate declined in tandem with the census. Even so, McLean had to lower its standards and hire untrained attendants on the wards. If the nursing shortage can be said to have had a positive side, it was that women were assigned to the men's wards for the first time in many years because male nurses were even harder to come by than female nurses. Thus did global warfare force the reintegration of the sexes upon the administration of a mental hospital in Belmont, Massachusetts, as farfetched a connection between cause and effect as one is likely to stumble upon. Meanwhile, McLean had to sell its cows because of the shortage of farm labor. "A sad affair," Wood remarked, lamenting the loss of a cherished tradition as well as an excellent supply of dairy products.

The most obvious casualty of the war was total push, which had been a labor-intensive program. Deprived of the full complement of experienced nurses, therapists, and psychiatrists, the experiment withered on the vine, and chronic schizophrenic patients retreated into their private fantasies. McLean's clinical program, which under Tillotson's direction had been seeking balances between psychological and physiological therapies, shifted strongly to somatic treatments which made lesser demands on professional time. ECT, a 5- to 10-minute procedure, became the treatment of choice for patients diagnosed as suffering from depressive illness, altogether 74 in 1944. Insulin, abandoned in 1941 in favor of ECT, was reintroduced in 1944 and administered in doses which did not induce coma but nevertheless seemed to benefit the patient.

Lobotomies were resorted to with somewhat more frequency. There were nine during 1944, all on patients said to have suffered schizophrenia for at least 10 years. A few of these patients were considered to have improved, and it was thought that a couple might be able to leave the hospital. Nothing, however, was said about what constituted "improvement" or what degree of independence the discharged individuals might be able to enjoy in the noninstitutional world. Howard noted that of the 80 or so lobotomies he knew about at McLean, none of the patients got worse. He estimated that about one-third remained the same, one-third improved but required continued hospitalization, and one-third were discharged "socially recovered."

A skeleton staff of well-intentioned, overworked, underpaid psychiatrists doled out such parcels of psychotherapeutic time as they could, but a lot of the ground that had been gained during the 1930s was washing away beneath their feet. Since it was wartime, administration and staff bore the reduced circumstances stoically on the assumption that they were temporary, and the cows would come home again after the war.

Right in the middle of this clinical nosedive, McLean suddenly acquired a talented neurochemist and began building a new biochemical research laboratory. It was a strange gift—a little like getting a dining room table when one has asked for a bed. Just how and why this research endeavor came to pass is difficult to pin down with historical precision because so many of the facts are fugitive, but a general picture emerges from bits and pieces of evidence.

The first event of consequence was the election in 1940 of Ralph Lowell to the Board of Trustees and his assignment to the McLean Committee. A member of boards all over town, Lowell took an immediate—and, as it turned out, abiding—interest in McLean. As he surveyed the place, he decided that the trustees ought to be doing more for it, and he evidently converted Francis C. Gray, chairman of the McLean Committee, to this opinion. It is probable that Cecil K. Drinker, former dean of the Harvard School of Public Health and professor of physiology at the Medical School, introduced Lowell and Gray to the notion that the something that ought to be done for McLean was a basic research component.

Lowell's sense that the trustees were neglecting McLean was supported by the historical record. During the nineteenth century and up through the move from Somerville to Belmont, the board had distributed its attention and favors more or less evenly between its two charges, McLean and Massachusetts General Hospital. But ever since the day they voted for the mandatory retirement of Edward Cowles, the trustees had been treating McLean like a troublesome stepchild; though individual trustees, usually the chairman of the McLean Committee, acted as advocates for McLean, the board as a whole tended to view it as an irksome budgetary item.

We have seen how during Tuttle's administration the trustees transferred executive power to the director of the general hospital and how they permitted the incipient research program to die of financial malnutrition. We have seen Packard begging better salaries for his staff and trying vainly to liberate McLean research from the "whims of the Trustees" by creating a separate endowment. We have seen Tillotson gently nudged aside so that Wood could be brought over from Fruit Street and installed in the director's office in Belmont. Though Wood was signing the checks, the limits of his power over the purse strings are suggested in a testy note he enclosed with a check set over to the treasurer's office. "Dear Mr. Weld:" it read. "A little manna from Heaven. This does go into the Director's Fund. It is mine to use as I ______ please. At the rate things are going it looks as though I will have to use it to help make up the deficit" (4).

Maybe it was natural that McLean should have slipped in the affections of the trustees during the twentieth century. Once the institution moved out to Belmont, it remained approximately the same size and, like the rest of psychiatry, could not claim any breakthroughs in the treatment of mental illness. Meanwhile, the general hospital expanded steadily, and the quality of medicine practiced therein made it one of two or three of the most prestigious hospitals in the country. The general hospital made much larger financial demands in part because during the twentieth century the cutting edge of medicine advanced with speed and required increasingly elaborate instrumentation and skilled personnel.

The MGH budget ran anywhere between four and five times that of McLean's; its deficits also exceeded McLean's many times over. It was, however, comparatively well endowed. As for the cutting edge of psychiatry, it was an inappropriate metaphor. Psychiatry moved amoeba-like, advancing a pseudopod here, retracting one there, and offering few clues to the general direction of its motion. Accordingly, the trustees' investment in MGH exceeded their interest in McLean. The human factor no doubt also played a role in their attitude. As Gregg had pointed out in his address to APA in 1944, mentally ill patients tended to arouse fear or horror more readily than sympathy in their beholders. There is no reason why trustees should have been exempt from this instinctive reaction. Overall, one gets the impression that they found McLean financially annoying and medically depressing, but morally and humanly necessary.

While there can be little doubt that the trustees concerned themselves seriously with the comfort and safety of McLean's patients, the manner in which they disbursed funds kept research and clinical programs at a bare minimum. Whether or not Lowell understood this background when he joined the board, he apparently recognized certain inequalities of treatment, as well as slippage in McLean's reputation, and committed himself to doing something for MGH's country cousin.

The second piece of the jigsaw puzzle that became the McLean research laboratories was the resignation in 1943 of biochemist Elmer Stotz, the man who had replaced Whitehorn in 1938. When Stotz, a good research scientist, defected to Cornell, the trustees faced the problem of whether to leave the biochemist's post vacant—an option they might have gotten away with under wartime conditions—or to search for a new person. By this time the seed of the research laboratory idea had been planted, and they deployed Drinker as a research consultant to assist in the selection of a new biochemist. Drinker, who had a strong emotional attachment to McLean, assembled an advisory committee consisting of Wood and Tillotson from McLean, Stanley Cobb, James Howard Means (the enlightened chief of medicine at MGH), A. Baird Hastings, Folin's successor as professor of biological chemistry at the Harvard Medical School, and Donald van Slyke of the Rockefeller Institute.

A third piece of the puzzle can be found in the cluster of scientific activities within the Harvard community that had direct or indirect bearing upon psychiatry. Harvard's broad umbrella covered a lot of territory, including the teaching hospitals, the School of Public Health, and various university departments, along with the Medical School. Among others under that umbrella were several people studying the epilepsies; Erich Lindemann and his sociological and crisis intervention studies; Myerson exploring the potentials of certain drugs, total push, and electroshock; psychologist H. A. Murray and his group working on experimental validation of Freudian hypotheses; Tillotson investigating aspects of metabolism as well as ECT results; and Cecil Drinker examining the physiology of psychoses. Stotz had represented biochemistry in this constellation of activities, and his absence was felt beyond McLean's borders, for that left no one involved in basic research in brain chemistry.

All of the pieces in the puzzle came together: an opening at McLean, a gap in the Harvard programs, the impulse of the trustees to do something for McLean, and a recognition within Drinker's committee that precious little basic research in neurochemistry was going on anywhere in the country and that to set up a program would put feathers in Harvard's and McLean's respective caps. The choice of a man to develop the program fell upon Jordi Folch-Pi. Though neither the first nor the last scientist to be interviewed for the position, he had the strong support of both van Slyke and Hastings. Folch, who was described by a former colleague as a "fiery Catalan," had come to the United States on a fellowship to the Rockefeller Institute in the 1930s and could not get back to Spain because of the civil war. At the Rockefeller Institute, Folch had worked under van Slyke's wing and become involved in the isolation and classification of blood lipids.* As this work proceeded, Folch began to concentrate his attention on brain lipids. Since lipids constitute about 60 percent

*Lipids are a complex group of organic substances, including fatty acids, neutral fats, waxes, steroids, and phosphatides, distinguished by being insoluble in water but soluble in alcohol, ether, and other fat solvents. Lipids are important constituents of cells as well as sources of body fuel.

of dry brain weight, his research tangent appealed to Drinker's committee.

Folch's work was indeed basic research by the most stringent contemporary standards. In an era when basic research was not established, or the need for it not taken for granted, setting up Folch and his team out at McLean was a bold concept, one that might not pay off. Folch's studies did not depend on mental hospital patients for research materials; they might have been conducted in any properly outfitted laboratory. The committee's plan, however, was to use basic research, which they fully understood as a long-term effort, as a nucleus for attracting researchers and spinning off other programs to link with clinical areas.

In the annual report for 1944, the trustees announced plans for the construction of a Scientific Research Department building at McLean

> where the cure of mental and nervous disorders may be studied and advanced. . . . This new Department will be devoted exclusively to the scientific research of brain and mental diseases, with a view to developing better methods for the treatment of mental and nervous disorders. The large percentage of the mentally disabled in the Armed Forces and the innumerable cases of similar permanent disability in civil life have made mental diseases a problem of first importance for the nation.

This statement, like so many others needed to defend the costs of basic research, foreshortened the distance between laboratory and sure-fire quick fix for mental illness beyond anyone's wildest dreams, but the public required reassurances.

Folch became director of scientific research at McLean on July 15, 1944, just as the cows were being sold. The war was still on, though the Allies were beginning to gain the upper hand; there were shortages on the home front; and a whole generation of kids grew up licking rationing stamps and pasting them into books. McLean's clinical staff hobbled along. In the midst of all this, the trustees acquired some funds for a new laboratory building, a feat accomplished primarily by Lowell, who secured money from the Hyams Trust, of which he also happened to be a trustee. This gift, to which the trustees added monies from Wood's carefully husbanded surplusses, financed the new laboratory for biochemical research, which was completed and dedicated on May 17, 1946.

There are few moments of high hilarity in the McLean chronicle, but the dedication ceremonies proved to be one of them. A large and distinguished audience, including over 200 representatives of the medical profession along with trustees, benefactors, and wives in stylish hats, had been assembled to listen to an even more distinguished panel of speakers extol the virtues of basic research on the brain. Drinker, Cobb, Herbert Gasser (director of the Rockefeller Institute, who gave a dazzling speech in which he quoted Poincaré's dictum that "an accumulation of facts is no more a science than a heap of stones is a house"), Wilder Penfield (a well-known Canadian neurosurgeon who studied epilepsy), and Edward Strecker, recently president of APA, all delivered dignified addresses. It was Folch who unintentionally provided the comic relief.

Folch had run into Lowell the day before the dedication ceremonies and brandished a sheaf of papers, saying "I've got my speech all ready for tomorrow." Lowell observed the thickness of the manuscript with consternation and reminded Folch that he had only been allotted 10 or 15 minutes to speak. But Folch was inflexible. Rather that abbreviate his remarks, he read off the entire text at machine-gun speed. His rapid-fire delivery, overlaid by a pronounced Spanish accent, left the audience flabbergasted. No one understood a word he was saying. David Crockett, the recently appointed director of research and development for the trustees, remembers scanning the stunned faces in the crowd while simultaneously trying to prevent himself from collapsing from his own chair in laughter.

In fairness it should be noted that few people in the audience, including the medical doctors, would have understood much of what Folch was saying even if he had spoken in perfectly modulated Oxonian tones. Only a small coterie of specialists knew anything about lipids at that time, and Folch used technical language. Folch turned out to be difficult to understand under ordinary circumstances. Even when he was not trying to beat the clock, he talked rapidly, and his accent got in the way of easy comprehension. Fortunately, Alfred Pope joined the McLean laboratory in 1946 as research associate in neuropathology.

While pursuing his own line of research, he developed a faculty for understanding what Folch was saying, both linguistically and scientifically. Accordingly, he often acted as Folch's translator/ interpreter, a role he accepted with grace.

The gamble on basic research at McLean paid off. Early in his career there, Folch perfected a simple procedure for obtaining a total brain lipid extract uncontaminated by nonlipid material. The paper he wrote describing this process became one of the most frequently quoted articles in biochemical literature, and the "Folch procedure," as it was called, eventually evolved into a verb: Now that lipid chemistry is commonplace, lab assistants know what it means to "Folch" a tissue. (Better to be immortalized by a verb than a disease—the usual fate of innovative members of the medical profession. Think of poor Alzheimer!) While developing this procedure, Folch discovered a new class of compounds which play an important structural role in membranes and consist of a closely linked combination of a protein and lipid units. He named these macromolecular constituents "proteolipids," and they became the dominant theme of his research over the next several years. These two pieces of work put the McLean laboratories on the map.

Folch's studies in neurochemistry and Pope's in neuropathology attracted more well-qualified applicants for training in basic research than the laboratory could accommodate, allowing them the luxury of picking the ripest from the crop of applicants. Grant money, if not exactly fulsome, flowed toward the research program in an increasingly abundant stream. The clinical aspect of the hypothetical two-pronged program was, however, slow to develop. While treating one another with respect, clinical psychiatrists and research staff exchanged no meaningful medical dialogue. The psychiatrists understood as much about Folch's proteolipids or Pope's investigations of the enzymatic architecture of the cerebral cortex as poets do about particle physics. And though Folch, as director of the laboratories, was a good McLean citizen, attended meetings with other heads of departments, and was interested in what was going on in the hospital, he had nothing to do with patients.

The gap between clinicians and researchers narrowed a little when Mark Altschule arrived in 1947 as director of internal medicine and research in clinical physiology. While overseeing the physical well-being of McLean's patients—it was he, for example, who judged whether a patient was physically fit to receive ECT—Altschule investigated the pathologic physiology of mental disease principally through studies of carbohydrate metabolism conducted during the early 1950s in various diagnostic classes of patients. He created a frail link between the laboratory and the psychiatric wards, thanks in some measure to his gift for language; he was capable of expressing abstruse concepts in accessible English.

By 1954 the research laboratories had seven full-time and two part-time people on their staff. Altschule in physiology had a full-time assistant. Grant money kept coming in, and the McLean research concern had a national reputation. The laboratories had become a little like the tail wagging the dog.

Over on the clinical side, the cows did not come home. In the same year that the laboratories were dedicated, Wood wrote in his annual report that he was depressed—he actually used the word "depressed"—that the hospital had not returned to prewar conditions. To some extent McLean confronted the same problems in the post World War II era that it had faced back in 1918. Once again there was a desperate nursing shortage for approximately the same reasons. There was, as well, a scarcity of psychiatrists. First, as Gregg had pointed out in 1944, psychiatry had a poor record of training and recruitment. Second, more and more psychiatrists were opting for private rather than institutional practice. Many younger men and women educated during the 1930s had trained in psychoanalysis with private practice quite specifically in mind. But even non-Freudians decided that office practice was more rewarding. The patients whom they saw were those they were more likely to be able to help; if they could not, or if the patient became dangerously ill, he or she could be referred to a mental institution. Psychiatrists could charge reasonable hourly rates for their services in offices. Altogether, many psychiatrists viewed private practice as less exhausting and frustrating, as well as more lucrative, than working with psychotics in hospitals.

This competition for professional time created the kind of supply and demand situation in which McLean had usually fared poorly. Packard's incessant pleadings for higher staff salaries and the numerous defections from the psychiatric staff during the 1920s were memories that had not yet faded. McLean wages in the late 1940s and early 1950s were still miserly. One man who spent a summer in Belmont as a junior psychiatrist around this period opined bluntly that the salaries "stank."

Wood, who usually produced laundry lists of events for his annual reports, abruptly changed his style in 1947 and addressed the hospital's financial problems aggressively. He began by citing the religious origins of hospitals and the charitable ideals that had formerly motivated the people who worked in them to relieve the suffering.

> Employees of many years of faithful service behind them still seem to retain the feeling of doing their various jobs because they enjoy their work and above all because they feel that they are doing their part to help others. Yet this group of people is becoming smaller every year and this attitude toward hospital work is disappearing with them. No longer does the feeling of satisfaction in a job well-done and the helping of others serve as a goal. Money seems to be the predominant aim of today and the hospital salaries cannot meet those of business and trades and there are too few people who will or can afford to work for less money just for the satisfaction of helping others.
>
> But the employees are not the only part of the hospital concerned. The hospital itself is encumbered with money problems. Costs have more than doubled and the deficits are all out of proportion, while the endowment funds grow smaller rapidly. The problem of money has become all important. How much can be charged for this or that service? How much more can be charged for rooms and nursing care? Where can this vicious circle end?

Wood observed the crassness inherent in the fact that "the first thing discussed with relatives is the financial situation."

McLean recorded its largest deficit ever during 1947. Over half the patients cared for during the year had paid less than the standard rate of $60 per week. Some of those patients came from socially well-connected families and had been admitted at reduced rates because, for example, the family had suffered some financial setback. Other patients, originally admitted at full board, had become long-term residents and after months or years represented an intolerable drain on the family economy. Rather than transfer such a patient to a state facility, the trustees sometimes chose to lighten the financial burden by lowering the charge. There was nothing new in the principle of reduced-rate patients. McLean had always had them. Never, however, had they represented such a large proportion of the population, an accumulation which occurred rapidly as medicine extended the life spans of people with chronic mental illnesses.

However much he may have respected the principle of and necessity for basic research, Wood was unhappy to see that insofar as new funds were being invested in the hospital they went to the laboratories, while clinical programs got nickel-and-dimed to death. That the laboratory operations were paid for primarily by grant monies unavailable for clinical care was a financial technicality he was in no mood to appreciate. Things were limping along in this unbalanced gait with no solution in sight when, in 1948, McLean got socked by scandal.

The proper telling of the story requires a brief retreat in time. Back in 1942, perhaps in an effort to entertain American GIs and, not incidentally, to increase circulation, *Esquire* magazine had published pictures of some scantily clad women. Hugh Hefner would have yawned, but the contents of the magazine came to the attention of the U.S. Post Office Department, which challenged *Esquire's* second-class mailing privileges. (The country is at war, and officials in Washington are worrying about second-class mailing privileges for *Esquire*?) The department held a hearing and summoned psychiatrists as expert witnesses. Dr. Benjamin Karpman, a senior psychiatrist at St. Elizabeth's, testified that the photographs were sexually stimulating and lewd. McLean's Tillotson, however, defended *Esquire* by taking the view that its pictures were "good clean pictures glorifying good figures and a tribute to American womanhood." The newspapers picked up this quote and ran with it. Tillotson came through this skirmish unharmed, and the story apparently sank into oblivion, there being more important events to command public attention.

Five years later, during the second week of October, a 28-year-old McLean nurse, Anne Marie Salot, filed a complaint with the State Department of Mental Health charging that Tillotson's amorous attentions were endangering her health. Salot, a very good looking brunette, had been a student in the McLean Training School for Nurses and later a lieutenant in the Navy

Nurses Corps, then returning to McLean as a member of the nursing staff. She and Tillotson had been romantically involved for some time before she registered her complaint, which included, in addition to her belief that her mental health was in jeopardy, the claim that she had been forced to resign from her job at McLean because of Tillotson's persistent advances. Within hours of learning about the accusations, which had been brought to Wood's attention by the commissioner of mental health, the trustees on the McLean Committee assembled in Lowell's Boston office to figure out what ought to be done. Later that evening, they demanded Tillotson's resignation, which he promptly submitted. He simultaneously withdrew from the faculty at the Harvard Medical School.

The fact of Tillotson's resignation and the reasons behind it passed unnoticed by the press. The Boston Braves had made the World Series, and the mind of the city was fixed on baseball (the Braves lost). However, in the latter part of November, Tillotson and Salot appeared before a special Middlesex County grand jury on morals charges. The courtroom teemed with reporters as both pleaded not guilty, but the jury thought the evidence sufficient to bind them over for trial. The press had a field day. The newspapers featured photographs of Salot, who was very photogenic. Tillotson was characterized as a "world-famous psychiatrist," a designation that the press did not base on his professional reputation but rather on the old testimony regarding *Esquire*. That episode was resurrected from the depths into which it had supposedly sunk and was repeated again and again in newspaper articles as though it were evidence of Tillotson's lascivious nature.

The trial took place on May 9, 1949, in a crowded, expectant courtroom. Tillotson appeared with his wife at his side, as she had been throughout the earlier proceedings. To the disappointment of the press, both he and Salot changed their pleas to guilty. They had no doubt realized that protestations of innocence would have subjected them to a long, highly publicized trial and further exposed them to the greedy imaginations of the public; a plea of guilty was hardly worse than the damage that had already been done to reputations, including McLean's. As it was, Tillotson's family had suffered terribly from the ordeal.

There being nothing to argue about, the trial began and ended on the same day. Tillotson was fined $750; Salot was fined $25 and placed on probation. When questioned by reporters after the sentencing about his plans for the future, Tillotson replied that although he had received three offers to head hospitals elsewhere, he had no intentions of leaving Massachusetts. "I plan to stay here and live down the unfavorable publicity attendant upon this case" (5).

He did precisely that. The State Board of Registration in Medicine reviewed the evidence in his case and, though it took time to arrive at a decision, suspended his license for three months—in effect, a mild slap on the wrists. Tillotson stuck by his word and eventually opened an office in his home in Belmont. There he built up a successful private practice.

From McLean's point of view, Tillotson dropped into a historical black hole. The 1948 annual report mentioned his "resignation" in a single sentence. By contrast, the installation of a new stained glass window in the chapel rated two full pages of prose. Though one would not expect the report to have dwelled upon the salacious details of his departure, a few words might have been said about his having run the clinical program for 16 years, often under trying conditions, or about some of his solid, if not earthshaking, research. Tillotson came in for equally rough treatment in the McLean chapter in the MGH history volume for that era, edited by Faxon; his name appears only three times, and then as a matter of necessity. Paul Howard, who worked with Tillotson for years, observed the injustice of neglecting his long professional career. But officially, Tillotson had become persona non grata because he had committed the unpardonable sin of tarnishing McLean's respectability, a quality which at that point in the hospital's history seems to have carried greater weight than a progressive clinical program.

The months immediately following Tillotson's departure set a new low watermark for McLean. The internal problems of money and staffing that Wood had enumerated in 1947 showed no signs of resolving themselves. Externally, McLean's good name was dishonored. Only the research laboratories can be said to have been thriving.

After Tillotson's departure, Paul Howard was designated acting chief psychiatrist, a title indicating the temporary nature of the position until the person is properly ordained as chief or a new person is brought in from the outside and installed in the chief's chair. Howard labored under the stigma of "acting," attached to changing titles, for seven years. Though Howard ignored the tenuousness of his role and acted deliberately within the limits of his power, the situation smacked of indecisiveness. McLean looked like an airplane caught in an endless circling pattern, unable to decide where to land.

During this seven-year interregnum, certain external developments affected the hospital. In 1949 Congress acknowledged the scale of mental illness as an economic and social problem and established the National Institute of Mental Health (NIMH). (There had been a National Cancer Institute since 1937 and National Heart, Dental Research, and Microbiology Institutes since 1948. Mental health might have had its own division earlier if the profession had pressed its case more forcefully.) Congress voted an initial appropriation of $8.7 million and continued increasing the federal contribution steadily each year, so that by 1955 NIMH funds were exceeded only by those assigned to cancer and heart disease. Some of this federal money eventually found its way to McLean in the form of research and training grants.

While benefitting from federal programs, the psychiatric world fared poorly in voluntary health fund-raising drives. Up through 1953, mental health drives fell way behind those for polio, tuberculosis, cancer, heart disease, crippled children, cerebral palsy, muscular dystrophy, and arthritis. In 1954, like a slow horse in a long race, mental health pulled a neck ahead of arthritis. But this was no close horse race. While the March of Dimes raised $51.4 million in 1953, the National Association for Mental Health scraped together $700,000. Fund-raisers observed the peculiar difficulties of attracting money to help the mentally ill, attributing them to the attitude of fear and suspicion that surrounds mental illness. (It is curious to recall, by contrast, how successfully McLean had raised money during the nineteenth century.) Even former McLean patients with charitable instincts could not be counted upon to donate money to the hospital. One particularly memorable man spent years at

McLean, died there, and designated cancer research at MGH as his beneficiary.

Thus, the modern financial picture began to emerge. On the one hand, NIMH, the National Institute of Neurological Diseases, and private granting agencies (conspicuous among them the Scottish Rite Committee for Research in Schizophrenia, a Masonic group which was a pioneer in supporting mental health research) provided "soft" funds for research and training or seed money for certain programs; on the other hand, the "hard" money was very hard to come by indeed, and the institution was poorly endowed.

The entrance of insurance companies into the medical business supplies another piece of the financial picture. Where psychiatric hospitals were concerned, insurance companies were most conspicuous by their absence. Whereas Blue Cross, the principal third-party payer in Massachusetts, had been helping to pay its subscribers' general hospital costs since the late 1930s, its policies did not cover mental illnesses. This lapse did not occur because insurance executives were dimwits who carried medieval images of insanity in their minds; they were, rather, hard-nosed bottom liners who studied the statistics. The data showed that mental patients often stayed in hospital for months, if not for years, and even if discharged might well require readmission within another year or two. During 1952 at McLean, for example, newly admitted patients with promising prognoses, who represented a mere 25 percent of the total population of the hospital, stayed an average of two months. The average length of stay for *all* patients at MGH was approximately 11 days! In short, selling coverage for mental illness did not look like a sound business venture.

Wood griped about Blue Cross approximately every other year and complained that state and federal hospitals received government support, whereas places like McLean had to depend exclusively on fees from patients. (His latter observation, while accurate, failed to take into account that most state hospitals struggled along on pittances by comparison with McLean.) Hospital costs were rising precipitously, especially in the area of wages. The buildings verged on antiquity and were a drain on the budget. Patient charges had to be adjusted accordingly.

Meanwhile, the combination of the Depression and Roosevelt's New Deal had effected some degree of economic leveling and reduced the number of families who could afford to admit a mental patient to a fancy hospital. Thus, many of the small private hospitals of McLean's ilk suffered severe financial problems during this period. A few institutions kept ahead of the money crunch by limiting their clientele to neurotics who could be treated relatively quickly, thereby ensuring a high rate of turnover and minimizing the likelihood of chronicity. McLean, however, ran greater risks by accepting psychotic and brain-damaged patients. Though financial credentials were criteria for admission, the money was known to run out before the patient was ready for discharge. Even so, the patient population, which had as recently as the 1920s included middle- and working-class people, had become by the 1940s almost exclusively affluent and/or well connected, as well as very provincial.

The picture that emerges of McLean during the last seven years of Wood's directorship and Howard's tenure as acting clinical chief is a mixed one: a hybrid of strict regimentation and humanism, of deprivation and indulgence. There was, for instance, the matter of money. The following directive was inscribed in Wood's looseleaf rule book, one of the more instructive treasures remaining in McLean's archives. Under the letter "M"—after Maids, Medications, Medicine cards, and Medicine closets—is the following entry about Money: "Patients are allowed to have money for purchases or entertainment only upon signed permission of the physician-in-charge. The balance of money is to be given to the supervisor when the patient returns from an outing." Staff members recall the irony of belabored discussions over whether or not patients, a few of whom were practically zillionaires and most of whom came from far more luxurious origins than any of the psychiatrists, ought to be allowed to carry around 50 cents in their pockets. Meanwhile, nurses made arrangements to have mink coats signed in and out of Filene's storage facilities according to season. The former steward explained further: "We catered to patients. If the patient did not like the lamb we served for dinner and asked for lobster, we gave lobster. They could afford it. Appleton House was the Ritz Carlton" (6).

Visiting hours were set between the hours of 1 and 5 P.M. except on Sundays. The nurses on the wards had orders to restrain visitors from speaking with patients other than the one they had come to see. "This is to protect the patient's privacy and to prevent any possibility of letters being mailed on the outside by visitors." McLean controlled the patients' mail by passing it on to their families for monitoring, a practice that no doubt protected various celebrities from crank mail originating from a mental institution. Regulations governed the storage of medicine, who had charge of which keys, the guarding of silverware or other implements that might be turned against the self or others in violence, the administration of various forms of therapy and narcotic drugs, and other matters directly pertaining to the safety of the patients and the rational administration of the hospital. A former director of nursing remembered a routine from the 1940s, when she was a fledgling nurse, according to which the ward nurses were supposed to have the patients up and out of bed by 7:30 every morning. She had one patient who refused to get up on command, and her supervisor dressed her down daily for her failure to make the patient comply. After several days of this, her patience finally gave out and she marched into the patient's room and said, "I don't give a damn if you never get out of bed!" Much to her surprise, the patient got up immediately (7).

The entry in Wood's rule book that best captures the antique, authoritarian spirit of McLean was directed to the employees on the subject of vacations:

> The Trustees grant two weeks vacation after one year of satisfactory service. The vacation is given to prepare the employee for the next year's work. It is not a bonus and it is not given for services rendered. In other words, we are not entitled to a vacation, it is given to us if we intend to remain in the service of the hospital. Anyone leaving the service of the hospital within three months after vacation will have his vacation money deducted from his last paycheck.

A real morale booster, that!

It is in Howard's accounts of the clinical service, which appeared in the annual reports, that one senses McLean's efforts to keep abreast, if not ahead, of progressive trends in psychiatry—progressive at that time being most closely identified with intensive psychotherapy that was accented, if not fully flavored, by psychoanalysis. The contrast in tone between his reports and those of his predecessor Tillotson is quite striking. Howard—whose curriculum vitae included two years in journalism prior to medical school and analytic training during the 1930s at the Boston Psychoanalytic Society and Institute under the guidance of Helene Deutsch (who herself had had one year of didactic analysis with Freud), as well as residencies at Boston Psychopathic Hospital, Boston City Hospital, and MGH under Stanley Cobb—had a capacity for empathy with patients remarkable even in a psychiatrist. He was flexible in his approach to mental illness and, accordingly, receptive to somatic treatments. He viewed them as elements in a comprehensive course of therapy that included individual psychotherapy as well as improvement of social life within the hospital:

> Modern concepts of personality disorder insist on the value of such personalized, dynamic hospital treatment. For beyond the dramatic alterations in the course of psychoses or neuroses brought about by physiological, medical and nutritional treatment, or by electric shock, insulin and lobotomy, lie the personality needs of each maladjusted person. One of the more cheerful aspects of hospital psychiatry today as compared with a few years ago, is the greater accessibility of patients for treatment of their disturbed attitudes by psychotherapy, some of the newer physiological influences having softened rigid psychotic symptoms or persistent anxiety.
>
> If the usual idea of getting the patient well by digging to the root of problems was enough, psychotherapists might operate rapidly; unfortunately, there is much more of nurturing the growth of the patient in a suitable emotional environment, and we all grow slowly. (8)

But Howard's ideals of individualized treatment within a protective, wholesome social framework were beyond the capacities of McLean, for despite his claim of a small patient load per physician (as opposed perhaps to state institutions), the professional staff was really very small. On an ordinary day, they could fit around one or two tables in the coffee shop. In 1953, for instance, Wood, Howard, Willis Bower (chief of the women's service), and J. Douglass Sharpe (chief of the Men's Service) constituted the senior staff. Four or five residents served under the service chiefs. A few staff psychiatrists, like Maria Lorenz, worked a few days a week at McLean; Irene

Pierce, the psychologist, was there two days a week. Most of these people lived in quarters on the grounds.

The daily routine began at 8 A.M. when the service chiefs met with their respective staff members to review the nursing reports of the past 24 hours and to discuss which patients would be receiving ECT or other special treatments. Around 8:30, the entire staff gathered in Wood's office to discuss any extraordinary occurrences from the previous day. They then repaired to the coffee shop for a break, during which they conducted a good deal of hospital business. After coffee, they dispersed to the wards in their charge to visit those patients for whom they were responsible. They reconvened in the administration building around noon and dined in grand style, joined by key administrative personnel. (This luxury fell before the economic axe around 1954; thereafter, the staff lunched more humbly in the cafeteria.) Twice a week Howard conducted a clinical case conference in the medical library; the eight or nine staff people involved in the clinical care of patients attended those conferences regularly (9).

The size of the professional staff, the orderly structure of the day's assemblings and partings, and residence on the premises made McLean more like a family than an institutional operation, with Wood reigning as pater familias and with most of the assets and deficits that go along with family membership. There was a certain coziness that came with intimacy, even among those inclined to disagree with one another. But there was not enough critical mass to permit the level of personal attention to patients—particularly the withdrawn, difficult to reach patients—that Howard and others would have liked.

Nevertheless, Howard tried some innovations. He was the first of McLean's modern clinical chiefs to recognize explicitly the therapeutic potential of several patients living together and to attempt to systematize group activities. Howard's older brother Edgerton was a psychiatrist on the staff at the Austen Riggs Center in Stockbridge, Massachusetts, where a number of adventuresome patient-management forms were tried (and some discarded). Riggs was an exciting place during the 1950s. Its director Robert Knight had turned it into a major center of psychoanalytic training and research. Erik Erikson arrived in 1950 and refined his theories.

Howard learned from his brother's experiences at Riggs and introduced a few modest reforms at McLean. In 1954 he organized the Patient Activities Association (PAA), a voluntary "club" that initiated and sponsored group activities by and for the patients. "It has the same therapeutic intent as the activities in an ordinary town, in which the citizens participate," Howard wrote (10). The second body, the Patient-Personnel Conference (PPC), consisted of seven patients plus five nurses, a psychiatrist, a psychologist, the administrator, and a recreational worker. Initially organized to explore the possibility of group meetings on the wards, the PPC quickly evolved into a formal channel of communication through which patients could express their opinions about hospital regulations, such as whether the men might be allowed to shave themselves or how patients might be able to move about the hospital grounds with greater liberty. Though the PPC did not have any authority to make or change rules, it did provide a mechanism for bringing patients' concerns to the attention of the staff and involving patients in the administration of the hospital. If there was more illusion than reality to the patients' powers within either the PAA or the PPC, that was irrelevant. Both staff and patients understood the force of illusion.

Perhaps the biggest problem that McLean faced during this period was the staggering number of chronic patients: a problem that neither Howard nor Wood seemed to be able to cope with. There were, first of all, a large number of geriatric patients with brain damage. In 1952 the hospital had 100 patients averaging age 77; 30 had been admitted with diagnoses of cerebral arteriosclerosis or senility. Though McLean superintendents since Luther Bell had grumbled about backlogs of chronic patients, the elderly among them had usually not lived very long after admission. Recent medical advances had altered that demographic picture. Modern psychiatry could do nothing for elderly brain-damaged individuals, but modern antibiotics extended their lives considerably. Patients who would have died of pneumonia in the 1930s pulled through with the aid of penicillin in the 1940s. McLean's nursing and medical staff tended these patients considerately. But no matter how the lily was gilded, this was custodial care. The only remotely cynical comment discernible in any of Howard's annual reports showed up in 1953 when he noted that senile patients did not take up psychotherapeutic time and helped pay the costs for patients who might get well. Yet even this was not always the case because some elderly patients paid reduced rates.

Francis de Marneffe, who arrived on the McLean staff in 1953, remarked upon a second, more disturbing class of custodial patients; namely, those who simply were not expected to recover, usually schizophrenics. Some of these patients seemed "relatively well put together" on the surface, but more probing conversation would disclose pathologies such as hallucinations; others were more obviously disturbed. Fifteen years earlier, Myerson and Tillotson would have tried to reclaim some of these patients through the total push program. In the early 1950s, however, the hospital held "no expectation that they were going to recover to the point that they would be able to be discharged from the hospital and lead independent lives." Therefore, the hospital provided a place for them to live, to be looked after, and to some extent to be entertained. It protected them from the consequences of their illness (11).

McLean at mid-century was a struggling organization, barely able to keep abreast of progressive treatment concepts, let alone serve as a model for other hospitals. Residents, having heard its clinical program was static, looked for more exciting, dynamic training opportunities. Institutions like the Menninger Clinic in Topeka, Kansas, Hillside in New York, Chestnut Lodge in Washington, D.C., and Austen Riggs in Stockbridge commanded much more professional respect than McLean. The Boston Psychopathic Hospital was enjoying a revival under the leadership of Harry Solomon and setting an example for intensive, individualized treatment of psychotic patients, discharge planning, and follow-up studies. By contrast, the McLean archives reveal this candid assessment of the place by a psychiatrist who had spent a summer there during the early 1950s.

> The hospital itself has wonderful grounds and potentially good facilities. If C. L. [Chestnut Lodge] only had what they have there! There is much that is not modern, of course, and in the care of major custodial patients that creates problems. The chief detractions are the type of patients they have there and the management of the hospital. Everything revolves around Dr. Wood. . . . The atmosphere is almost medievalistic or feudalistic in that respect. . . .
>
> There is no real therapy as we know it, as far as I can ascertain. The chief formulae seem to have been shock, encouragement, reassurance and sublimation through activities. Because of the high rates and the luxuriousness of the place, aristocratic clientele is found, consisting of patients whose families don't want them to get really well, and want them out of the way. Most of the patients looked to me like social rejects of a blunted sort mixed with annoying neurotics. Dull and stupefied, or pestiferous. A premium is placed upon outward cooperativeness. And the same goes for the personnel . . . generally, I thought the whole institution geared to the moronic level presumed to characterize the patients. There are some good nurses of course, and probably some good attendants; but most of the personnel seems made up of former inmates of mental institutions where they didn't get well through dint of insights. I suspect that it is a notch above state hospitals in the area, but it certainly is far from being in the same class with a psychoanalytical institution. It houses too many presumed chronics. . . .
>
> . . . Pay is at a stinkingly low level because it is presumably offset by altruistic satisfactions and loyalty rewarded. . . .
>
> . . . Given some good administration at the top, supplemented by some vigorous decisions, and given guidance in the real essentials in cases of functional illness, I think the institution could again be built up, and indeed it might once again set an example. . . . There is certainly a need; but I think it would take a man with intense doggedness and perseverance to attack it.

This devastating indictment (from a psychoanalytically biased observer) found the sore spots in McLean: the load of chronic patients, the poor salaries, the outdated mode of administration, the sense of rolling along in an old rut. Thanks to the presence of a few skilled psychiatrists, McLean still helped some people back to the community. But as the number of chronic patients, geriatric and otherwise, accumulated and no one offered a fresh vision of the hospital, the rut threatened to become deeper and entrap the place in a purely custodial role—a role it had tried to avoid from its inception.

CHAPTER

10

Alfred Stanton: Fermentation

If some of the difficulties which encumbered McLean during the postwar decade were idiosyncratic to the institution, the primary one, the rising numbers of chronic patients, was generic to all mental hospitals that did not turn their backs on the very ill and the elderly. Those relatively few patients fortunate enough to be in private hospitals at least had the advantages of pleasant accommodations, visits from psychiatrists, good nursing care, and diverting activities. The great majority of chronic mental patients languished in crowded, poorly staffed state institutions where they sometimes did not see a doctor for weeks. Whatever problems chronicity posed for private hospitals were magnified many times over in public institutions. The path to solutions seemed blockaded by shortages of funding, skilled psychiatrists, and scientific knowledge.

A glimmer of hope appeared in the early 1950s thanks to the imagination of a French surgeon, Henri Laborit. Laborit was using a new drug, chlorpromazine, a compound belonging to the phenothiazine family, to calm his patients before administering anesthesia. He observed its soothing and unusual effects and suggested that it might have some application in mental disorders. Several French psychiatrists experimented with the agent. Some noticed that it increased the efficiency of barbiturates in the sedation of psychotic patients; others observed that it was sometimes useful on its own. Chlorpromazine (under the trade name Thorazine) came into use at Worcester State Hospital in 1954 and was being tried on a grand scale in the New York State hospital system, where some 30,000 patients were immediately placed on drug therapy. The following year, McLean psychiatrists began to prescribe Thorazine very cautiously. Though it would take some time to sort out the appropriate applications of Thorazine and the chemical analogs which rapidly came onto the market, the initial impact upon the atmosphere in the wards was spectacular. Patients who had been violent, agitated, and dangerous became placid.

Antianxiety drugs such as meprobamate (Miltown) and chlordiazepoxide (Librium) also appeared in the mid-1950s. Meanwhile, physicians using an agent in the treatment of tuberculosis noticed its euphoric effects upon their patients. The drug, a hydrazine compound, proved useful in the treatment of some depressed mental patients by acting as an inhibitor of a brain enzyme, monoamine oxidase. This class of drugs was soon followed by the tricyclic antidepressants, drugs based on the same theory of physiological activity.

Though chemically different, the antipsychotic, antianxiety, and antidepressant drugs had one thing in common: They made mental patients behave better and often feel better. As management tools, they were unquestionably more reliable than any of the earlier somatic treatments in becalming hyperactive, suicidal, excited, disoriented, or dangerous patients in mental hospitals. The drugs frightened patients and their families far less than Metrazol, insulin, or ECT, let alone lobotomy. Drugs could be doled out in benign little pills or liquid doses. While they had some side effects, they posed fewer medical risks to the patient than the shock therapies or psychosurgery. (However, they resembled the shock treatments in the inscrutability of their action, though they became slightly less inscrutable as researchers learned more about how they worked.)

The psychiatric profession, particularly that segment of it which treated institutionalized patients, accepted the drugs gratefully and prescribed them generously, but did not delude itself that they cured mental illnesses. The medications were perceived, rather, to be useful on two levels. They could quell the florid symptoms of disease in individual patients, who subsequently became more receptive to psychotherapy. The multiplication of these effects by tens or hundreds made the management of hospital wards infinitely easier, especially for the nurses and attendants who passed so much of their time in the company of patients, while making the experience of hospitalization less traumatic for the patients.

About a year after drugs made their entrance into psychiatric practice, the federal government made an attempt to come to grips with what it belatedly recognized as a national problem. In 1955 the 84th Congress passed Joint Resolution No. 256, "providing for an objective, thorough, and nationwide analysis and reevaluation of the human and economic problems of mental illness," otherwise known as the Mental Health Study Act of 1955. The resolution began, "whereas some 750,000 mentally ill and retarded patients are now being hospitalized on any given day," and proceeded through a litany of whereases that identified mental illness as a social problem of huge dimensions. Mental patients occupied 47 percent of the hospital beds in the country. The direct economic costs of mental illness to taxpayers, including pensions to veterans with psychiatric disabilities, exceeded $1 billion per year and were increasing by more than $100 million per year. Only one-third of the patients admitted to state hospitals, which carried roughly 80 percent of the national patient load, were discharged within the course of a year. Mental illness was frequently implicated in other national epidemics such as alcoholism, drug addiction, juvenile delinquency, truancies, family dissolutions, suicide, and work-related problems. Groping for an adjective that would do justice to the scale of the problem of mental illness, Congress settled on "staggering."

Joint Resolution No. 256 created the Joint Commission on Mental Illness and Health as a study group under the leadership of Kenneth E. Appel, a former president of the American Psychiatric Association, and Leo H. Bartemeier, chairman of the Council on Mental Health of the American Medical Association. They assembled a team of agencies and individuals, principally psychiatrists but including clergymen, psychologists, sociologists, nurses, biologists, educators, anthropologists, and lawyers.

The Joint Commission sponsored wide-ranging studies from which, after five and a half years, the staff prepared a final report and submitted policy recommendations to Congress.

That report, a book-length document, disproved the conventional wisdom that committees are doomed to design camels. Thanks in large part to the efforts of Jack Ewalt, who was staff director during the project, the final product was a careful, well-written, and often moving study. As a bird's-eye view of psychiatric practice, research, and education in the late 1950s, it can't be beaten. The report laid out the story with clarity and candor. It referred to the "incredibly small fund of knowledge about the causes and cures. [Mental illness] is a field where much-qualified guesses abound and the few hard facts achieve prominence by their very scarcity" (1).

The Joint Commission remarked upon the changes wrought by drugs in the treatment of hospitalized patients:

> Unquestionably, the drugs have delivered the greatest blow for patient freedom, in terms of non-restraint, since Pinel struck the chains off the lunatics in the Paris asylum 168 years ago. The most noticeable effect of the drugs is to reduce the hospital noise level. Bedlam has been laid to rest. . . . In the surprising, pleasant effects they produce on patient-staff relationships, the drugs might be described as moral treatment in pill form. (2)

Though unified in the opinion that drugs were management rather than curative agents and extremely guarded in its optimism, the Joint Commission observed that for the first time in history, the mental hospital population had declined. In New York State alone, the census dropped from 91,000 in 1954 to 89,000 in 1959, a demographic trend that the study correlated with the number of patients receiving drug therapy.

Instead of displacing psychiatrists, medication actually increased the demand for them by bringing hitherto remote patients within striking range of psychotherapy. Locally, active membership in the Boston Psychoanalytic Institute rose from 66 in 1953 to 133 in 1963 and again to 227 in 1973, and there were many psychotherapists who did not belong to the institute. While it is true that some analysts committed to a psychogenic theory of mental disorder scoffed at drugs, such rigidity of attitude did not characterize the Boston group. In the opinion of

George E. Gifford, Jr., psychiatrist and chronicler of the Freudian-inspired psychotherapies in New England, the long, strong tradition of dialogue among psychiatrists, members of academia, and hospital physicians produced a more flexible approach.

> Fortunately strong medical eclecticism decreased polarization between the physiological and psychological schools, and instead encouraged cooperative study. The pioneer research of Walter Bradford Cannon on the physiological correlates of emotion brought together the psychological and organic approaches. The investigations of Otto Folin, John C. Whitehorn and William G. Lennox [who studied the epilepsies with Cobb] developed more completely such symbiotic viewpoints and, most important, diverse approaches were tolerantly supported by hospital administrators. (3)

That the coming of age of psychoanalysis and its intellectual progeny occurred in tandem with the development of the modern psychotropic drugs was not really contradictory. Even though the medicines suggested more strongly than ever a biochemical substratum to mental illnesses, the identification of essential causes remained a chicken-and-egg riddle. Did a person's biochemistry go haywire because of psychic insult? Was there a fundamental flaw in the system? Other elementary questions, most of them older than Methuselah, resisted resolution. A study cited in the Joint Commission's report observed that professionals "differ on what persons 'are' when they are emotionally disturbed or mentally ill, on how they get that way, on what is wrong with them, on who should be placed in that category, on why they stay that way, and on what should be done about it . . ." (4). Medicines and psychotherapy both had limitations, particularly in the treatment of deeply disturbed, hospitalized patients. Yet drugs relieved some of the worst symptoms of disease, and psychotherapy helped patients adjust to the pressures of the real world. Accordingly, the natural inclination was to use all weapons in the arsenal, however imperfect their record of performance, and train them simultaneously on the target.

In the early 1950s, when the need for drastic measures at McLean began to make itself obvious, pending administrative turnovers presented the trustees with opportunities to make changes without spilling any blood. With Stanley Cobb scheduled to retire as chief of the MGH Psychiatric Service in July

1954 and Wood's departure slated for July 1956, the trustees decided to review the entire spectrum of psychiatric services in their charge. A vague plan was hatched for combining the two entities and creating a new department called "The Mental Health Services of the MGH." This proposal envisaged, among other things, the full, free exchange of staff and patients between the two institutions, as well as a tightly knit residency training program. Naturally the administrative structure would require a complete overhaul. Since nothing came of this plan in the long run, it is pointless to itemize its finer details. However, the idea hung in the air for a couple of years and influenced the selection of personnel (5).

Stanley Cobb was succeeded by Erich Lindemann, a German-born psychiatrist and analyst who had been on the MGH service since the late 1930s. Lindemann had earned nationwide professional respect through his studies of families who had lost relatives in the terrible Cocoanut Grove fire in 1942. He became increasingly concerned with heading off psychological disasters through crisis prevention and intervention. His interests propelled him out of his office at MGH into the community. At the time of his appointment as chief at MGH, he was the driving force behind the creation of the Wellesley Human Relations Service, a prototype of the modern community mental health center. He was an inspired man whose ideas excited others. However, he had little talent for the nitty-gritty of administration. Nevertheless, with a foggy vision of a unified psychiatric service hovering overhead, a search began for someone to fill Wood's position at McLean, someone who could work effectively in partnership with Lindemann.

The name of Alfred H. Stanton, chief of the closed ward section of the Boston Veterans Administration (VA) Hospital, was placed into candidacy in 1954. Since the position at stake was that of psychiatrist-in-chief at McLean (a new title for what would be both the clinical and administrative head), as well as a tenured associate professorship at Harvard Medical School, the rituals of search were elaborate. As medieval knights once had to prove themselves worthy of fair maidens by performing a series of heroic tasks, so such candidates had to overcome a series of academic and political obstacles.

Stanton's curriculum vitae fared very well in the prevailing climate which identified progressive treatment of mental illness with psychoanalytically influenced therapy. Born in 1913 and raised in the shadows of St. Elizabeth's Hospital, where his father worked as a nonprofessional, Stanton had studied medicine at George Washington University and then taken an internship in neurology. In 1940, while receiving his training analysis at the Washington-Baltimore Psychoanalytical Institute, he became a resident in psychiatry at Chestnut Lodge Sanatorium, one of the very few mental institutions in the country at that time which practiced intensive psychotherapy with schizophrenic and other psychotic patients. There, Stanton came under the spell of Harry Stack Sullivan, a leader of the "interpersonal" school of psychiatry, who conceived of mental disorders as arising out of disturbed cultural and personal relations. If the architecture of Sullivan's approach was of original design, the substructure upon which it was based was psychoanalytic and in practice represented an application of psychotherapy that extended beyond Freud's expectations.

During World War II, Sullivan delivered an extensive series of clinical talks at Chestnut Lodge. "At times I can visualize the scene," wrote Dexter Bullard, the medical superintendent,

> and recapture the moods of both Sullivan and the group, which included Mabel Cohen, Edna Dyar, Frieda Fromm-Reichmann, Douglas Noble, Robert Morse, David Rioch, Alfred Stanton, Edith Weigart, Ben Weininger, and Mabel Wilkin. The setting was the recreation room of my house, on the grounds of Chestnut Lodge. The staff would assemble after lunch, before an open fire in cold weather; the Great Dane would lie down on the hearthrug, and Sullivan would begin. . . . At times the dog would be used to illustrate a point, and on these occasions Sullivan might take time out to pat his head, as if asking his opinion too. Needless to say, there were times when the discussion became as spirited and acrimonious as, may I say, learned. (6)

Nourished by exposure to Sullivan's provocative discussions, Stanton joined intellectual forces in 1947 with Morris Schwartz, a sociologist, and began a three and one-half year study of the inner workings of a leading mental hospital. They set up shop on a disturbed ward and observed in fine detail the manner in which administrative practices filtered down and influenced the behavior of the patients. Their findings documented the hypothesis that the way the hospital functioned played a substantial role in the patients' conditions. Seemingly innocuous incidents, such as a mix-up in communication that resulted in a patient receiving one set of instructions from a nurse only to have them contradicted two hours later by the psychiatrist, could precipitate grave clinical consequences. The experience of hospitalization could, in effect, laminate a secondary set of emotional defects upon the disorder for which the patient had been admitted.

Stanton's and Schwartz's analysis of the ward as a social unit was published in a book, *The Mental Hospital*, one of the most persuasive works in its generation of psychiatric literature and a piece of thoroughly gripping writing. The manuscript had already been set in type when Stanton's name came before the McLean search committee. Stanton, meanwhile, had moved from the Washington-Baltimore area to Boston, where he served first as chief of the closed ward section at the Cushing VA Hospital, and later moved on to the Boston VA Hospital.

In mid-1954 Stanton was invited to review the psychiatric programs at MGH and McLean and to present his recommendations for future developments. After spending many hours in conversation with Wood, Howard, and Lindemann, Cobb's heir-designate but not yet in office, as well as poking around McLean, Stanton drafted a report which, if not as brutal as the assessment quoted at the end of the last chapter, addressed many of the same issues. "The reputation which has come to my attention is a mixed one," he wrote.

> The most widely held opinion among the profession and the ancillary professions is that the psychiatric services of both hospitals are in a sort of state of suspended animation. Dr. Howard's "Acting" position, and Dr. Cobb's impending retirement are given as reasons, but I suspect they are rather symptoms. As one physician put it to me two years ago, he felt defensive about referring a patient to McLean on the principle that nothing would be done, but he would not dream of sending the patient elsewhere locally. Partly McLean shares this reputation with the other large voluntary mental hospitals of the eastern seaboard with which it is informally associated. These hospitals have all been felt to be largely static since the depression; they should, on the basis of their independence and general position, be in the very center of straight psychiatric research, and they are not. As a group they have largely failed in taking the intellectual leadership which their structure and history makes their

> responsibility. Of the group, McLean is in as defensible a position as any, but it fails to match the psychiatric activity that now occurs in certain general hospitals, 'psychopathic type' hospitals, and even several small private hospitals and large state hospitals.

Stanton then began to itemize McLean's problems: The research program, he said, was "seriously skewed" in favor of chemical and physiological studies at the expense of the psychological and social sciences, a bias which hurt clinical practices. The hospital had too few psychiatrists to provide intensive psychotherapy. There was no group therapy whatsoever. "Group therapy has achieved such a place in so many hospitals that a hospital which fails to use it must defend this choice." He remarked that the psychology department was understaffed—it consisted of one person working only two days a week—and that there were no social workers or vocational counselors or rehabilitation experts.

> One other problem seems to me conspicuous on the basis of informal talks with various members of the staff; there is nothing so hard on morale as the suspicion that better clinical work is being done elsewhere and that nothing is being done to approach the best clinical practice. This is precisely the feeling that has been reported to me from several sources—and it requires vigorous action.

Stanton advanced a two-pronged program. He gave top priority to improving clinical treatment by a major staffing-up which he believed could be achieved in part relatively inexpensively by retaining psychiatric staff on a half-time or even hourly basis, while increasing the number of residents and letting them do the bulk of psychotherapy under proper supervision. (Residents came dirt cheap in those days.) He also advocated the addition of clinical psychologists, social workers, and other categories he had noted among the missing. Stanton's second proposal was "A Serious Research Program"; namely, the building of psychological and social science studies to balance the biological research already in place.

Stanton's vision of a more distant future held the development of a comprehensive medical program and of outpatient psychiatric services at McLean and, vaguely, "the substantial unification" of the McLean and MGH services (7).

Altogether, this was the most comprehensive, visionary set of recommendations to reach a McLean Board of Trustees since the 1880s, when Cowles outlined his views of what the hospital should be. Stanton was not prepared to settle for halfway measures. As he noted in a later memo to Lindemann, "it must be emphasized that it leads somewhere. It would not be human to start a ferment going in a hospital and then lead it merely into a morass of generalities or wistful hopes that it would be nice if . . ." (8). Stanton knew too that his suggestions would be costly and stated that they could not be paid for merely by income from patients. However, except for offering strategies for expanding the psychiatric staff, Stanton did not address the problems of finance.

Lindemann supported Stanton's views, as did Harry Solomon, ranking professor of psychiatry at Harvard Medical School and medical director of Boston Psychopathic Hospital, whose thoughts had been solicited by Ralph Lowell, by then chairman of the trustees' McLean Committee. Beginning with the general principle that "the McLean Hospital should stand first of all as a superb treatment center for the mentally ill, on a par if not superior to any other similar hospital in the country. This is not true at present," Solomon outlined a program very similar to Stanton's. In one respect he went even further, suggesting that the laboratory research under Folch's direction would be more properly located in the medical school, "thus freeing this fine building for work more closely related to the problems of the hospital." "The upgrading and development of the institution must be a continuing process," Solomon concluded. "It requires inspired leadership and great support from the Trustees. I believe that internal leadership will be well given by Dr. Stanton" (9).

The trustees accepted Stanton and his proposals for McLean. The Search Committee approved his nomination. The moment of hesitation in the otherwise smooth courtship came from Stanton's side. He paused to wonder whether he really wanted the political and executive chores that belong to modern institutional administrators. But the lure of a Harvard professorship dangled within his grasp. Lindemann, too, had had such qualms when offered the MGH position: As he later confessed to one of his colleagues, "one did not turn down a Harvard professorship lightly" (10). Like Lindemann, Stanton accepted.

Stanton arrived at McLean in October 1955 as psychiatrist-in-chief. He was, as well, associate professor of psychiatry with tenure at Harvard Medical School. Wood had another eight months as director, and while continuing to go through the motions of attending trustee meetings and representing McLean at various functions, he was a lame duck. Howard, who had labored so long with the stigma of "acting" before his various titles, stepped aside gracefully and accepted the designation of associate psychiatrist-in-chief. He was enthusiastic about Stanton's appointment and eager to work with him.

Stanton had been raised as a Quaker, and his religious background revealed itself as morality of a very high order. The staff at McLean immediately perceived him as a man of "tremendous integrity who had very high expectations, . . . somebody who believed the world could be improved—that one could, in fact, make a difference, and that it behooved us to make a difference in the lives and treatment of our patients" (11). One colleague referred to him as a "moral crusader disguised as a social scientist" (12). Such highly principled people seldom give lightly of friendship and confidence, and so it was with Stanton. At McLean he depended principally on an inner circle of people whom he drew tightly around himself, leaving those who fell outside its perimeter to consider him remote, even a little cold, yet worthy of their respect.

Stanton was a learned man who tended the garden of his mind thoughtfully. His discussions of cases were little masterpieces of nimble intellect. His intelligence enjoyed exercise, and people who knew how to read him could see the shadows of boredom cross his countenance when he got trapped by some long-winded, cliché-ridden presentation. His own propensity for laying out all sides and dilemmas of an issue, though stimulating at case conferences, was not conducive to administrative efficiency. He had a philosophical rather than an instrumental approach to problem solving. He had spent three and one-half years observing how the fallout from casually made decisions in the front office altered patients' behavior on the wards. That experience, coupled with a keen sense of the unpredictability of the long-range consequences of human actions, compelled him to careful consideration.

In the presence of good talk, Stanton was a first-rate listener. Benson Snyder, a psychiatrist (not at McLean) who lived three houses down the road in Wellesley Hills from the Stanton family, remembered how "Alfred" had listened to and encouraged his ideas for analyzing the psychological and social dynamics of a major university. Snyder's concepts jelled, and he wrote *The Hidden Curriculum*. He also remembered Alfred as a warm friend and a good sailing companion.

Stanton the inner man was very hard to reach. He was a complicated person with interior hiding spaces. Anecdotes about him do not always fill in the picture, but sit off to one side like pieces from a jigsaw puzzle that have somehow strayed into the wrong box. Yet certain constants run through all descriptions: intellectual honesty, democratic instincts, the capacity to evoke strong—if not always positive—feelings in the people close to him, and patience and skill as a psychiatrist. He loved clinical work, being on the wards, and working with patients.

Stanton rejected a straightforward medical model of mental illness in favor of a concept of multiple etiology which he explained as follows:

> Overcrowding is a predisposing cause of plague, but the organism is the specific cause; if there is no specific cause, there will be no plague. The concept of multiple etiology is different. Here the notion is that the illness occurs if and only if two or more agents are active; both (or all) are necessary conditions for the illness. It requires both the infective agent, and the host susceptibility for infectious diseases to exist. Remove either and the condition is controlled. Now in psychiatry we have reason to believe that not only does this latter condition pertain, but an even more promising one may be true—that the multiple agents need to be continuously active. If this proves to be the case, the situation will be like that of a table—cut off any one of the legs and the table falls. It is aside from the point to argue that one or the other leg of the table is the "true cause" or the most "basic" or "deep" or "fundamental." . . . Those who have worked with grossly psychotic patients in intensive psychotherapy, while they may disagree on almost everything, seem to me to agree that it is frequent that patients may—in the middle reaches of treatment—become acutely and grossly psychotic as a response to something the therapist said or did, something which is sometimes rapidly identifiable, with a rapid subsidence of the gross psychotic reaction. Under such circumstances it is tempting to think of the word "schizophrenia" as a transitive verb with the therapist as an object. . . .

> A second point is allied to this first one: if illness is a more or less continuous construction, so are activities characteristic of health.

Stanton viewed the psychotherapist's obligation as supporting the "intact area of function" in the patient's personality by defining a respectable role for the patient. "Like other roles in our social order, it contains advantages and obligations; like many other roles it is defined as a transient role rather than a way of life" (13). As the word "transient" implied, Stanton did not accept the premise of chronicity in any mental disease category. He interpreted the fact that some mental patients became chronic as a failure in the treatment program rather than an unavoidable course of illness.

With respect to schizophrenia, Stanton's primary interest, his views put him in direct opposition to Kraepelin's turn-of-the-century description of the disease and at odds with Freud's pessimism regarding its treatment. Stanton's understanding of mental illness and of the relationship between patient and psychiatrist came directly from Sullivan. Though interested in the biological aspects of disease and respectful of the investigations of basic researchers, he believed, along with many of his peers at the time, that intervention at the psychological and sociological levels held greater promise for patients than medicines. Drugs might be helpful in making a patient receptive to psychotherapy, but he preferred not to use them until all alternative avenues had been explored and resulted in dead ends.

The originality of Stanton's thinking and his legacy to the field of psychiatry lay in his refinement of the concept of patients as social beings temporarily residing in the specific subculture, or ecosystem, of the mental hospital. His ecological perspective addressed contextual complexity, the interdependence of people and their surroundings, and the possible consequences of changes in the environment on its inhabitants. The view illuminated the specific adaptations made by individuals to the constraints imposed by the environment. Every element of the ecosystem had therapeutic or pathologic potential.

Stanton's ideal hospital was a therapeutic community in which social exchanges and activities reinforced the psychotherapist's support of the healthy aspects of the patient's personality. The general hospital model could not serve this purpose. "We have all learned, I hope, to be skeptical of the assumption that the best model for a psychiatric hospital is the general hospital," he observed. General hospital medicine attended to disease elements and left the healthy systems to themselves. A person entering a general hospital surrendered to the role of "sick patient," a role which Stanton saw as damaging to mental patients because it perpetuated the psychological constructions of illness. One notes with interest that Stanton's arguments against the general hospital model were in precise opposition to Cowles's logic in favor of it: Cowles had believed the "sick patient" role gave the patient hope by implying a return to health; Stanton contended that the role exacerbated the symptoms of disease.

Stanton's recognition of the complexity of the social context had disadvantages of which he was fully aware. "The ideal institutional treatment, then, will probably be somewhat different for every patient, and the ideal institution is likely to be different for different types of patients" (14). He further acknowledged that psychiatry had little experience and research data to apply with confidence to such a design. The development of a therapeutic milieu in an institution the size of McLean suggested intensity of observation, communications networks, coordination, and fine tuning on a sophisticated level. Nevertheless, Stanton was determined to try.

Stanton's first appointment to the McLean staff was a social worker to communicate with patients' families and help with discharge planning. He then moved quickly to build up the psychiatric staff by introducing a fee-for-service system which permitted psychiatrists to get paid for psychotherapy on an hourly basis. This meant that McLean patients were charged for their therapy sessions over and above the weekly rate, a practice which was working successfully in other private hospitals. It also meant that McLean could attract psychiatrists who did not have to work for the slave wages of yore. Stanton managed to persuade a couple of psychiatrists who had worked with him at the VA to transfer to McLean. One of them remembered his introduction to McLean as a kind of cultural shock. Accustomed to working with ex-soldiers in a veterans' hospital, he was unprepared for the luxury of the place, the upper-class social attitudes of patients and their families, and the sense of resignation among the patients which reflected the custodial role into which McLean had lapsed. Most of all he was startled by the number of presumed chronics, those people remarked upon earlier who were simply not expected to get well. He, like Stanton, believed many of those patients to be capable of regaining a measurable degree of mental health and returning to the community.

Stanton also began expanding the Psychology Department and using psychologists as therapists over the objections of those psychiatrists who held fast to the position that only certified physician-psychiatrists ought to be treating patients. Stanton prevailed and set up a system which allowed psychologists to do therapy with a psychiatrist responsible for the overall treatment program. The establishment of a clinical psychology program had pragmatic advantages because it put McLean in a competitive position for social and behavioral science grant monies which were becoming available. The American Psychological Association would not give training accreditation to a department which did not offer training in therapy, and grantors were reluctant to give research funds to unaccredited programs. Stanton, desperate for ways to supplement his budget, prodded his staff to apply for grants. Meanwhile, the appointment of two social anthropologists constituted the embryo of a Social Science Department and represented Stanton's effort to launch his "serious research program."

The numerical increase in McLean's professional staff during the first five years of Stanton's tenure was phenomenal: The Psychiatry Department increased from 13 to 62 (including all full- and part-time active staff; note that the number of residents jumped from two to 20). The Psychology Department went from one to seven; the Social Work Department went from zero to seven; and biological research gained a few people. Other departments such as nursing, activities therapies, and medicine remained approximately the same in size.

These numbers do not even begin to describe the changes in the clinical program. First, Stanton effectively redefined psychotherapy at McLean. "He expected that all patients admitted to McLean would, in fact, receive psychotherapy," de Marneffe remembered,

> and psychotherapy was very rigorously defined as sitting down with the patient in an appropriate setting, such as an office, and conducting psychotherapy for 50 minutes two, three, or four times a week. It had to be scheduled. . . . This was different from what it had been when, in the course of making rounds, we as psychiatrists or residents had sat down for 15 or 20 minutes with a patient to talk about what he or she was doing. At the time we had called *that* psychotherapy, but under the Stanton regime it certainly would not have been considered adequate. (15)

Most patients received some type of drug therapy prior to or in tandem with psychotherapy. Shock treatments were practically nonexistent; only ECT was still administered occasionally, on the order of two or three patients a year. Lobotomies were no longer performed. A number of patients were in group therapy in addition to private sessions with their psychiatrists or psychologists.

Equally significant to Stanton's way of thinking were what he called "the changes in the warp and woof of hospital procedures" in line with his concepts of milieu therapy. A system of clinical treatment was put in place in an effort to ensure continuity of care for the patient, along with good communications among all staff members involved with that patient. A staff psychiatrist administered each case, worked up the newly admitted patient, arrived at a diagnosis and therapeutic plan, supervised and worked with the nurses, psychologist, and social worker, and arranged for laboratory studies and psychotherapy with another person; the staff psychiatrist also managed the resident assigned to his ward and conducted weekly meetings of ward personnel.

Visiting hours, previously a few hours a day, were extended from 10 A.M. to 10 P.M., seven days a week. Psychiatrists prescribed liberties to leave the ward or the grounds much more liberally and with much less red tape than previously. (Stanton had an allergic reaction to the buzzword "privileges" as applied to freedom to visit the grounds or the town. He used to say that the mental hospital was the only place he knew where fundamental constitutional rights were referred to as "privileges.") Telephones were installed on the wards, and patients were permitted to carry small sums of money, to shop for other patients, and to visit other wards. Patient organizations and hall meetings became more animated, and there were more evening activities—movies, music, talent shows, and so forth. A small day-care program was started, initially for discharged patients, with the expectation that it would eventually expand services and accept non-McLean patients. A volunteer group was organized. For a couple of years, patients were occasionally permitted to keep caged pets in their rooms; this, however, proved to be a bit too much. "Yeah," recalled one staff member, "for a while there we tried everything!"

No aspect of the patient's existence at McLean was considered trivial. Stanton offered an example of how the alteration of a small detail, coupled with insight into a patient's residual competencies, altered the clinical course for one man:

> Mr. R. had watched television intently from a point about four feet from the screen most of the time for years. He had been chronically schizophrenic for many years, and was glued to the television both by his own routine inclination and by a belief among the nurses that many years ago he had thrown an aide out the window. Dr. [X], noting that someone always turned the set on for him, turned it off, indicated that he would have to turn it on himself from now on if he wanted to look at the television. Although thoroughly angry, Mr. R. from that time on turned on the television set. In the course of his protests, Dr. [X] (who had taken the trouble to know that decades ago Mr. R. had completed a college major in meteorology), asked Mr. R.—who never talked to anyone except to the nurse on routine matters—whether he would take the responsibility for posting weather predictions daily for the ward. Mr. R. answered for a month that he wouldn't say yes and he wouldn't say no. He then consented. A few weeks later, he was elected secretary of the ward meeting and, later, delegate to the central patients' committee, submitting with agonizing concern a short, clear written report of the meeting to his own ward group. A student nurse, active in this program, had to leave the ward on rotation, and Mr. R. turned later to his physician and told of missing her, with tears in his eyes and an appropriate emotion. Only a few weeks before, no one living had ever seen any emotion other than the irritation characteristic of blocked feelings. (16)

The observation that milieu therapy was moral treatment in modern costume would hardly be original. The Joint Commission on Mental Illness and Health wrote that:

> To Pinel's principles for the treatment of psychotics twentieth-century psychiatry can add little, except to convert them into modern terminological dress, contribute more systematic thought on the significance of various symptoms, intensify the doctor-patient relationship through scientific knowledge of psychological mechanisms, treat the patient as a

> member of a social group which expects him to behave in accepted ways. . . . (17)

J. Sanbourne Bockoven noted in 1956 that "It is . . . a little humiliating to realize that modern psychiatry is fast approaching a point of view similar to that of moral treatment as it was practiced by the founders of the American Psychiatric Association well over one hundred years ago" (18).

Stanton's remarks about supporting the intact area of the patient's function echoed Wyman's 1822 annual report, in which he described the asylum's rules, regulations, and diversions as "breaking up wrong associations of ideas, and inducing correct habits of thinking as well as acting." Yet comparing moral treatment to milieu therapy is a little like comparing a Model-T Ford with a new Mercedes. In the intent to design an environment in which mentally ill people might get well (a project in social engineering), Stanton benefited from a century and a half of experience as well as a more sophisticated model of human behavior. He had drugs to dispel hallucinations and becalm the excited; he did not have to strap them into chairs. The staff worked hard to reach withdrawn people, to help them regain social skills, and to prevent them from becoming dependent on the hospital. Sometimes the therapeutic design succeeded. Sometimes it failed.

Statistical comparisons between vintage Wyman moral treatment and milieu therapy are impossible with reference to results. Aside from the problems raised by the mismanagement of numbers in the early nineteenth century, there are too many variables and unknowns to allow for confident measurement. Even the statistical data published in Stanton's annual reports make for slippery footing. Judgments concerning degrees of improvement were still subjective; one may well wonder, for instance, what distinguished "moderate" from "slight" improvement. Extremely low estimates of "recovery"—only 13 of 346 patients discharged in 1960, for example—were in some part a product of a policy whereby patients were discharged as early as the psychiatrist-administrator believed they could negotiate the community; the patients were expected to improve further by continuing psychotherapy on an outpatient basis.

Other figures showing a more rapid rate of turnover during Stanton's tenure than during Wood's reflected changes in the composition of the patient population.

Early in Stanton's administration, the Social Work Department evaluated all McLean's chronic patients and recommended moving many who could not be helped and were carried on the books at reduced rates to nursing homes or some other facility so as to make room for patients who could pay and would be more susceptible to treatment. Figures from 1955 give some idea of the magnitude of the financial problem: The hospital's cost per patient per week was calculated at $140; the *average* weekly charge was $126 (19). Stanton reacted uncomfortably to the suggestion, especially as it pertained to individuals in frail physical health. Though he accepted the logic of the argument, he executed it reluctantly. From time to time, he intervened to rescue some long-term patient from a nursing home. Nevertheless, during 1956 and 1957, a total of 46 patients diagnosed as suffering chronic brain disorders were discharged from the hospital; of that number, 35 were prey to "disorders of late life." The passage in 1956 of an amendment to the Social Security Act providing more aid to states to support the elderly in nursing homes made this discharge policy somewhat more palatable to Stanton, though he never was at ease with it.

Meanwhile, McLean began admitting younger patients. The admissions office was receiving more and more application forms on behalf of adolescents, and though poorly prepared to receive them, the staff nevertheless chose to take them in. This squared with the conscious effort to reverse the trend towards a custodial role in favor of a higher rate of successful treatment and turnover. One of the few principles that psychiatrists had agreed upon since the early nineteenth century was that the patients most likely to profit from therapy were those suffering first attacks of mental illness, people in whom the patterns of disordered thought and behavior had not been so deeply engraved as to resist all attempts to modify them.

As the percentage of patients over the age of 60 dropped from more than 50 percent in 1952 to 43 percent in 1957 and to 32 percent in 1960, the number of adolescents admitted climbed. In 1952 there had been a few adolescents scattered about

McLean's wards; in 1960 individuals under the age of 20 accounted for 15 percent of all admissions (49), and this trend accelerated during the 1960s. It was coupled with an explicit policy of encouraging the admission of the "sickest available patients" (20). Seriously ill schizophrenics composed an increasingly sizable fraction of the population.

It bears noting that—along with staffing-up, changes in clinical and administrative procedures, and the gradual transformation of the patient population that occurred during the first five or six years of Stanton's administration—the education program was overhauled. Structured training was introduced for medical students and residents in lieu of the old throw-'em-in-the-water-and-see-if-they-can-swim form of apprenticeship. An increasingly liberal supply of NIMH training grants, Stanton's personal reputation, and rumors that the McLean program had improved attracted more applicants. But the anticipated coordination with the MGH residency program did not materialize. As John Nemiah, who was then running the MGH training program, wrote diplomatically, "the joint program, though well coordinated on paper, was perhaps less successfully implemented in practice owing to the ten miles of city traffic that separated the two institutions and to an equally inhibiting distance in ideologies and practice" (21). Stanton's even more polite reference to the "tyranny of geography" dodged the central issue altogether; namely, a prevailing opinion at MGH that McLean's approach to mental illness was too psychoanalytic. After a while MGH took to sending its residents to the state institution at Danvers for their exposure to patients with prolonged mental illness. Geographical piffle: Danvers was more than three times the distance to Belmont. McLean, meanwhile, rotated its residents to the Beth Israel Hospital, the Peter Bent Brigham Hospital, and the Boston VA.

Overall the program that Stanton developed for McLean resembled the Joint Commission's recommendations for the institutional care of seriously ill mental patients:

> The most important requirement for an intensive treatment center is a well-trained and competent staff at least as large as the number of patients served. This staff should have a good-sized complement of skilled psychiatrists who know how to work comfortably with a clinical team

> including a variety of professional and subprofessional persons who can assist them in the treatment of patients. Such workers would include occupational, recreational, and physical therapists as well as psychologists, social workers, nurses and attendants.
>
> . . . The psychological atmosphere of the ward in which the patient is to live during the period of treatment must be carefully scrutinized and properly organized in a way that at once offers the protection he needs and yet provides a gentle but firm stimulus toward resynthesis of his personality and his progress toward independent existence. (22)

That this and other recommendations concerning inpatient treatment conformed to the program Stanton was trying to put in place at McLean was not very surprising in view of the fact that the commission had retained Stanton's one-time coauthor, Morris Schwartz, to undertake the survey of patient care for the report.

The Joint Commission's opinion represented the progressive elements of mainstream psychiatry, circa 1960. By the time its findings were off the presses, the process of fermentation Stanton had started at McLean was sufficiently advanced to restore its reputation as one of the institutions in the country that might serve as a model for inpatient care.

Stanton's program placed certain strains upon McLean. One of the most obvious of them, at least to the trustees, was the accumulation of the hospital's deficit at a nerve-shattering rate. The word "deficit" may have some readers shifting uneasily in their chairs and flexing their minds to leap over some boring paragraphs in anticipation of prose drier than dust. But an important issue is at stake: There is a perceptible relationship between the organization of psychiatric practice and how it is paid for. Money is a necessary, if not sufficient, explanation of McLean's modern configuration. Though this relationship existed in some measure throughout McLean's history, it achieved great importance after World War II. Also, while similar observations have been made about all of medicine—see, for example, Paul Starr's *The Social Transformation of American Medicine*—the financial dynamics related to psychiatry had certain variations, such as the limitations of third-party payments and the involvement of public monies in state institutions.

The onset of the modern deficit at McLean, as distinguished from Cowles's deficit at the turn of the century, predated Stanton. Even with the parsimonious practices of Wood's administration, hospital expenses began to outrun receipts in 1952. The fiscal year ending September 30, 1955, showed a net deficit of $132,600. The simple explanations for such sadly unbalanced ledgers were two: increased wages for employees plus the high cost of maintaining a decrepit physical plant on the one hand and, on the other, the large numbers of patients carried at reduced rates. The trustees hoped that Stanton's program, with its goal of preventing chronicity and producing a more rapid turnover of patients, would eliminate the merciful but costly practice of reduced charges and balance the books.

The trustees believed McLean ought to be able to manage, if not turn a profit, on the income from patients. This expectation—confirmed by George Putnam, the current McLean trustee—had deep roots in the original rules of admission to the asylum, wherein it had been stated that "compensation will be demanded for the board of all patients, . . ." a regulation which could be enforced because of the law that made the towns responsible for the indigent insane within their precincts. Thus, such paupers as were admitted during McLean's early years had their charges paid by townships.

Later, the development of the state mental hospital system funneled off publicly supported patients, leaving McLean with private paying patients. In theory, then, the hospital ought to have supported itself and did so for extended periods, from the 1840s to the 1880s, for example, as well as many years during the 1920s, 1930s, and late 1940s. The custom of subsidizing some patients at reduced rates also had historical antecedents dating back to the sliding fee scale and the Appleton fund. Its perpetuation in a postwar economy of soaring medical costs was economically, if not morally, unsound. The general hospital, by contrast, had always accepted charity patients, had provisions for free beds, and ran a regular deficit. But MGH was endowed, circa 1961, to the tune of about $20 million, a time when McLean's endowment stood at around half a million.

As Stanton had warned in his initial survey, McLean could not run, let alone implement the programs he outlined, on patients' revenues alone. Between 1956 and 1961, the annual budget jumped from approximately $2 million to $3.1 million, with hearty deficits in each year. Though McLean acquired some funds in the form of research and training grants, no stable source of income was secured. In fiscal 1960 the net deficit came in at $144,500. In an attempt to offset it, the trustees raised the basic room and board rate from $30 to $38 per day. That translated into $13,870 per year without psychotherapy at a time when $10,000 was considered a decent annual income. (The lowliest McLean employee, paid at the minimum wage rate of $1.15, would have earned $46 a week or about $2,400 a year.) During the same year, the hospital occupancy rate fell off by 8 percent from 1959 to 79 percent, a low census which Stanton attributed to the more frequent use of day-care and outpatient services by discharged patients who previously would have stayed longer in the hospital. But, he admitted, "The census is subject to unpredictable and terrifying swings" (23).

Meanwhile, McLean was still carrying more than $350,000 in free room and care, not for theoretically untreatable patients, as in the past, but usually in cases "where a longer period of treatment is required than had been anticipated in the relatively hurried appraisal at the time of admission" (24). Note that by this time Blue Cross was covering "nervous and mental disorders" at the rate of $12 per day for up to 60 days of hospitalization (25).

Financial difficulties posed serious obstacles to Stanton's ambitions for establishing social and behavioral science research at McLean. Folch, Pope, and their colleagues in the scientific research laboratories continued to raise grant money successfully, but social science initiatives did not attract funds as anticipated. Stanton observed that the criteria for methodological soundness in the behavioral sciences were controversial even within disciplinary boundaries, that grant applications got turned down at a rate of about 60 percent, and that McLean kept losing senior social scientists practiced in research development to more secure niches in academia.

A good deal of behavioral and social science research went on at McLean without any support at all, a situation that said a great deal about the dedication and intellectual curiosity of the researchers, as well as about Stanton's ability to attract kindred spirits. But the number, range, and scale of these efforts fell well below Stanton's definition of a serious research program. On the whole, it seems he had overestimated the potential for outside funding, as well as the trustees' ability to dredge up other means of support. So the deficits continued to grow, and by the end of 1961 the trustees were staring at 10 straight years of red ink on the McLean books.

Given Stanton's priorities, the magnitude of the task he set for himself at McLean, and the financial difficulties that littered his path, it is not surprising that he began to feel restive about five years into his administration. In December 1960, Willis Bower gave notice of his intention to accept a position as superintendent of the Colorado State Hospital in Pueblo. By that time Bower had become Stanton's general-purpose right-hand man, acting as a cross between clinical coordinator and administrative aide, with no special title. In effect he had the best grasp of institutional organization of anyone on the staff. Stanton, who had relied heavily on Bower's administrative talents, asked Francis de Marneffe, then clinical administrator for Codman House I, to assume his role. Stanton's choice surprised a number of people on the staff, but none more so than de Marneffe himself, for he had never belonged to Stanton's entourage. The immediate point of this story, however, lies in Stanton's caveat to de Marneffe that a decision to accept Bower's duties amounted to a de facto choice of an administrative rather than an academic career (26).

The warning revealed a big part of Stanton's personal frustration. He could feel administration consuming more and more of his energies. He had not accomplished any genuine research since his arrival at McLean. At age 47, he was stuck on the academic ladder at the rung of associate professor. The contrasts between his own career and Lindemann's did not elude his attention. Whereas Stanton was mired in administration, Lindemann managed to escape his office and devote much of his time to community-oriented research, leaving the mechanics of the MGH Psychiatry Service largely in the hands of subalterns. Thus, Stanton's message to de Marneffe originated in his own discovery that a man could not expect to do both, at least when the institution to be administered was as complicated as McLean. (Many scholars, in and out of medicine, have found themselves wriggling in some administrative trap. Modern institutional dynamics have made the scholar/manager an endangered species. No doubt a few representatives survive, but they are hard to sight, harder to capture, and have never been known to breed in captivity.) de Marneffe did not share Stanton's qualms about administration. He had found his limited experience of it enjoyable and accepted Bower's obligations with pleasure.

Unknown to de Marneffe, Stanton had notified Ralph Lowell by letter, in September 1960, that he wished to shift back to research. He had asked to be relieved of all administrative responsibilities by the summer of 1962. He permitted himself to be advanced as a candidate for a professorship sponsored by the Foundation Fund for Research in Psychiatry, hoping that the chair would be given to Harvard and that he would become its occupant.

When he learned in the spring of 1961 that the decision had gone elsewhere, Stanton was devastated. He confided to Lindemann that he felt more agitated than he could remember in his "grown up life." "I have worked in various hospitals, done administrative work which I hated, given up most of my clinical work which I love, in the interest of a distant goal—having a hospital in which the type of research in which I am interested could be done." Stanton was driven further to despair by a series of negative decisions by the National Science Foundation and NIMH on social science research proposals originating from McLean. "This series of interrelated (?) body blows have just about terminated the social science program of research at McLean," he noted (27). Crushed, Stanton signaled the trustees that if an attractive research position came up somewhere else, he would take it. But whether he left McLean or stayed in a redefined role, the institution was due for another shuffle of the administrative deck.

In the fall of 1961, the trustees dispatched young John Knowles to Belmont to size up the situation and suggest what steps might be taken to rectify the financial picture while providing for an orderly administrative transition. Knowles had just been appointed director for medical affairs at MGH and stood first in line to inherit the vacant general director's position. The trustees may have been testing him by seeing what he would do with McLean. Knowles, who had a quick mind and the benefit of a first-rate administrative assistant, made fast work of his assignment. Instead of issuing a back-breaking document, he compressed his recommendations into four and one-half pages. He identified McLean's financial problem as primarily one of a declining inpatient census, recommended some short-term "realistic economies," made some suggestions for increasing the admissions rate, and advised increasing the day-care rate while extending outpatient services to non-McLean patients. There was nothing particularly novel in any of that.

Knowles had studied the report of the Joint Commission on Mental Illness and Health. It was, after all, the most authoritative and current overview of psychiatry in circulation. Accordingly, he endorsed the clinical course that Stanton had set for McLean and his advice aimed at preserving that direction and insuring continuity. According to his version, "Dr. Stanton would delegate the necessary authority and power to Dr. de Marneffe as Director of Clinical Service and Mr. Prekup as Administrator . . . they would cover these two areas of the hospital between them, reporting ultimately to Dr. Stanton and the various McLean Committees. . . ." This division of labor would liberate Stanton for research, an idea which Knowles appeared to favor, or in the event of Stanton's departure provide for stable governance (28).

In the midst of these discussions about administrative restructuring, McLean experienced an unusually high number of suicides. During an eight-month period between September 1961 and March 1962, six patients succeeded in taking their own lives. There had, in fact, been a total of 12 suicides since 1957, but the last six had occurred at an alarming rate. By contrast, though there had been several attempts, there had been no accomplished suicides from 1950 to 1957 or from 1944 to 1949; one had to reach back to 1929 to discover a comparable incidence: eight deaths between 1929 and 1932. In March 1962, Stanton ordered a review of all the suicides during his administration in an attempt to prevent further deaths.

Since so many patients in the care of a mental hospital have suicidal ideas, a suicide is dangerous because it may encourage them, and each successful attempt increases the likelihood of others. The phenomenon of clusters of suicides had been remarked upon both in other institutions and in society. A rash of suicides such as broke out at McLean in 1961–62 upsets the patients. In a profound way it demoralizes the staff, from psychiatrists on down to mental health workers. When a young resident killed himself later in the spring of 1962, though no straight line could be drawn between his death and the previous patient suicides, many of the staff instinctively read his action as a barometer of the hospital's mood. If anxiety could have been isolated and quantified like Folch's lipids, it would have been measured in unusual amounts among the McLean staff during the spring of 1962. They were depressed by the suicides and concerned about impending administrative changes. Stanton by then had indicated his intention to stay in Belmont, but it was not clear what his role would be.

The trustees' decision finally turned out to be a variation on Knowles's suggestion. As of July 1, 1962, there was to be a new order: Stanton would remain as psychiatrist-in-chief but he would delegate patient care responsibilities to an as-yet-unnamed director of clinical psychiatry. de Marneffe would hold the title of director of hospital affairs. He would act as the chief executive officer responsible for developing and recommending policy and for the coordination of McLean's several departments; he reported directly to the trustees and he carried the hospital's license to operate.

On paper the changes did not appear to make too much difference. Stanton would continue to set clinical policy and the new clinical director would report to him. de Marneffe, it seemed, had acquired a title and more formal authority to carry out the responsibilities he had inherited from Bower. That the shift in power had been something more than superficial became evident in December when de Marneffe moved into what had always been the principal office on the ground floor of the administration building. The trustees officially appointed him director in January 1963. The administrative restructuring upset some of the staff, especially people close to Stanton who had been unprepared for the change and some of whom felt abandoned. But the shock wave subsided; most of the staff adapted; and people went back to the difficult business of hospital psychiatry.

CHAPTER

11

McLean in the Age of Aquarius

Trying to tell the story of any institution during the 1960s without reference to political and social turbulence would be like describing the U.S. economy in the 1970s without mentioning Arab oil. A few banks and insurance companies may have succeeded in insulating themselves against the blustery weather of the decade, but universities, hospitals, government agencies, manufacturers of consumer products, churches, and other organizations whose viability depends on public perception had to pay attention. The weather was particularly inclement in the Boston area, which held an irregularly high concentration of youth because of its numerous colleges and universities.

In the early sixties the young people—well, *most* of them were young—joined the crusade against racial discrimination in the South, then turned their attention to the war in Vietnam, and eventually challenged just about every form of conventional authority that fell in their path. Some of their targets were poorly selected. Some of their information was inadequate or wrong. Some of their actions, in contradiction to their slogans, were violent. Some of their causes were silly. Yet, however flawed, the activist movements of the sixties stimulated reflection about social conformations and rules that had been taken for granted for decades.

Institutions, insofar as they can be said to "think," reexamined themselves and their social missions. To some extent program developments at McLean during the sixties reflected the ferment in the social context. To pass them off merely as consequences of treatment concepts or of financial determinants would oversimplify the forces which acted on the hospital. The opening of an Out Patient Clinic with below-standard fees was one example of McLean's attempt to engage changing values by extending services to classes of citizens it had neglected for generations.

The revisionist spirit of the sixties seized the psychiatric profession and produced some heretical theories. Scottish psychiatrist R. D. Laing explained poetically that schizophrenia was not a disease at all but an appropriate adaptation of highly sensitive individuals to an insane environment. Thomas Szasz rejected the medical model of mental illness and argued that psychiatric problems were expressions of difficulties of living rather than illnesses. Freud took some hard knocks, notably from feminists who protested his theory of penis envy. In 1968 Szasz proclaimed psychoanalysis "as moribund and irrelevant as the Liberal party in England" (1). French historian Michel Foucault attracted attention when he wrote *Madness and Civilization* in 1965, a book which identified psychiatrists and mental institutions as agents of authoritarian social systems, suppressing the free expression of the "mad" (2).

The sixties also witnessed the proliferation of unconventional ways of dealing with psychological discomforts, some of which mainline psychiatrists would have diagnosed as mental illnesses. Psychodrama, sensitivity training, and encounter therapy groups split off from standard psychiatric settings. Other modes were modeled on Alcoholics Anonymous or Oriental religions. People who would have consulted a psychiatrist in the 1950s went off in search of a guru in the sixties and became vegetarians. Transcendental meditation became fashionable and was run as a profitable business. The old Reichian orgone box was taken down from the shelf and dusted off. There were efflorescences of gestalt, nude, and primal scream therapies, as well as rolfing. Some of the treatments advertised during the sixties seemed to an observer with historical perspective to be twentieth-century rehashes of spiritualism or the flimflammery of the nineteenth century with its all-purpose tonics.

No matter how peculiar they appeared, these efforts to address psychological distress offered alternatives and competition to conventional psychiatry. Their enormous appeal during the sixties provided an indirect measure of popular dissatisfaction with orthodox treatment. By contrast, the attacks on medicine during the sixties were leveled at the institutions and organization of practice: the conservative American Medical Association, the vanishing family practitioner, the impersonality of the high-tech hospital, the unavailability of good medicine to the poor, high costs, and so forth. Long-haired hippies who broke their arms went, however sullenly, to the emergency ward. They did not try to set their shattered bones with extra portions of brewer's yeast.

Evidence that professional psychiatry could not speak in a unified voice confused the lay public. Sensational trials featuring impeccably credentialed psychiatrists delivering conflicting testimony concerning some defendant's sanity embarrassed the profession. (Orthopedists often did the same thing in courtrooms, as in "whiplash" cases, but the press did not pay much attention to such civil proceedings so the public did not become totally disenchanted with orthopedists.) Gadflies like Laing and Szasz, buzzing around the professional fringes, found sympathetic audiences because they wrote well and hit an exposed nerve.

There was also gathering unrest close to the heart of psychiatry, in academia. Remarking on arguments that raged for nearly three years around the selection of a successor to Erich Lindemann at the MGH Psychiatric Service, Leon Eisenberg—who emerged as the successful candidate—commented: "The debate about the schools of psychiatry was bitter and wearing. After all, a committee searching for a chief of Medicine doesn't have to decide among an allopath, a homeopath, a naturopath, or what have you; that nonsense was settled with the birth of scientific medicine in the last half of the nineteenth century" (3).

As the sixties drew to a close, the debate escalated around the question of just what constituted "scientific" psychiatry. Though all parties to the quarrel dignified the principle of science, they differed widely over the elements of that science.

Hard-core psychoanalysts trying to maintain professional dominance represented one extreme of the argument, a new generation of biologically oriented psychiatrists trying to gain legitimacy represented the other. As their altercation intensified, positions solidified, and harsh, irrational charges were exchanged. This political climate made life uncomfortable for the many psychiatrists who occupied the middle ground. Neither adversary offered them persuasive evidence to permit total commitment to either a purely psychosocial or a purely biochemical model of mental disorder.

Above all, however, the sixties belonged to youth and so in large measure did the history of McLean during the decade. The admission of increasing numbers of adolescents remarked upon in the last chapter continued. By 1967–68 admissions in the 13- to 20-year-old group ran at 32 percent, the largest of any single age group. By that time, nearly one-third of the patients were teenagers, a demographic fact that changed the character of the hospital.

McLean was one of the earliest institutions to welcome adolescents, but others followed suit within a few years. The abrupt appearance on the psychiatric scene of teenage patients raises the question: Where had they been before? They were not in mental hospitals, either public or private, in significant numbers before the 1960s. Past and present McLean staff members, as well as other psychiatrists, offered some conjectures. It was observed that adolescence, the period of transition between childhood and adulthood, is in some respects a modern phenomenon. In earlier centuries, children metamorphosed abruptly into grownups. The ancient Jewish ceremony of the bar mitzvah confers the responsibility of manhood upon the 13-year-old male, and the Christian rite of confirmation also symbolizes initiation into maturity. In her study of the Middle Ages, *A Distant Mirror*, Barbara Tuchman paused to alert readers to the extreme youth, by contemporary measures, of many of the key actors on the medieval stage. Romeo and Juliet were teenagers; the idea that they wished to marry (and become parents) did not shock Elizabethan audiences in the least. Closer in time, Luther Bell and some of the other founders of the American Psychiatric Association assumed mature duties at ages when men of our own generation are college undergraduates. Modern adolescence, by comparison, is a prolonged period which, in the view of some psychiatrists, generates special sets of psychological and sociological pressures which have created a new category of psychiatric casualties.

One observer, who was at McLean during the 1950s, 1960s, and 1970s, recalled that most of the teenage patients admitted to the hospital in the late 1950s had been in the throes of what is sometimes called "adolescent turmoil." They were the neighborhood troublemakers, the tire-slashing boys or the promiscuous girls who in an earlier generation would have been packed off to military academies or boarding schools with strict disciplinary codes. That, at least, would have been true for McLean patients who came from affluent families. Delinquent adolescents from less-advantaged homes had other destinies, such as reform school. The pathological profiles of McLean's adolescent patients changed during the sixties. They were more seriously ill; there were more potential suicides, schizophrenics, and drug abusers among them.

The ruptures in culture and family which marked post World War II America have been widely observed: the rising divorce rates, the mobile family (which, for children, means frequent changes of schools and friends), confused theories of parenting and, as the sixties progressed, the erosion of trust in traditional forms of authority. People who remember the upheavals of the sixties may also remember frequent references to "alienated" youth. Mental hospital statistics demonstrated that some young people were indeed alienated in the nineteenth-century medical sense of the word.

These various explanations of the sudden rise in adolescent patients overlap one another and hinge on the notion that widespread mental illness among teenagers is of recent vintage. One cannot quarrel with data that show adolescents constituting a far greater fraction of mental hospital population than ever before. However, there is evidence in the historical record to suggest a higher incidence of adolescent illness than contemporary psychiatrists suppose. Charles Folsom's *Mental Diseases*, published in 1886, shows people under the age of 20, including preteens, accounting for less than 10 percent of admissions to all Massachusetts asylums. But Folsom was well acquainted with the mental disorders of adolescence:

> In early life chiefly the degenerative or the hereditary type of insanity occurs, or some modification of it. The prevalent forms coming next are insanity of puberty and adolescence and the curious morbid psychological developments of lying, stealing, running away from home, all sorts of perversity of action and thought—impulse overpowering reason; often resulting in cure if wisely treated, but not seldom ending in various forms of so-called moral insanity, suicide, epilepsy, hysteria, primary insanity, prostitution, and offenses against the laws. It is largely a matter of accident rather that a result of any established principle whether such boys and girls are sent to reformatories and prisons or to insane asylums. (4)

The author thereby offered his opinion that mental hospital statistics did not accurately reflect the incidence of mental illness among teenagers.

A random reading of McLean's old case records substantiates Folsom's observations. The 18-year-old girl discussed by Hoch, Cowles, and colleagues during a case conference reported earlier in this book was said by her father to have suffered two attacks of illness prior to her admission to the hospital. Patient Number 7160, valedictorian of her high school graduating class and a brilliant freshman at Radcliffe, had isolated herself for four years in her home and in the secret life and language of her mind before her admission to McLean, in 1888, at the age of 21. Yet another young woman endured intermittent sieges of anorexia for seven years. Her weight dropped to 80 pounds and she nearly starved to death before her parents applied for help at McLean. These and other case histories, plus suggestive gaps in the biographical information on other patients, signal the probability of a greater frequency of serious mental illness among teenagers than revealed by admissions statistics. The answer to the question "where were they before?" implied by these old McLean case histories is "at home" with families for whom the idea of an asylum was horrifying under any circumstances, and unthinkable for a child. Eventually, drained of all hope and energy, they gave up and yielded the child, by then perhaps 20, to a mental institution.

It is, after all, difficult to demonstrate that the conditions of human existence are objectively worse (or better) now than in any other era. More than 2,000 years of Western literature (Sophocles, Dante, Blake, Hawthorne, Tolstoy, Dickinson, Yeats, and Gide, to name just a few, along with the venerable Shakespeare) plus the superb studies of recent generations of historians, particularly the French *annalistes* and American scholars such as Oscar Handlin, document the persistence of the struggle for human survival and dignity against all manner of obstacles. What is measurable is the impact of the birth rate on the demographic profile of post World War II America. The children of the "baby boom" became the adolescents of the sixties, and they made up a larger percentage of the total population than ever before. Yet even this fact does not adequately account for their even sharper rise as a percentage of psychiatric patients.

One additional observation helps fill out the explanation. It was noted that families who had once considered their troublesome children disciplinary problems, going through a stage they would outgrow, shifted their concept of what might be wrong with their children and began applying for medical, rather than educational or law enforcement, assistance. At the same time, society's expectations of appropriate behavior in adolescents underwent some changes.

McLean had never discriminated against adolescents, and the moments in its history when there were no teenagers in residence were rare and accidental. Since youngsters were so few in number, no special provisions had been made for them. They received the same accommodations and treatment as their adult counterparts. By 1959, however, the youth population was of sufficient mass to challenge the hospital's collective ingenuity. It had become evident that the time-honored occupational and recreational activities—pottery classes and softball, for example—did not adequately engage the kids' attention between psychotherapeutic encounters. Furthermore, many of the patients, nearly all of their parents, and the McLean staff were concerned about the interruption in education. Several weeks or months of hospitalization might set a teenager back a year in school. The social workers, prodded by anxious families, were stretched thin trying to arrange private tutoring sessions, the results of which were more often unsatisfactory than not. In 1959 the superintendent of the Belmont school system agreed to accept McLean patients in his public schools if they could attend full time. A few tried. They all failed.

Frustrated by the miscarriage of the Belmont experiment and concerned for the patients, various staff members persuaded Stanton that McLean should develop its own educational program so that adolescents could get on with their natural work of schooling. Since there were no educational experts on the staff, McLean directed inquiries to the Department of Education at Boston University and the Harvard Graduate School of Education, which supplied programmatic assistance. These events transpired as de Marneffe was assuming Bower's responsibilities, and development of the school was his first big administrative assignment.

By September 1961, the hospital opened a high school in Arlington House, an empty building on its grounds. The school had one full-time teacher, several part-time teachers, and 15 students. Arrangements were made with the Belmont school system so that the students could receive academic credit for completed course work. While trying to maintain as much of a regular pedagogic atmosphere as possible, the school's program and structure acknowledged the special needs of the students, most of whom had had severe academic and social difficulties in ordinary public or private schools.

The Arlington School flourished. In 1966 it was able to open its classrooms to non-McLean adolescent patients being treated in the Out Patient Clinic when the State Department of Education extended financial support under Chapter 750 of the Public Law. By 1968 the Arlington School had a full-time faculty of nine, six part-time teachers, a librarian, and support personnel; 55 patients were enrolled in the full program. McLean tapped the rich pool of artistic and academic talent in the Boston area and found writers, scholars, and musicians willing to volunteer for special programs: Novelists talked about writing; a Boston preclassical music group performed a recital of Renaissance songs and dances; a high-tech scientist gave a lecture-demonstration of the NASA spacemobile. The Arlington School offered courses in "urban studies" and "scientific models," materials which did not usually show up in ordinary curricula. In June

1968 the school held its third commencement and awarded high school diplomas to 10 students. In 1970 it was accredited by the New England Association of Schools and Colleges. It continues to thrive today and has added college-level courses to its curriculum.

The Arlington School could not be mistaken for a regular school, but for many of its pupils it worked better. As one of its grateful graduates put it, "We didn't have that jive nothingness that pushes most kids through high school. You can't tell a whole bunch of potential suicides that they must have a high school diploma."

The school was McLean's most original development on behalf of its adolescents. There were others: The Activities Therapy Department, which administratively combined occupational and recreational therapies, organized a youth group, staged "happenings," and arranged other events geared to teenagers. Adolescents participated in work programs—as receptionists or painters, for instance—at the hospital. Music therapy, a long McLean tradition, changed its tune from string quartets and jazz to the pop/rock and folk beats of the sixties. When the influx of youth began in the late 1950s, psychiatrists who could claim expertise in the treatment of adolescent disorders were scarce. McLean established a training program and received NIMH support for a residency in adolescent psychiatry. Teenagers prompted the initiation of family therapy. The Social Work Department expanded enormously in response to the large adolescent population and the intense demands of families for assistance in discharge planning.

There was at least one programmatic casualty along the way. The Patient-Personnel Conference fell into disarray and was discontinued toward the end of the sixties. Like their peers in the outside world, McLean's teenage patients were too anarchic in spirit and too impatient for change to endure "establishment" dialogue. They needed to invent their own forms of expression, and the hospital tried to provide ways they might do so. It also bears noting that as the number of adolescent patients increased, so did the incidence of "burnout" in the nursing staff, particularly among young nurses prone to identify with their youthful patients.

Affluent, rebellious local adolescents sometimes referred to McLean as the "Alcatraz of the East," but by the mid to late sixties, the hospital had acquired a first-rate national reputation for the treatment of adolescent disorders. A psychiatrist in Houston, Texas, Shervert Frazier, confidently referred a very sick young patient there. He observed that the hospital had done an excellent job with her.

The reasonable speed with which McLean came to grips with the needs of its new class of patients suggests that the redesigned administrative apparatus set in motion in the summer of 1962 acted with efficiency. Stanton willingly relinquished his executive responsibilities. He kept the title of psychiatrist-in-chief and continued to set the overall clinical policies of the hospital, but was busy incubating research projects. The dependable Howard administered the treatment program until someone could be found to fill the new position of director of clinical psychiatry.

de Marneffe settled into the director's quarters. Born in Belgium in 1924, de Marneffe had escaped his native country in 1940 on the order of the government, which evacuated all young males after the Nazi invasion so as to avoid their being conscripted or sent to labor camps by the Germans. He made his way to relatives in Oxfordshire, finished schooling in England, started medical studies at Kings College in London, interrupted his professional education to sign up with the Royal Air Force, and completed his medical degree at Westminster Medical School in 1950. He then set off on a voyage of self-discovery in North America. After some intellectual uncertainty and thousands of miles of wandering, he wound up in Boston as a resident on Cobb's service at MGH in January 1952. The chief resident then was Peter Sifneos, who had done two years of residency at McLean and whose accounts of the institution attracted de Marneffe. He decided to complete his training in Belmont. He arrived there in January 1953 and was assigned to spartan living quarters on the second floor of the administration building. A decade later, he had graduated downstairs to the director's office. Though chiefly occupied with administrative responsibilities, he continued to treat patients in psychotherapy. His presence at McLean more than 33 years after his arrival as a resident spoke strongly of his attachment to the institution, as well as of

McLean's propensity for evoking loyalty in its staff. This intangible quality has struck a number of people forcefully.

The administrative structure of which de Marneffe became a key element resembled the one in place during the 1930s and 1940s when Wood was director and Tillotson was psychiatrist-in-chief. It was a formula which had worked satisfactorily in the past. However, the conditions of administration had changed drastically since the 1940s. The days when McLean's staff could conduct business seated comfortably around a table or two in the coffee shop had long passed, and the duties of administration, both clinical and executive, had proliferated and grown more complicated.

Within the hospital, there was a much larger staff, more departments and programs, and greater sums of money at stake, all of which presented the chief executive officer with problems of manpower, internal communications, program implementation and articulation, and resource allocation. Simultaneously, McLean's relationship with the external world became more complex. Though chartered by the Commonwealth and accountable to it from its inception, McLean had for more than a century fulfilled this obligation through simple formalities—the filing of annual statistical data with the State Department of Mental Health, for example—and pursued its development independently. The presence of four appointees of the governor on the Board of Trustees was considered sufficient safeguard that McLean would live up to its pledges of high standards of care.

Throughout de Marneffe's tenure, however, the requirements of numerous accrediting agencies, the intensification of state scrutiny, judicial decisions, and third-party payment systems placed the hospital under a regulatory microscope, publicly accountable for aspects of its operation ranging from the gender and racial composition of personnel to the civil rights of patients to the charges it set for treatment. No longer could McLean construct a new building just because the administration and trustees believed it needed one: The hospital had to file a determination of need certificate with the Commonwealth and persuade legislators that its need was indeed justified.

The new regulatory environment and an increasingly litigious society thrust de Marneffe into public arenas which other directors had not been required to enter. Sometimes he felt more like a labor lawyer than a psychiatrist; other times, more like a politician or a public relations man. At all times, however, his chief role was advocate for McLean and its patients. Altogether it was a difficult job, and though de Marneffe attacked it with enthusiasm, he came to see some drawbacks. As he wrote after about a dozen years in office, "If the psychiatrist-executive chooses to rise to these new responsibilities, he will no doubt experience some frustration. His activity will not always achieve results immediately. The satisfaction that comes from one's contributions making a real difference may often have to be deferred" (5).

One satisfaction came de Marneffe's way rather quickly. At the time of his appointment, one of McLean's principal administrative problems was financial. He accepted the glove the trustees flung at his feet and set out to balance the budget, with an able financial adviser acting as his second in the challenge. During 1963, the first full year of the restructured administration, the hospital recorded a surplus. Although it was a mere $2,495, it was the first surplus McLean had recorded in more than a decade. The next year yielded a surplus of almost $63,000. During the first 10 years of de Marneffe's directorship, if all surplusses and deficits are calculated before "treasurer's income," McLean came out $40,000 in the black.

Better financial management and a few other factors contributed to this improved picture. Insurance coverage for mental illness became more realistic, especially when Blue Cross came out with its Group Master Medical plan in the late sixties. By 1969, 80 percent of McLean's patients were covered in some measure by third-party insurers, including Medicare. Meanwhile, the trustees raised the basic daily rate every year from 1965 to 1970, during which time it doubled and went from $40 to $80. Rate hikes on this scale were not unique to McLean. MGH recorded analogous rises in charges, as did general and private mental hospitals across the country. At McLean the development of day-care and other transitional programs provided some additional income. Simultaneously, with the gradual attrition of the old long-term chronic patients, "free services" diminished as a percentage of the budget. Confident that

McLean's financial wild horse had at last been lassoed and tamed, the trustees heaved a collective sigh of relief.

The economic success did not occur at the expense of programmatic development. The process of fermentation started by Stanton in the mid-1950s continued throughout the sixties. The opening of the Arlington School and other programs for adolescents have already been discussed, but there were other initiatives which must be mentioned, if only briefly. To put them in some perspective, note that many of the programs McLean set in motion during the sixties were based on concepts which had already been developed at other, usually public, institutions.

For example, Boston State Hospital diversified long before McLean. Its outpatient department dated back to 1950. In the early sixties, it had a halfway house, a day-care center, a night-care center, an adolescent service, an alcohol program, a rehabilitation service, a screening program, a child psychiatry program, a home treatment service, an addiction center, and general practitioner and family care programs to complement its inpatient facilities, which treated both acute and chronic patients. It conducted energetic research in psychopharmacology. Boston State and other public mental hospitals served principally low- to middle-income patients, many of whom depended entirely on insurance to pay their medical bills and some of whom had no insurance at all until Medicaid came along to provide a little support.

Public institutions were therefore under tremendous pressure from their constituents and regulating agencies to develop effective short-term treatment methods, preventive programs, and less costly alternatives to full hospitalization. They had neither the personnel nor the facilities to provide long-term intensive psychotherapy and diverse activities; their patients could not afford to pay for extended hospitalization; and the state budget could ill afford those expenses. Given the convergence of these forces, it is not surprising that public institutions should have originated many of the treatment options that were later adopted by private hospitals.

McLean, of course, served a very different constituency and took pride in its identity as a private, protective, secluded retreat in which psychiatrists, psychologists, psychotherapists, activities therapists, nurses, social workers, and educators could work intensively with each patient—for several months or more if need be. That the hospital chose to develop new inpatient facilities and partial care programs and to extend its services to new categories of patients during the sixties was in part a natural extension of the "open hospital" concept embraced by Stanton and in part a response to the social activism of the decade.

In 1963 McLean dedicated a new Rehabilitation Center, financed in part by federal construction funds acquired under the Hill-Burton act. Since laboratories, nurses' residences, and private cottages cannot reasonably be reckoned as clinical buildings, the Rehabilitation Center was the first new building for patients to have been constructed since 1906! In 1964 McLean opened outpatient services to the general public. Clinical fees were deliberately set low to provide care to people who could not afford the rates of a private psychiatrist. By 1970 the McLean Out Patient Clinic was treating nearly 1,000 patients a year—individually, in groups, or in family clusters—and had become the principal mental health resource in the Cambridge-Arlington-Belmont area. It offered training programs for residents, psychology interns, nurses, clergymen, social workers, and volunteers working in community programs where they were apt to encounter psychiatric difficulties.

The patients who presented themselves to the clinic came much closer to representing the socioeconomic composition of society at large than did McLean's inpatient population, which, even with the extension of insurance coverage, remained predominantly privileged. Instead of acting as an instrument of democratization, the Out Patient Clinic created a two-tiered society at McLean. Outpatients and inpatients seldom crossed institutional zones. Those outpatients ill enough to require hospitalization had to be referred to other less costly institutions. The clinic did, however, generate some good will in the community and help to modify the popular image of McLean as a place which catered exclusively to the rich.

McLean took other initiatives during the sixties, which, like the clinic and more liberal policies with respect to off-grounds liberties for inpatients, altered its stance vis-à-vis the external world in the spirit of the "open" hospital. The concept of the mental hospital as sanctuary gave way to a philosophy of treatment aimed at reintegrating patients into the community as swiftly and fully as possible. In 1960 McLean set up its first transitional service, a Day Care Center for McLean patients far enough along in their treatment so as not to require full-time hospitalization, yet still too fragile to be tossed back into the world. Towards the end of the decade, a follow-up study of 104 patients who had passed through the center produced some encouraging data: Only 28 of those patients were under institutional care. Nine had died (five by suicide), but the remainder—almost 65 percent—were living successfully in the community. Since the study group included a high percentage of chronic schizophrenics, the statistics were impressive.

Against this background, in 1970 the Day Care Center began accepting carefully selected patients and offering them an alternative to total hospitalization, guided by the notion that for those individuals day care would be more effective than a locked ward. Day care also had the advantage of being cheaper. There was, however, a financial hitch: Insurance companies which covered 60 days of full hospitalization would not disburse a dime for day care. Therefore, a patient who might have been better off in a day program but who needed insurance benefits would have to choose inpatient treatment (6).

The Out Patient Clinic and Day Care Center operated on McLean's grounds and turned the hospital's face towards the community. The opening of Berkeley House, a halfway facility in Boston's Back Bay, inserted McLean into the heart of the city. The Victorian brownstone townhouse, when filled to capacity, became home base for 23 people, mostly former young McLean inpatients, who worked, went to school, or attended the Day Care Center in Belmont during the day.

Back in Belmont, McLean expanded along another front. In 1965 the hospital identified its desire to treat children below the age of 13 (the minimum age for admission) as part of its long-range development program. The interest in young children followed naturally from the hospital's intense involvement with the disorders of adolescence. It was suggested that a McLean program might get started by linking up with one of the existing pediatric departments elsewhere within the Harvard system, such as at MGH.

It was also obvious, however, that an outlay of capital would be required to set up appropriate treatment facilities. Surplusses notwithstanding, there were no piles of money lying around in wait for such an opportunity. Then McLean got lucky. At about the same time that it proposed the child psychiatry program, a substantial amount of capital became available through the Hall-Mercer Fund, a legacy administered jointly by trustees of the Pennsylvania Hospital and McLean-MGH trustees. Traditionally, part of the income from this fund had been used to support the MGH Psychiatric Service, and the initial suggestion for investing the capital was for the development of a child psychiatry program at MGH. However, David Crockett, who coordinated fund-raising projects, was feeling a trifle sheepish about the second-rate treatment McLean usually received in fund drives. He knew about the McLean proposal and introduced the trustees to the notion of steering the Hall-Mercer money towards Belmont. An agreement was reached in 1967, and McLean began planning a $2 million center, financed half by the loan of Hall-Mercer money on a favorable interest basis and half by matching federal funds, to house a child psychiatry program. The building was dedicated in 1973. Predictably, the diversion of the Hall-Mercer money to McLean did not sit well with the MGH Psychiatric Service; it was one of those events which illustrated the structural awkwardness of their relationship and contributed to ill feelings.

This sprint through the programmatic history of McLean during the sixties would fall short if it failed to remark upon the demise of the School of Nursing in 1968, 85 years and 1,945 graduates after its organization by Cowles. The school closed for most of the same reasons that forced the MGH School of Nursing to terminate its program in 1981: high cost of operations, difficulties in recruiting students, and the clear preference of prospective nurses for degree, rather than diploma, programs in a credential-conscious market. These problems were cropping up in 1964 when the director of nursing requested her assistant to study the situation. The study, neatly condensed into three pages, concluded that "the three year diploma program in nursing at McLean Hospital, steeped in tradition, has had a long and glorious past, but it can no longer fill the needs of the hospital" (7). The report did not cling to sentiment: The tents, it said, must be folded. Having confronted the new realities of the nursing profession, the school graduated its last 23 students in June 1968. McLean does, however, continue to offer specialist training to graduate nurses.

A briefer tradition came to an end in 1968 when Ralph Lowell resigned his position as chairman of the trustees' McLean Committee. George Putnam, who had been a member of the committee since 1963, was appointed as the new chairman. He recalled that the other trustees seemed to be apologetic about burdening him with the McLean chairmanship and said he would not have to hold the job down for very long. He also understood that he had free rein to encourage developments provided the hospital broke even.

The positive elements of McLean's evolution during the sixties—its reputation for fine work with adolescents, programmatic diversification, and balanced books—were to some extent undermined by two difficulties which refused to yield to solution. By contrast with the obvious improvement in McLean's financial position, there occurred a gradual decline in the average daily inpatient census. In 1962 the occupancy rate was 74 percent, calculated on 278 available beds. The figure inched upwards to 83 percent in 1965, but economy dictated the closing of Codman II and a reduction in the number of beds by 22, making for more cost-efficient deployment of hospital facilities. Over the next six years, even though the census percentages appeared healthier, McLean was in fact suffering a shortage of patients; in 1971 the hospital shut down nine more beds.

Ironically, about three times as many patients tried to get into McLean as were admitted. In 1969, for instance, the hospital accepted only 26 percent of the people for whom inquiries were made. Moreover, owing to seasonal variations in the census and complicated admissions procedures, prospective patients often had to endure long waiting periods prior to hospitalization. Eventually, it became clear that McLean's lengthy admissions processes and criteria contributed to the census problem by alienating referring psychiatrists and by turning away potential patients.

The population statistics for the period struck a dissonant chord. On the one hand, McLean had stabilized its financial position while expanding its clinical programs; on the other hand, it was clearly operating below capacity. The trustees, Stanton, de Marneffe, and the head of the Social Science Department (who routinely analyzed the statistics) were all concerned about the census figures and for a time somewhat mystified by them. But in 1970 the social scientist arrived at an explanation by concentrating his attention on admissions data. He observed that during that year patients diagnosed as schizophrenic accounted for 52 percent of all admissions and that the number of patients with other psychotic disorders was also on the rise, while diagnostic categories such as neuroses or personality disorders were decreasing. "In combination these figures are quite compelling: McLean is increasingly specializing in the treatment of schizophrenia and other psychoses and away from the treatment of less incapacitating illnesses such as neuroses" (9).

The analysis of admissions data had, in fact, disclosed a pattern of selection which had evolved from Stanton's principle that "the hospital encourages the admission of the sickest available patient" coupled with his ecological view that "the ideal institution is likely to be different for different types of patients." Influenced by Stanton, the McLean community had arrived at a tacit agreement about McLean's area of expertise; that is, what the hospital was and was not good for. The narrowing of focus resulted in diagnostically discriminatory admissions practices. As an isolated phenomenon, the pattern of specialization was not necessarily problematic. But when placed in the context of census rates, long-term economics, and McLean's sense of its mission, it became an issue.

Prompted by the low census, in 1971 de Marneffe, encouraged by Putnam, commissioned Ralph Hirschowitz of the Harvard Laboratory of Community Psychiatry to undertake a study of the hospital and the community. Hirschowitz was asked to conduct his research in the spirit of a market study and to address the questions: What patients has the hospital treated traditionally and how well? What patients has the hospital not treated and why? What patients might it treat in the future? The objective of the study was to assist McLean in identifying a broader spectrum of potential patients and to advise the hospital on how to attract them.

Hirschowitz's final report, based on a seven-month investigation of the hospital and its various constituencies, both actual and potential, was quite a large document. He and his team observed the hospital's organization as a whole and the operation of its several components. They also interviewed outside psychiatrists, former patients and their families, and people in the greater Boston area who had never had any contact with McLean. The result of their work constitutes as wide-ranging a collection of local opinions about McLean as is available for any single period in its history. A few brief passages convey the flavor of the study and suggest some of the issues that McLean faced as it moved into the 1970s.

Hirschowitz described dynamics within the institution which, in his opinion, prevented it from acting effectively in the marketplace. Though a number of criticisms addressed structures and procedures, he identified the origins of these problems in attitudes and traditions. The report—which did not mince words—aimed critical darts at "orthodoxy," "role clinging," "ultra-stability," "routines and rituals [which] no longer fit the needs of changing consumers," and "traditionalism." Clinical practices came under fire, especially the tedious admissions procedures. Referring psychiatrists were quoted. "It's hell to get a patient in." "It's an absolutely impossible place, it's impossible to get a patient in without endless red tape." "I once tried to get a patient into McLean Hospital whom I was satisfied was in a classical crisis and simply needed a place to rest up for a couple of weeks and receive some appropriate reality-oriented crisis intervention. I was told that the patient would have to stay in for at least six weeks and that such short-term treatment was not available" (9).

The report noted that McLean's reluctance to treat short-term patients, along with its tendency to keep its patients hospitalized for long periods of time, ignored the limitations of insurance coverage and other financial realities with which most people had to cope. Hirschowitz's views in this respect were best summarized under the heading of what he called the "dirty hands" myth:

> There is an elitist posture of some McLean staff members which suggests that consideration of economic matters violates "professional dignity." The pragmatic need to engage in business or politics is either ignored or attempts are made to delegate these aspects of administrative tasks to less "pure" staff members. The attempt to ignore considerations of economic expediency has wide and unfortunate ramifications. For example, attempts to meet the needs of new, and poorer, consumers have been described in the Hospital's informal organization as "quick and dirty psychiatry."
>
> A further consequence of the "dirty hands" myth is "splitting" in the executive suite. Because of the reluctance of some clinical administrators to engage themselves in issues of economic survival and growth, the burden of fiscal policy setting and control has fallen upon the shoulders of the administrator and the Director. Since resource allocation decisions are then regulated by them, they have become split off as the enterprise's "bad guys." This frees clinicians at the apex of the organizational hierarchy to play more supportive "good guy" roles. This splitting of functions between administrative and clinical directors is evident at all levels, so that a financially responsible party talks "services" with clinical staff but "money" with nonclinical staff (10).

Patients and their families provided the research group with the least reliable opinions about McLean. Most patients refused to be interviewed. Among those families willing to talk about the hospital, evaluations correlated with the degree of improvement in the patients. In a couple of instances in which a patient had fared poorly at McLean and subsequently improved in another institution, the families blamed McLean. Some parents of adolescent patients felt the staff did not keep them fully informed about the child's condition. On the whole, however, if the patient had done well—and many of them had—the family's responses were positive.

"Concerned citizens," represented primarily by volunteers who worked with patients in the hospital, were found to be surprisingly naive about how McLean functioned, what psychiatrists really did, and how they did it. At the same time, the volunteers believed McLean was a fine hospital. They expressed a nearly unanimous wish that it would share its expertise (whatever it was) with the community via newspaper columns, consultation with local health clinics, 24-hour hot lines, and a walk-in crisis center.

Lastly, the Hirschowitz report dealt with that "segment of the public which does not care about McLean Hospital and rarely has firm opinions about it."

> These "non-concerned citizens" are not an informed public; their opinions are based upon "folklore" or local community myths about McLean Hospital; if they reside far away from the Hospital they may have no information at all. The general lore about McLean Hospital has three themes: the haven for "spoiled little rich kids"; the place for the "crazy" members of rich and famous families (a theme embellished with names, true and false—"They say ______ was there"); and the place to which the scions of aristocratic New England families send their grandparents to die in states of exaggerated opulence. (11)

The Hirschowitz report ended with a long section of recommendations, including an elaborate restructuring of the hospital which was never implemented.

While producing a fascinating compendium of opinion along with some useful structural insights, the market study was off center in certain crucial respects. While taking potshots at "elitism" and "traditionalism," Hirschowitz missed McLean's deeper identity as a private hospital committed to offering the best in patient care, a commitment that entailed a high staff-patient ratio and generous physical facilities, both costly items. Hirschowitz's view of the marketplace placed McLean in competition with local community mental health centers, general hospital psychiatric services, and public institutions such as Boston State Hospital. McLean could not expect to compete for their patients without compromising its standards and altering its identity at the risk of its reputation and its existing constituency. Rather than suggest changes based on the firm core of principled dedication in the McLean tradition, Hirschowitz advised what he admitted were "radical" reorganizations which McLean might perceive as "threatening." Whether McLean felt threatened or not, it apparently considered Hirschowitz's radical plan unwise and did not follow it.

However, some of the other observations in the report were taken seriously: the clog in the admissions pipeline, poor communications with local referring psychiatrists, and the need for a better diagnostic balance in the patient population, including more people who could be treated on a short-term basis. More experimentation, diversification, and innovation were implemented during the 1970s, though not necessarily in ways Hirschowitz had recommended.

After the census problem, McLean's other difficulty during the sixties concerned clinical administration. While de Marneffe had assumed the duties of chief executive officer with the gusto of Teddy Roosevelt charging up San Juan Hill, the distribution of patient care responsibilities did not proceed according to the plan outlined in 1962. Stanton was stranded in a netherland, halfway between clinical administration and research. A year and a half passed with Howard, the associate psychiatrist-in-chief, performing the routine clinical chores while a candidate was sought for the position of director of clinical psychiatry. Given the natural limitations of the slot (Stanton retained the title of psychiatrist-in-chief), a long line did not form itself in pursuit of the job.

Eventually, in the fall of 1963, the hospital recruited attending psychiatrist Samuel Silverman, who ranked as an assistant professor at Harvard Medical School. A well-intentioned man with a good reputation as a psychoanalyst, clinician, and supervisor of residents, Silverman quickly became unhappy in the position and resigned after a year and a half. Clinical duties reverted to Stanton and Howard. The former begrudged time away from his research; the latter, as readers by now ought to expect, slipped philosophically into his old role. Luckily he did not have to play "musical offices" with every change of title or function.

The longer this condition of irresolution persisted, the more unsatisfactory it became. Then in 1967, Stanton, reassured that his tenure and a research position at McLean would be secure, told the trustees that he would relinquish the title of psychiatrist-in-chief to make way for a first-rate clinical administrator. The ritual ad hoc search committee was duly appointed with representatives of McLean, MGH, and Harvard Medical School among its membership. This committee could not arrive at a consensus concerning an individual candidate or the terms of appointment. After a year and a half of stormy deliberations, it was disbanded.

In 1969 Stanley Eldred graciously assumed the director of clinical psychiatry position knowing perfectly well that the failure of one search committee did not mean the search had ended.

Stanton returned his energies to orchestrating the clinical research program. The trustees and the dean of the Medical School, Robert Ebert, resolved the search quandary by appointing an outsider, Douglas Bond (son of the aforementioned Earl Bond), former chairman of psychiatry and dean of the Medical School at Case Western Reserve, to cast a neutral eye on the situation. Bond was supposed to assemble a review committee, but he cut through the bureaucratic jungle by handling the matter directly and individually.

Among other things, Bond recommended the academic separation of McLean from MGH, an arrangement which would give the psychiatrist-in-chief at McLean academic parity with the chief of the MGH Psychiatric Service, as well as with the chief psychiatrists at other Harvard teaching hospitals. This had not been the case in the past—Stanton had been Lindemann's academic subordinate—and had been one of the principal issues over which the original search committee had stumbled. Bond's advice was accepted, and the search committee was reassembled under new leadership. The revised committee functioned smoothly and swiftly: The new ground rules removed the most serious impediments to rational search, and the new chairman, Paul Russell of the MGH Surgical Service, was an excellent diplomat. The committee agreed on the selection of Shervert Frazier, professor of psychiatry at Columbia University and deputy director of the New York Psychiatric Institute (the old New York Pathological Institute). Frazier arrived as the new psychiatrist-in-chief and a full professor at the Medical School in 1972.

That same year marked the formal retirement of Paul Howard after 34 years of service to McLean. With the possible exception of Whitehorn, no other individual outside of a full-fledged head of staff had ever won so much affection and respect within the McLean community. His retirement was marked by a dinner at the Harvard Club with tributes in which the word "humanitarianism" was appropriately overused. The hospital recognized him as an institutional resource, set aside office space for him, and continued to call upon his long experience. At this writing he is chairman of the Institutional Review Board, a committee which reviews the ethical implications of clinical research proposals.

CHAPTER

12

A Hospital for the 1980s

This volume spans 175 years in the history of one private psychiatric institution. That period recorded three outstanding developments in the approach to mental illness: moral treatment, which substituted a medical for a metaphysical interpretation of insanity and placed the treatment of the afflicted on humanitarian grounds; Freudian theory, which provided a dynamic map of the mind that guided psychiatrists to a more profound understanding of the psychology of mental life in illness and health; and biomedical intervention, beginning with the shock therapies of the late 1930s followed by the introduction of psychotropic drugs in the 1950s. McLean stood in different relationships with each of these three developments. The hospital was unquestionably a pioneer of moral treatment. If not exactly in the forefront in the application of psychoanalysis and the dynamic therapies which evolved from Freud, the staff was receptive to the concepts; the psychoanalytically based treatment of schizophrenics and the therapeutic milieu of Stanton's era renewed McLean's reputation for leadership in the early 1960s.

With respect to medical treatments, however, McLean always seemed to be slightly out of step. Cowles's biochemical hunches had been on the right track at the wrong time. The turn-of-the-century technology had not been powerful enough to substantiate them. Hindsight now permits the observation that he marched ahead of the pack. Half a century later, when chemotherapy started to take off, the spirit of psychoanalysis dominated the McLean clinical program, and the hospital fell out of step again and slipped behind the leaders. Throughout the 1950s and 1960s, Mark Altschule was the lonely voice of clinical physiology at McLean. He pursued his research with single-minded intensity, conducting clinical tests with McLean patients or, when they were not available to him, patients at the Children's Hospital and the Metropolitan State Hospital. As early as 1954, before Stanton's arrival, he concluded that evidence from metabolic and other tests indicated "that the psychoses are diseases and not merely states of mind, and that a purely psychodynamic approach to etiology and therapy is not valid" (1).

McLean's implementation of Stanton's program drove Altschule deeper into intellectual isolation. As director of internal medicine until 1968, he observed the traffic in the pharmacy and was prone to provocative statements in his section of the annual reports. In 1965 he observed:

> Great increases occurred in the giving of the antipsychosis drugs and tranquilizers. The amount of this change is so striking as to suggest a change in the prevailing ideas about the nature of mental diseases and more particularly how these disorders are to be treated. A study of the phenomenon might, however, reveal that there has been no conscious recognition of any such change in the prevailing ideas and that the increased use of the drugs in question is owing to the operation of unconscious factors.

McLean at this time identified itself as a "psychoanalytically oriented" hospital. A report on the treatment of adolescents during the period noted that "the hospital atmosphere was generally responsive to dynamically oriented and milieu techniques as a method of reaching adolescent patients, and resorted to medication somewhat reluctantly but out of necessity in more difficult situations" (2). This was the "chemical straightjacket" view of drugs: Patients sometimes required restraint but should be released as soon as possible from the modern incarnation of straps and muffs so as to get on with the real treatment of dynamic psychotherapy.

While McLean adhered to this view, drugs were exerting powerful influences on the deployment of research energies as well as on social policy. The Joint Commission on Mental Illness and Health had remarked upon a correlation between shrinking patient censuses in state institutions and the prescription of drugs almost immediately after Thorazine came into large-scale use in the mid-1950s. The commission believed that drugs could be used to manage severe illnesses on an outpatient basis and strongly urged the development of community mental health centers as "a main line of defense in reducing the need of many persons with major mental illness for prolonged or repeated hospitalization."

The mental hospital population continued its decline steadily into the sixties. That the 1956 Social Security amendment providing financial aid to states to support the elderly in nursing homes might be partially responsible for the downward curve was a possibility generally overlooked in the excitement. Attention centered on the drugs which, though not touted as cures, nevertheless extended the hope that mental inpatient institutions might eventually be phased out. If the gross symptoms of mental disease could be subdued, then patients did not need to be in hospitals, or so the reasoning went. They could live in the community and receive whatever treatment they needed as outpatients. The theory was both morally and financially appealing. Accordingly, in February 1963 the Kennedy Administration advanced the Community Mental Health Center Act. The legislation was designed, in the president's words, to replace "the cold mercy of custodial isolation" with "the open warmth of community concern and capability" (3). A liberal Congress responded by allocating construction funds for community mental health centers (CMHCs) in 1963 and again in 1965. As the centers opened, state institutions discharged more and more patients. According to the bureaucratic logic that insists on capturing complicated human and organizational experiences in a single word, this process acquired the ugly name of "deinstitutionalization."

The community-based plan had two fundamental flaws. The first was built into the legislation. Congress authorized construction monies but did not supply continuous funding, so federal support ended in 1965. It had been supposed that, as state hospitals emptied out, the states would be able to shift money that had gone for inpatients to the CMHCs. But the old facilities did not empty out enough; operating costs rose (state mental institutions, like McLean, were generally old buildings, expensive to maintain); and state budgets were otherwise stretched thin by entitlement programs such as welfare. Thus, the CMHCs operated on slender budgets with personnel insufficient to meet the demands placed upon them. Boston's principal CMHC, a handsome building named in honor of Erich Lindemann, early visionary of community-based psychiatry, stands as a symbol of legislative shortcomings. Funded under the 1963 act, it was one of the most expensive structures on a per-square-foot basis erected in Boston at the time, and it was never completed. By the 1970s it was understaffed, and such staff as there was was underpaid and overworked.

The second problem was that some of the patients discharged from hospitals when their florid symptoms subsided under the influence of drugs proved incapable of living in the community, taking their medicines according to schedule, and reporting to the mental health clinic at specified intervals—all of which they had to do in order to maintain mental stability and survive in the community. (McLean psychiatrists would have predicted this problem. They may have lagged behind in psychopharmacology, but they had a lot of experience with very ill patients.) These former mental patients joined the Bowery-variety vagrants, to whom the public had long been accustomed, on park benches, in church vestibules, libraries, and subway stations, constituting a new subculture of homeless, helpless people.

That segment of the public which did not cross paths with deinstitutionalized patients on a regular basis was made aware of their situation by the communications media, and opinions about community care soured. The optimism of the early sixties turned to skepticism and then to denunciation. Psychiatrists were blamed for having exaggerated the powers of drugs and for overselling the concept of community clinics. However, a careful review of the psychopharmacological literature, while unmasking a few ideologues, reveals that most of the claims were reasonably measured. The temper of the times must be taken into account.

Lay advocates of CMHCs seized those fragments of scientific evidence that shored up their moral position and ignored the rest. Dorothea Dix had used the skewed statistics of moral treatment to sell nineteenth-century politicians on the idea of asylums. A century later, civil libertarians used drugs to sell the concept of the community clinic. Both reform movements were driven by humanitarian concerns as well as by convictions about proper treatment. The rhetoric surrounding the CMHCs had as much to do with civil rights as with psychiatry. The possibility that all mental patients could not enjoy, tolerate, or even survive the same degree of liberty as healthy people got lost in the absolutism of reformist arguments. The CMHCs were doomed to disappoint because they had been built on unrealistic premises with short-sighted financing.

While funding the building of community centers, the federal government also began diverting more and more research funds in the direction of drug investigations. Huge numbers of projects were launched with the support of NIMH, along with the hearty endorsement and financial cooperation of the pharmaceutical industry, for which psychotropic drugs meant huge profits. A new species turned up in the psychiatric fauna: the psychopharmacologist. By 1960 the American College of Neuropsychopharmacology (ACNP) had organized itself. This new generation of researchers slowly learned a lot, if by no means all, about the latest additions to the apothecary's shelf.

Once psychotropic drugs came into clinical use, investigators approached them from three basic perspectives. First, they worked in laboratories at defining the precise mechanisms of action in the central nervous system, efforts which, in conjunction with basic biochemical and neuropathological studies such as those conducted in McLean's research laboratories, gradually advanced understanding of how the brain functions.

Second, clinical researchers ran experiments designed to improve the efficacy of drugs, to develop better guidelines for how much of which medication to use for what symptoms, and to minimize the side and toxic effects. Some of this research could be conducted on laboratory animals. The disastrous interaction of the monoamine oxidase inhibitors (antidepressant drugs) and cheese, for example, was tested on well-fed rats. However, there are no schizophrenic rats, and experimentation with humans, of necessity, proceeded hesitantly and delicately. New chemical compounds were synthesized and tested, but the hope of discovering faster-acting, curative drugs did not materialize. Research did not produce any miracles, only a more confident grasp of the medicines at hand.

The appearance on the American market in the late 1960s of lithium was an event of singular consequence for the theory and practice of psychiatry with respect to psychotic illnesses. Ironically, this uniquely effective element had been an ancient remedy for insanity. It is known that physicians in the age of Hippocrates used to send mental patients to take the waters of certain hot springs in northern Italy. Modern chemical analyses of those waters revealed high concentrations of lithium. The drug's recent history began in the late 1940s when an Australian, J. F. J. Cade, experimented with lithium on animals, remarked upon its quieting effects, and then extended his tests to manic patients, among whom he noted dramatic responses in 1949. His reports excited European psychiatrists, and lithium moved into clinical practice on the Continent and in England, where it was prescribed for the treatment and control of manic-depressive illness. One McLean researcher observed that lithium was slow to reach the United States first because psychiatrists worried about its toxic effects and second because of a "lack of commercial interest in this inexpensive, unpatentable mineral and, consequently, lack of industrial support to demonstrate the efficacy and safety of its use" (4).

Lithium ended the practice of prescribing Thorazine and its chemical relatives to all psychotic patients, for it soon became clear that manic-depressive disorders could be controlled with proper administration of lithium, in much the same way that diabetes can be controlled with insulin. This fact helped bring about a new diagnostic rigor and clarified some of the distinctions between schizophrenia and manic-depressive illness, reducing, if not eliminating, the confusion between the two conditions which had existed since Kraepelin.

Working along other clinical fronts, psychopharmacologists discovered how to control or prevent the toxic effects of certain medications, how to increase or decrease dosages safely, how to recognize when a drug was not achieving the desired results, and when to abandon its use and try something else. Through all of these efforts, by the end of the sixties chemotherapy had graduated from the class of chemical straightjacket to that of therapeutic ally.

Third, researchers ran a number of studies to evaluate the performance of drug therapy compared with other forms of treatment. In 1970, Philip R. A. May, clinical professor of psychiatry at the University of California at Los Angeles, summarized several investigations which had focused on results of the treatment of schizophrenic patients.

> Experimental evidence from controlled research studies indicates that when the powerful effect of antipsychotic drugs is considered, the results of hospital treatment are equally good at all levels of milieu care, except under circumstances of virtual neglect or gross deificiency.... With drugs, not only can we help [patients] stay out; we can also help more patients out of hospitals more quickly and without any loss in quality of result. (5)

In every study May cited, drugs, rather than milieu or psychotherapy, proved to be the significant factor in the improvement of schizophrenic patients. He did not dismiss the role of psychotherapy, but stated his belief that the benefits of long-term, formal psychotherapy had been exaggerated and ought to be supplanted by psychotherapeutic "management" in the hospital, supplemented by formal counseling after discharge.

May's paper appeared in a volume called *Changing Patterns in Psychiatry*, an anthology revolving around research in psychopharmacology and the impact of drugs on treatment. The studies conveyed a sense of vitality in psychiatry such as had not been in the air since the salad days of moral treatment. Save for an allusion to *The Mental Hospital* in the introductory historical chapter, McLean was invisible in the volume. There was, however, ample evidence of activity in the Boston area. Two authors of chapters represented Harvard Medical School and the Massachusetts Mental Health Center, another two Boston State Hospital, and two more, one of whom was Milton Greenblatt, commissioner of the Massachusetts Department of Mental Health, the Tufts Medical School. If psychopharmacology was the new cutting edge of clinical psychiatry, as more and more people believed it was, then McLean had fallen behind.

As the shortcomings of community mental health centers made themselves noticeable in the early 1970s, the dream of assigning mental hospitals to the archeological heap began to dissolve. Discharged patients wandered city streets, metaphors for the inadequacies of both psychiatry and social policy. At the same time, biological research and treatment presented promising avenues of attack on a problem which was getting worse and more costly every year. Federal research funds migrated from social and behavioral studies such as Stanton had championed to biologically based investigations.

The search committee that selected Shervert Frazier as McLean's new psychiatrist-in-chief in 1972 worked against that backdrop and took as one of its principal objectives the resuscitation of the biomedical perspective in Belmont at all levels of the hospital's performance: clinical care, training, and research. Frazier's professional background, character, and flexible approach to mental illness suggested that he might indeed be able to accomplish all of these things.

Frazier had studied medicine at the University of Illinois, spent a few years in general practice, and then gone on for advanced training, first in internal medicine and later in psychiatry, as a fellow at the Mayo Clinic in the 1950s. During the 1960s, he went to Texas. He was head of the Psychiatry Department at Baylor University and psychiatrist-in-chief at Ben Taub General Hospital in Houston from 1962 to 1968. He also became commissioner of mental health for the state of Texas. From the Southwest, Frazier had a distant impression of McLean as one of a half dozen or so "Ivy League" mental hospitals—along with the Menninger Clinic, Sheppard-Enoch Pratt, and the Institute for Living, for example—that did very good treatment. As mentioned earlier, he had once referred a very ill young woman to McLean for treatment and had been satisfied with what the hospital had done for her. He had read Stanton's and Schwartz's *The Mental Hospital* and thought it a fine piece of work.

Frazier moved from Texas to New York in the late sixties. He was a professor at Columbia University and deputy director of the New York Psychiatric Institute, an institution with a long, unbroken tradition of research. Thus, Frazier came to McLean with strong academic and clinical credentials and respect for basic research, as well as experience in the politics of community psychiatry gained as a commissioner in Texas. He also had a lot of energy and good instincts about how to set large-scale changes in motion.

Frazier did not subscribe to any party lines in the ideological debate between psychoanalysts and psychobiologists. Though a trained psychoanalyst, he had studied and practiced internal medicine, and his concepts of mental illness were eclectic. His views on etiology appeared in capsule form in the first paragraph of a chapter, written with Benjamin Seltzer, in the *Harvard Guide to Modern Psychiatry*:

> Behavior can never be divorced from its anatomical substrate in the brain, but neither can it be treated as a pure neurological phenomenon without reference to learning and the environment. Many psychiatric syndromes previously thought to be functional, such as general paresis and the avitaminoses, have been found to be organic in nature. On the other hand, even though increasing evidence points toward a biological basis for schizophrenia and depression, the psychodevelopmental model of these conditions may remain quite valid. (6)

Frazier's adaptation of Pascal's wager to psychiatric theory reassured the existing McLean staff that he respected the psychosociological perspective and that he was not about to lead the hospital into revolution but, rather, into a phase of rapid evolution. It also bears noting that, because he conceived of himself acting most effectively in academic and clinical areas, he did not covet the responsibilities of chief executive officer and found the administrative structure that placed de Marneffe in charge of those functions agreeable.

Three developments in particular marked Frazier's tenure as psychiatrist-in-chief at McLean: the expansion of biomedical research; the establishment of "specialty units" for the treatment of patients with clearly identifiable disorders and the conduct of clinical research and training; and the arrangement of contract services for the state. The contract services, while of value to the hospital, were somewhat peripheral and will be described after those developments which were closer to its heart.

By contrast with Stanton, whose model for McLean had been a social science research laboratory in the interest of determining the ideal therapeutic milieu, Frazier took his clues from his experiences at the Mayo Clinic, coupled with the implications of biomedical research during the 1960s, and worked with the model of a university hospital. That model differed in certain respects from the one Cowles had invoked in the 1880s because it rested on a recent body of empirical evidence indicating that different forms of mental illness responded to different therapies which, in turn, suggested complementary research initiatives. The data available to Cowles had not justified treatment variations, nor were the research techniques of his time highly specialized; psychiatry then was a specialty in itself, not yet further subdivided into even more refined areas of expertise. By the 1970s, however, there were a great many subspecialties, both in practice and in laboratories, ranging from child psychiatrists to psychopharmacologists. In Frazier's view, a good academic psychiatric hospital, like a good teaching general hospital, collected the best specialists, investigative and clinical, thereby offering treatment options as well as rich research and training programs.

Frazier proved to be a remarkably effective catalytic agent. He had the good sense not to tamper with the basic identity of McLean as a first-class private institution. Instead of trying to place it in competition with community mental health centers—as Hirschowitz's report had suggested—Frazier's program built on the hospital's strengths: the existing core of basic research, the tradition by which staff members rather than residents ran the clinical programs (a pattern which encouraged stability of personnel with high levels of ability and long experience), and the pleasantly surprising (surprising to a newcomer, that is) reserves of loyalty that were evident among all categories of McLean's personnel.

Within this context, Frazier acted as a master planner, establishing a framework within which individuals could design specific components according to general guidelines. He recruited excellent people and gave them opportunities to be creative and to implement their own programs. Since the plan was conceptually sound by virtue of engaging the hospital's sense of mission as well as progressive trends in psychiatry, it succeeded as a whole. Since the design of its several parts entailed risks, it is not surprising that a few efforts floundered or that, given the relative independence of individual programs, there were some administratively clumsy overlaps. Frazier took the mishaps in stride and moved on to the next piece of business, confident that his basic model was the correct one for McLean.

Though developments on the research and clinical levels occurred more or less in tandem and simultaneously with certain changes in hospital procedure, it is simplest to treat them topically. Research, of course, had been a presence at McLean since the turn of the century and particularly since the establishment of the biological research laboratories in 1946. However, while the laboratories had succeeded as a disembodied enterprise, they lacked the size to engage in clinical research and weld connections to the patient care program. Stanton, though respectful of the labs' efforts, remained remote from them and took no steps to encourage biomedical research at the clinical level. When McLean explicitly set out to correct this situation in the early 1970s, it was able to take advantage of a couple of circumstances in the local psychiatric community. The first piece of luck came as a consequence of the Harvard Medical School's decision to sever its ties with Boston City Hospital. This rupture left Jack Mendelson, who had been running studies of alcoholism at Boston City Hospital, without academic affiliation, and word passed along the grapevine that he was looking for a new home for his program. McLean quickly invited him to move his study to McLean, combine it with the fledgling drug abuse research program, and become director of an expanded Alcohol and Drug Abuse Center.

The second event was even more unexpected and gratifying than the first. To establish a rigorous psychobiological research program, McLean needed an individual around whom such a program might coalesce. With this objective, Frazier appointed a small search committee at McLean under Alfred Pope's chairmanship. Seymour Kety, a senior research scientist at MGH, was invited to sit on this committee and share his expert knowledge of people working in neurobiology. However, by the end of the first meeting Kety indicated that he might consider transferring his own research program from Fruit Street to Belmont. That effectively ended the search.

Kety then headed the psychobiological laboratories of the MGH Psychiatry Service, having come there in 1967 with Eisenberg. Prior to that Kety had been the first scientific director of the National Institute for Neurological Diseases and then Phipps professor of psychiatry at Johns Hopkins, after which he had returned to research at NIMH. There he developed a model for discriminating between genetic and cultural factors as causes of schizophrenia. He used Danish hospital records to compare the psychiatric status of children adopted in infancy who became schizophrenic as adults with the psychiatric status of the adoptive families. His findings demonstrated that biological inheritance was a significantly stronger predictor of schizophrenia than the psychosocial environment. At MGH, Kety assembled a talented research team and pursued this line of inquiry, expanding his data base and taking various cuts through the information to see what might be discovered about genetic/cultural overlaps in the schizophrenic disorders.

During his seven years at MGH, Kety put up good-naturedly with research facilities far less grand than those depicted to him prior to his arrival. Also, he knew that Eisenberg was planning to leave MGH, so the future of the Psychiatry Service was uncertain. Thus McLean's plans, which included new research laboratories, were irresistible. By 1977, four key people on Kety's team had transferred to McLean's new Mailman Research Center, leaving the MGH psychobiological research component badly decimated.

"With the opening of the Mailman Research Center, McLean now has the world's most outstanding research center in the neurosciences in the private sector," the 1977 annual report stated. Lest readers become architecturally disoriented, the center consisted of two new floors of laboratories ingeniously superimposed upon the old biological research laboratories. To build them, McLean raised $3.28 million in three years from 3,800 private donors and foundations, of which $1 million came from The Mailman Foundation and $250,000 from the Kresge Foundation. It thereby pulled off the largest single fund-raising venture in its history. The feat challenged the conventional wisdom that money could not be raised on behalf of the mentally ill; it proved that private resources could be tapped if one had a well-articulated program, knew whom to approach for money, and how to ask for it.

When the new structure was completed, the original bottom floors were named in honor of former trustee Ralph Lowell, who had so long encouraged basic research at McLean; they continued to house the work in biochemistry and neuropathology. Folch retired as director, and his post passed to Pope. Kety and his colleagues took possession of the upper two stories, the Laboratories for Psychiatric Research with subsections in genetics, neuroanatomy, neurochemistry, neuropharmacology, psychology, and a clinical unit. The Mailman Center, the Alcohol and Drug Abuse Research Center, research in the Hall-Mercer Children's Center, and Stanton's group studying the effects of psychotherapy on schizophrenia added up to a diversified, solid research program.

The Mailman Center was dedicated in October 1978 with great fanfare. First Lady Rosalynn Carter, honorary chairperson of the President's Commission on Mental Illness, arrived to the standing ovation of 1,300 guests scantily defended against the raw elements by a tent. She spoke earnestly of the Carter Administration's commitment to biomedical research in mental illness and of her own determination to "get across to the public . . . the crucial nature of basic research into the causes of mental illness." She cited a bleak statistic: The federal government was spending $17 billion dollars a year on mental health care; only one half of one percent went for support of basic research (7).

The weather was disagreeable, but it was a fine day for McLean. de Marneffe, observing that the Mailman Center had been funded, staffed, and completed on schedule and within budget, quipped, "As I look back over five years, we seem to have defied Murphy's Law—everything that could have gone wrong went right!" (8).

The development of specialty treatment units ran parallel to research. One by one McLean established an array of services to treat populations of patients distinguished either by diagnosis or age group. These clusters provided exceptional opportunities for clinical research, training, and accumulating expertise. The

Adolescent and Family Treatment and Study Center was set up for nonpsychotic teenagers whose families were willing to involve themselves in intensive therapy. The Appleton Treatment Center worked with alcoholics. A behavior therapy unit treated individuals with phobias, eating disorders, obsessive-compulsive behavior, psychogenic pain, and certain kinds of depression. Very regressed, manic, or suicidal patients were admitted to the intensive care unit. There was an Older Adult Service for geriatric patients and the preexisting children's unit.

Three sections of the Acute Care Service, called clinical evaluation units, while treating patients who had been selected according to specific diagnostic criteria, collaborated with researchers at the Mailman Center. An affective disease program, concentrating on depressive illness, was intertwined with the psychopharmacology program. Standard drug therapy regimens were scrutinized. Patients in the affective disease program who had not done well with conventional medications had access to experimental drugs—sometimes with encouraging results. Researchers investigated the biochemical aspects of depression. The conduct of research and the use of medication not yet on the market occurred only with the written consent of patients or, in the case of minors, of their families, and a patient could withdraw from the project at any time.

Anyone who has shared the life of a person afflicted with mental illness will not be surprised by the willingness of patients to try untested therapies. One former patient, clinically depressed for two years and unresponsive to several drugs, had a prior history of kidney stones, one of the most agonizing medical conditions known. Once, in middepression, he said, "I would trade this any day for a friendly kidney stone." Imagine, then, the elation shared by patients and staff when some treatment-resistant volunteers responded well to new antidepressants in McLean's affective disease program.

The specialty units admitted only limited numbers of individuals, and the majority of McLean's patients were assigned to the "generic" halls, in which diagnostic categories and age groups mixed. Nevertheless, since the staff designed individual treatment programs for each patient, care on the generic halls was not necessarily different from that on the specialty units.

The premise underlying McLean's clinical program as developed during Frazier's dozen years as psychiatrist-in-chief was that different forms of mental disease required different forms of treatment. The results of biochemical intervention tended to validate the hypothesis: Classes of illnesses responded to drugs of different chemical structure—the schizophrenias to neuroleptics, depression to antidepressants, bipolar illness to lithium. That some conditions failed to respond to drugs at all, or that the overall success of medication as a treatment (as in, say, schizophrenia) left much to be desired, was less suggestive of flaws in the theory than of gaps in scientific knowledge. Also, despite more rigorous diagnostic criteria, the manifestations of mental illness were still infinitely various, unsusceptible to laboratory analysis, and often very difficult to categorize.

The premise of special treatment for special diseases extended to psychological treatment of the emotional and social deficits associated with mental illness, teaching patients to recognize the warning signals of an approaching storm in the climate of their minds, and retraining to eliminate maladaptive practices. Accordingly, McLean offered several forms of psychotherapy: group, family, couples, behavioral, cognitive, and most universally, individual, with the latter varying widely according to the therapist and his or her perception of the patient's needs. Although some psychiatrists still practiced the more classical Freudian-inspired form, the rigidly scheduled psychoanalytic hour of the Stanton era gave way to more informal encounters. Some psychiatrists saw their role as counseling the patient on managing disease and life as affected by disease. It should also be noted that for all these changes in the clinical program, the principles of milieu therapy as implemented by Stanton—greater freedoms, rehabilitation, as much contact with the exterior world as possible—remained in place.

Hindsight permits the roots of differentiated treatment to be traced back to the shock therapies of the late 1930s when, after a flurry of experimentation, they were found to be effective with certain depressed patients. But the notion was slow to mature. Shock therapy had obvious drawbacks, and no one understood how it worked when it was successful. Such development of the theory as might have taken place was interrupted when the

Freudian school came to dominate institutional psychiatry. Psychoanalysis focused on individual pathology, not on disease categories. By contrast, the model developed at McLean during the 1970s recognized common elements specific to certain classes of disease while acknowledging that the same disorder precipitated individual life problems, given the originality of every human life. In acting upon the model in the creation of specialty units and in custom-tailored treatment programs, McLean probably went farther than any other mental hospital in the United States.

The renovation of McLean along academic lines helped to a certain degree to resolve the census problem that had plagued the hospital during the sixties. The revitalized training program attracted good residents, who in turn dispersed themselves throughout the country carrying glowing reports of McLean with them. Word traveled fast along the residents' network and did more good (or, potentially, harm) for the reputation of the institution than newspaper articles or what former patients said. But residents' gossip alone would not build McLean's census. Frazier, as mentioned earlier, was an astute politician. He went all over the country and even abroad, attending symposiums, giving speeches, and generally putting McLean's name before the public. Staff members were encouraged to do the same, to go to conferences, to publish papers, and to increase the hospital's exposure to professionals and the lay public. de Marneffe pushed community public relations aggressively. McLean began publishing a quarterly, the *McLean Hospital Journal*, and circulating it free of charge to mental health professionals. It would be hard to calculate which of these efforts paid the best dividends; no doubt it was their combination that worked so effectively.

In 1971 McLean had operated with 248 beds. In 1973 there were 275 and in 1976 there were 328—with the census running at 84 percent and financial surpluses in the hundreds of thousands. The hospital made nearly half a million dollars in 1980 and again in 1981; in 1982, when the census stood at 87 percent, McLean turned a profit close to $1 million. While the number of beds increased by 80 between 1971 and 1976, the number of patients admitted per year more than doubled, from 423 to 1,119. The accelerated turnover resulted from McLean's solicitation of short- and intermediate-term patients, more effective drug treatment, less frequent resort to long-term psychotherapy during hospitalization, and certain changes in the diagnostic profile of the patient population. The diagnosis of schizophrenia, the most intractable of mental disorders, applied to 42 percent of the patients admitted in 1971, and diagnosis of major affective disorders (that is, depression or manic-depressive illness) applied to only 3 percent. Ten years later the two diagnostic categories were represented in reverse proportions, with the major affective disorders, which stand a reasonable chance of responding promptly to medication and counseling, accounting for 47 percent of admissions and schizophrenia for only 6 percent. Though in some part a product of the deliberate policy of admitting shorter-term patients, the transposition of numbers also reflected more diagnostic precision; in retrospect, it is likely that many patients admitted as schizophrenics during the sixties were suffering a bipolar illness. Diagnostic statistics in other categories also showed alterations during the 1970s: There were more patients with alcohol and drug dependency problems, and there were a few epileptics. Overall, there was a better balance and broader spectrum of illnesses to complement the research programs. The age pattern also shifted slightly from adolescence to young adults as the baby boomers came of age.

These developments have taken place too recently to allow for perspective and critical evaluation. Certain statements, however, can be made in confidence. It is obvious that McLean improved the efficiency of clinical administration and treatment, brought the length of hospitalization more in line with health insurance coverage, and made inpatient care available to more people. The process of reversing the custodial role, started by Stanton, was fully accomplished. Census rates climbed and stabilized at a satisfying level. The hospital achieved a sound financial position. More importantly, it reacquired an excellent reputation for treatment, education, and research. But when it comes to judging where McLean's multifaceted program is placed on the path towards the apparently distant goal of cure and prevention of mental illness, common sense flashes warning signals, for such judgments involve too much foresight. It is safer to leave the business of prediction in the hands of fortunetellers and meteorologists.

Nevertheless—and mindful of how cautious one must be in using the word "progress"—McLean's records do suggest signs of progress. Some of those signs are subtle. For example, Seymour Kety recently remarked in a radio interview that better understanding of the genetic factors involved in schizophrenia had relieved families of the load of psychological guilt implied by the psychoanalytic model of the illness. The story of one patient illustrates his point:

> For the fifth time in eight years, Mary, a 30-year-old chronic paranoid schizophrenic, arrived at McLean Hospital. Her father, who accompanied her, tried to preserve his optimism, noting that this was the first time she had come willingly. Mary had been discharged about a year earlier at the insistence of her parents, despite the reservations of her treatment team and a guarded prognosis. Their plans for her had rapidly fallen apart, and Mary had spent several months traveling, living at home and fighting with her parents, and finally in other hospitals. Upon her return to McLean, she said she was "totally disorganized" and "didn't know how to put it together."
>
> Mary was hospitalized for two months. During this time she resumed individual therapy, was stabilized on medication, and generally reconstituted. She began to work at the Thrift Shop, and enrolled in a course at a local college. She was viewed as improved, and was discharged, this time to a highly structured residential setting with a hospital based day care program.

A representative of McLean's evaluative service unit visited Mary and her family several months later. Though frustrated by her continued dependence on the hospital and troubled in social relationships, Mary still hoped to finish college and said, "I have not give up on myself." She also reported that she was getting along much better with her family. Her father confirmed this view. "We feel better educated in the illness," he said. "We had been in the dark for so many years" (9).

The demystification of mental illness, schizophrenia and otherwise, the willingness of psychiatrists to explain the knowns and unknowns of various disorders, and the effort to set goals for patients that acknowledge realistically the perimeters (if any) suggested by the disease, all seem to represent progress over such raising of false expectations as occurred so many times in the past. Furthermore, Mary, who probably would have been hospitalized indefinitely in the era before psychotropic drugs, was treated as an inpatient for only two months and now enjoys some measure of liberty in an environment that helps maintain her in a stable state. If Mary's condition falls far short of the ideal of cure, her social circumstances are much better than they would have been in the past, and her family has been substantially helped.

McLean's management of a severely depressed, suicidal woman admitted as an emergency patient demonstrates how sharp diagnostic skills and specialized experience can make a difference. The woman had previously been treated on Cape Cod and discharged from a hospital there with a diagnosis of paranoid schizophrenia, "recovered." McLean reviewed her history and symptomatology, revised the diagnosis to manic-depressive illness, and treated her with lithium plus individual therapy. She was discharged after 45 days. When seen in follow-up, she said she had come to McLean "trapped in my own illness," sure she would end up as a patient for life. Instead she was taking her medication regularly, seeing her therapist, and negotiating the rough spots in her life. Her husband and children, instructed as to the nature of her illness, were warm and supportive (10).

These two examples, along with other remarks in this chapter, may mislead the reader to the belief that all McLean patients receive drugs as part of their treatment. Since the hospital's approach is flexible, however, this is not so, as in the instance of a 27-year-old nurse admitted with a 10-year history of chronic debilitating headaches, nausea, other somatic symptoms, anxiety, and depression. She had been unable to work for several years and complained of difficulties in her marriage and in raising her two small children, as well as of the financial strains her family experienced because she could not work. Her history included numerous medical and neurological examinations, four years of psychoanalysis, four previous hospitalizations, and a long list of painkillers and psychotropic medications. When admitted to McLean she was taking large doses of diazepam (Valium), Thorazine, and propoxyphene (Darvon). The hospital's treatment program, supervised by a psychologist, began with the gradual withdrawal of all medications, followed by careful assessments of conditions prior to headaches and monitoring of moods during a seven-day drug-free period. The patient then began one week of behavioral therapy, involving training in progressive relaxation plus cognitive restructuring and assertiveness training. She was discharged after a week of therapy, but continued as an outpatient; a short course in parent skill training and couple therapy were added to her regimen. A year and a half after the end of treatment, she was headache free, no longer taking medication, and had found regular part-time work (11).

The stories demonstrate how three patients, suffering different disorders, received very different treatments. Of the three, only the last may reasonably be considered "recovered." The nurse must keep taking her lithium, much as a diabetic takes insulin, but she is not chronically impaired. Mary has improved as much as current understanding of schizophrenia permits, but her troubles are not over, and she will probably never be able to function as a healthy woman.

Moving from McLean's center—the care of inpatients—outwards, one finds that traffic in the Out Patient Clinic doubled between 1970 and 1980. Transitional and partial hospitalization programs started during the sixties were augmented during the seventies. The Partial Hospitalization Service, however, ran aground around the end of the decade for financial reasons. Insurance coverage did not extend to partial programs, and McLean's services could not compete with community-based centers. Despite valiant efforts to salvage the operation, the drain on the budget was such that the hospital decided to terminate partial hospitalization in 1982. A new system of limited day care, through which patients could purchase special services, picked up part of the slack. Transitional facilities, such as Berkeley House in Boston, continued their work.

The provision of contractual services to external institutions, which McLean began in 1975, enhanced the hospital's training program by offering experience in forensic psychiatry, broadened the financial base, and helped alter its popular image as an exclusive, fancy institution. Contract programs also allowed McLean to hire more psychiatrists and psychologists and gave it a more powerful voice at the Harvard Medical School.

The first of the contracts went into effect when McLean, in response to inquiries from state officials, began operating the psychiatric service at Bridgewater State Hospital, an institution for the criminally insane, and established an "Institute of Law and Psychiatry." The Bridgewater program was one of Frazier's pet projects. He had a special interest in violence, dating back to his days as mental health commissioner in Texas, and he frequently attended Bridgewater patients personally. McLean eventually extended psychiatric care to prisoners in other correctional facilities in the state. The hospital also contracted to provide psychiatric and medical assistance to the Metropolitan State Hospital in nearby Waltham and offered consulting services for businesses and schools.

McLean's widespread reputation for excellence and financial success precipitated an unexpected complication in its history. On the last Monday in May 1983, George Putnam called de Marneffe and told him that a for-profit hospital chain, Hospital Corporation of America (HCA), was interested in buying McLean. de Marneffe thought Putnam was joking and laughed. Putnam, however, was absolutely serious. The trustees had already discussed the possibility in general terms with HCA representatives. HCA already owned 25 psychiatric hospitals, was negotiating the purchase of several more, and wanted to add the prestigious, Harvard-affiliated McLean as its flagship facility; the corporation was, therefore, prepared to make some concessions to the trustees' initial demands. When de Marneffe passed this information on to Frazier a few weeks later, the latter was flabbergasted.

Very quietly over the next few months, the trustees and HCA drafted a preliminary proposal consisting of the following principal elements:

First, HCA would buy McLean from the MGH Corporation for a sum in the neighborhood of $60 million.

Second, HCA would invest another $35 million in building renovation and construction at McLean, a figure which approximated the costs of bringing the antiquated physical plant up to date according to the estimates of a 1981 long-range planning study.

Third, HCA would endow five professorships at McLean for a total of $6.25 million.

Fourth, HCA would maintain the extent of free care at current levels.

Fifth, teaching and research funds would be maintained at current levels at a fraction of the budget.

Sixth, when ownership of McLean passed to HCA, a nine-member Board of Trustees would be established under the leadership of the dean of the Harvard Medical School. Harvard and MGH would select six trustees and HCA would appoint two representatives to the Board. These trustees would be responsible for all academic and policy decisions. They would not, however, have final approval of the budget for patient care.

Seventh, there would be a buy-back provision under which HCA would sell McLean back to the MGH Corporation at a favorable price in the event HCA should decide, for whatever reasons, that it no longer wanted to operate McLean under the terms of the agreement.

The trustees and HCA conducted their discussions with a discretion that the State Department or the Central Intelligence Agency might envy. Only de Marneffe, Frazier, and eventually the assistant director for fiscal affairs at McLean knew about the proposal. Therefore, trustee chairman Francis H. Burr's public statement that the trustees were engaged in negotiations with HCA caught the McLean staff completely off guard. The announcement came on Monday, August 1, when a number of senior staff members had set off on vacation. A few heard about the possible sale for the first time on their radios or read about it in the Boston newspapers. Many of them felt outraged. A number of other faculty members at the Harvard Medical School, including the influential Arnold Relman, editor of the *New England Journal of Medicine*, and physicians at other teaching hospitals shared their anger.

At the same time that Burr made his announcement, Dean Daniel Tosteson of the Medical School named a Faculty Advisory Committee, chaired by MGH neurologist Joseph B. Martin, to study the proposal and report back to him within two or three months. Frazier and Kety represented McLean on this committee, which listened to opinions from several quarters and conducted its deliberations *in camera*. As McLean staff trickled back from their vacations, de Marneffe held several meetings with them. He tried to address their concerns. He pointed out that he, too, had initially considered the proposal preposterous but upon inspection had come to believe it contained several advantages for McLean.

In spite of de Marneffe's efforts, staff objections solidified. The staff were, first of all, infuriated by a process carried on entirely behind their backs. They were further agitated by rumors in the press that the proceeds of the sale of McLean were to be turned over to MGH and saw the trustees as acting in a conflict of interest. Staff who held joint appointments with Harvard believed the terms of the sale endangered McLean's affiliations with the Medical School. They did not trust HCA, a profit-motivated enterprise, to continue to support the academic programs at the hospital. Reassurances that the academic issues might be ironed out did not convince the staff. Researchers worried about grant support. The buy-back clause did not produce a sense of security: If MGH used the $60 million for its building program—as many believed would happen—then where would the trustees get the money to buy back McLean in the event HCA wanted to sell?

Opposition external to McLean began to gather momentum. Teaching hospital traditionalists, among whom Relman was one of the more eloquent spokesmen, took to high moral ground and argued that teaching hospitals in particular ought not be influenced by monetary considerations. (No one seemed to notice that profit, or at least balanced budgets, had influenced the management of McLean for more than a century.) Faculty members on other teaching hospital staffs worried that if MGH trustees could sell McLean to HCA, their own board members might begin striking similar deals with for-profit corporations.

According to rumor, the Faculty Advisory Committee was initially inclined to approve the HCA offer. Ultimately, it recommended against the sale. Burr revealed the decision at a press conference on October 28, remarking that the sale was off, but that the status quo could not continue. The committee's formal report, dated November 1, stated that:

> in the judgment of the Committee, most of the negative reasons are not based on an assessment of the specifics of the proposal and/or of the previous performance of the Hospital Corporation of America. Rather, the reactions seem to flow from a set of values strongly held by many members of the faculty.

The committee dignified those values. One non-McLean member admitted in private conversation that he thought the proposal had been reasonable but that he had cast his vote against it because he knew how most of the McLean staff felt about the sale. "If my own staff opposed anything that violently," he said, "I wouldn't vote against them. It would be too demoralizing. A hospital, after all, is the people who work in it." The committee's vote effectively impaled the MGH-HCA proposal, if not the prospect that McLean (and maybe other Harvard teaching hospitals) might find other formulas short of outright sale for relationships with for-profit corporations.

The proposal to sell McLean to HCA served as an object lesson in the politics and economics of contemporary medicine. It stimulated nationwide debate and prompted academic medicine to take a closer look at how for-profit corporations operate and what might be learned from them and to reconsider what kinds of alliances might be advantageous to both parties without running roughshod over patients. But McLean had not enjoyed being at the center of this attention. The HCA saga embroiled the hospital in controversy for three long months. Bitter feelings lingered after the sale had been called off. The staff, long conscious of McLean's country-cousin position vis-à-vis MGH, had for the very first time challenged the trustees.

Once the tempest had died down, McLean was left with the problem of finding capital funds to implement the building program. Burr appointed a Long-Range Planning Committee, including representatives from the trustees, MGH, the Medical School, and five people from McLean (de Marneffe and Frazier among them) to search for solutions. The staff was purposefully kept abreast of its deliberations, as well as those of other committees handling sensitive policy issues.

This most recent chapter in McLean's history closed in late 1984 when Frazier accepted an invitation to become director of the National Institute of Mental Health. He moved from his dignified office in the yellow-brick administration building in Belmont to more spacious, but less handsome, quarters on the top floor of a 17-story building in Rockville, Maryland. There he continued to look back to McLean with affection and pride. He retained his professorship at Harvard.

Epilogue: Obscurity at the Center

As these final pages are being written in late winter 1986, McLean prepares to celebrate the 175th anniversary of its charter. From an administrative point of view, there are some other shoes yet to be dropped. The search committee for a new psychiatrist-in-chief has not completed its work. The committee is or is not closing in upon a candidate, depending on one's source of information. de Marneffe, after 23 years in the director's chair, occasionally waxes philosophical: Perhaps the new psychiatrist-in-chief should also be the chief executive officer. He has sometimes been uncomfortable with the division of authority.

The Long-Range Planning Committee is involved in negotiations with American Medical International (AMI), Inc., another for-profit hospital. The discussions have yielded an agreement that McLean and AMI form a satellite joint venture to operate nonhospital activities such as contract, drug-screening, and community residential programs. The initial AMI outlay of $8 million, to which McLean will add $3 million, will provide $11 million which, with the addition of borrowed funds, will help finance new construction. Eager to avoid another political disaster, de Marneffe and the committee have kept the McLean community informed of the process. The staff is complacent. They are veterans of the HCA war; the AMI arrangement, which does not lay a glove on teaching, research, or treatment of patients at the hospital, poses no threat.

The senior staff has changed a bit during the past few years. Frazier moved to NIMH. Jordi Folch-Pi, who put McLean's basic research program on the map in the 1950s, died in 1981. Seymour Kety and Alfred Pope retired in 1983. The latter maintains a presence in the Lowell Laboratories, where he is a mine of experience and historical lore. Final disposition of the laboratory directorship awaits the appointment of a new chief of staff, for institutions, like well-tooled machines, must mesh gears if they are to run smoothly, and no one knows what the new psychiatrist-in-chief will bring as priorities. Alfred Stanton died in 1983. During the last decade of his life, he engaged in research on the effects of psychotherapy on schizophrenic patients, specifically comparing "exploratory, insight-oriented therapy" (that is, psychoanalytically influenced therapy) with "reality-adaptive, supportive" therapy. As one of his admiring colleagues observed, it was a courageous project because Stanton questioned his own theories. Before he died, Stanton knew the results: The study demonstrated no appreciable differences between the two psychotherapeutic forms.

Howard, who has acted subtly as connective tissue through more than four decades of McLean history, remains active. If anyone can be said to represent the conscience of the hospital, it is he. He links the past with the future. He has for years done the best he can with available resources, resisted ideology, paid attention to new modes of treatment, and applied those which seemed to benefit McLean's patients. Lately he has the impression that psychiatry at McLean and elsewhere is more polarized than it used to be. The biomedical stalwarts and the heirs of Freud show occasional tendencies to rhetorical violence.

The extremities are atypical. On the whole, McLean psychiatry represents a compound of the three great developments that have occurred during its existence. Moral treatment remains in place, both as an attitude toward patients and in the form of a structured environment and stimulating activities. Though few psychiatrists or psychologists on the staff practice orthodox psychoanalysis, fewer still would deny that their comprehension of conscious and unconscious behavior, of how the mind thinks and feels, has been informed by Freudian theory. The place of biomedicine, both in the laboratory and in the treatment of patients, is now firmly established. What currently distinguishes McLean from other mental institutions is the extent to which these concepts have been organized around the model of the academic hospital.

I undertook this project two years ago with the conviction that patients were the "real" heros of McLean's history. The hours I spent reading case histories disabused me of this naive notion. Patients, however plucky and courageous they may be, are victims of puzzling disorders. As I followed the evolution of psychiatry through decade after decade during which so little happened which made any difference to patients, I concluded that this history had no heros at all.

Eventually, I had another change of heart. McLean's past is populated with heros, named and unnamed: all those people—attendants, nurses, psychologists and, above all, psychiatrists—who have been companions to patients and tried to heal them. I place psychiatrists at the top of the list because from October 6, 1818, when McLean admitted that first, wonderfully satisfying patient, a physician-psychiatrist has held the ultimate responsibility for the treatment of all patients.

Psychiatrists do not conform to the standard model of medical heros. They are not the William Mortons, Jonas Salks, or Christiaan Barnards who make headlines. They remind me, rather, of Dr. Rieux, the protagonist of Albert Camus's *The Plague*. In the novel, which the author based on a real experience, an epidemic of plague breaks out in Algeria during the 1940s. Though lacking medical resources, Rieux stays and works to fight it night and day. ". . . Every evening mothers wailed, . . . with a distraught abstraction, as their eyes fell on those fatal stigmata on limbs and bellies; every evening hands gripped Rieux's arms, there was a rush of useless words, promises, and tears; every evening the nearing tocsin of the ambulance provoked scenes as vain as every form of grief. Rieux had nothing to look forward to but a long sequence of such scenes, renewed again and again." In another passage the doctor responds to an interview, saying simply, ". . . I assure you I've no more than the pride that's needed to keep me going. . . . For the moment I know this; there are sick people and they need curing . . . what's wanted now is to make them well. I defend them as best I can, that's all."

As I rerun the images of McLean's and other institutional psychiatrists through my memory, from 1818 through to the present, I cannot imagine one of them who did not at some instant feel like Dr. Rieux. They all recognized limitations on scientific knowledge and on effectiveness of treatment. They all experienced failure more often than the practitioners of most professions. They witnessed the baffling phenomenon of spontaneous remission with the distracting realization that it had occurred independently of their ministrations. They watched flares of hope light up a dark sky and burn out. But they did not walk away from the mentally ill. They stayed and defended them as best they could. That, in my mind, makes them heroic.

Of all the individuals in these pages, Luther Bell represents that heroism most vividly. Through his writings and what others wrote about him, I came to believe I knew him and understood how he used his political, administrative, and research energies to paint a sheer veneer over a deeper layer of frustration. He was haunted by what he called the "obscurity at the center" of mental illness.

Though modern research psychiatrists, who may very well turn out to be the heros of future volumes of psychiatric history, appear to have drawn back the veil of mystery a fraction of an inch, the center remains in shadow. As a McLean scientist told a *Time* reporter in 1979, "We are not going to find the causes and cures of mental illness in the foreseeable future." Medical science is likely to discover a cure for acquired immune deficiency syndrome (AIDS), for which a specific virus has been isolated, long before a cure for schizophrenia. Psychiatry labors under the handicap of what Frazier acknowledges as "a vast amount of ignorance about how the brain works." Psychiatrists have recognized the hereditary factor in mental illness for well over a century, but the genetic culprits elude identification. The role of learning and environment, as causes or triggering devices, cannot be pinned down with scientific rigor. Society and psychiatry still argue over definitions of mental illness.

Among private institutions, McLean now enjoys respect as a leader and a reputation such as it had in the past, a reputation relinquished and regained. It has the most comprehensive research program of any private psychiatric hospital in the country. On October 6, 1985, 167 years after a young man was placed under Rufus Wyman's care in the Asylum in Charlestown, McLean admitted Patient Number 38,461 to its hospital in Belmont. The hospital will do its best for that patient, which is very good indeed. But given the state of the art, and depending on the patient's illness, that best may not be good enough.

Notes and References

Chapter 1

1. Rush, 1812, pp. 13–27.
2. Haslam, 1809, pp. 210, 236–237.
3. Pinel, 1806, pp. 113–114.
4. Deutsch, 1938, p. 82.
5. Services at the Laying of the Corner Stone of the Massachusetts General Hospital in Boston, July 4, 1818.
6. Deutsch, 1938, p. 66.
7. Myers, [1929?], pp. 10–11.
8. Amory, 1947, p. 168.
9. An English translation of Pinel's 1800 treatise appeared in 1806. The other seminal tract, Tuke's *Description of the Retreat at York,* was not published until 1813.
10. Armour, [undated], p. 3.
11. Eaton, 1957, pp. 47–48.
12. Amory, 1947, p. 225.
13. Bowditch, 1872, p. 10.
14. Eaton, 1950, pp. 9–11.
15. Wyman, Morrill, Jr., 1913, p. 32.
16. "Address of the Board of Trustees of the Massachusetts General Hospital to the Public," 1814.

Chapter 2

1. Bowditch, 1872, p. 37.
2. By contrast, the trustees engaged a nonphysician as the first superintendent of the general hospital.

3. Parkman, 1817, p. 24.
4. Pinel, 1806, p. 184.
5. Bowditch, 1872, pp. 97–98.
6. Little, 1972. This book contains Folsom's diaries with excellent footnotes and commentaries by the editor.
7. Bell, Luther, Annual Report, 1842.
8. Bowditch, 1872, pp. 381, 384.
9. Bell, Luther, Annual Report, 1842.
10. Wyman, Morrill, Jr., 1913, p. 32.
11. Drinker, 1947, p. 6.
12. Wyman, Rufus, 1830, pp. 5, 7. I recognize a school that argues that societies have defined insanity as a way of restraining those individuals who do not conform with social and political norms and thereby threaten their stability. This school might use Wyman's definition as ballast for its position. I do not wish to engage in a broad debate here because the issues are serious and complicated. However, I would counsel anyone tempted to cast Wyman's statement in that light to read the early case records of the McLean Asylum detailing the mental anguish and frantic behavior of Wyman's patients before bending his words in an unnatural direction.
13. "Massachusetts General Hospital Asylum for the Insane 'Rules of Admission,'" 1818.
14. Bowditch, 1872, p. 44.
15. Wyman, Rufus, 1830, p. 9.
16. Dain and Carlson, 1960, p. 284.
17. Boorstin, 1983, p. 463.
18. Pinel, 1806, p. 114.
19. Tuke, 1813, p. 136.
20. Kaplan, 1980, p. 83.
21. Little, 1972, p. 46.
22. Bowditch, 1872, p. 379.
23. Wyman, Rufus, Annual Report, 1822.
24. Wyman, Morrill, 1877, pp. 13–14.
25. Little, 1972, p. 29.
26. Tuke, 1813, p. 96.
27. Bowditch, 1872, p. 383.
28. Wyman, Morrill, Jr., 1913, p. 33.
29. Wyman, Morrill, 1877, p. 24.
30. Bowditch, 1872, p. 57.
31. Ibid. p. 62.
32. Ibid. p. 75.

33. Ibid. p. 101.
34. Ibid. pp. 188–189.
35. Bell, Luther, "McLean Asylum for the Insane," 1838.

Chapter 3

1. Lee, Annual Report, 1835.
2. Bell, Luther, "McLean Asylum for the Insane," 1838.
3. Bowditch, 1872, p. 126.
4. Bell, Luther, "McLean Asylum for the Insane," 1838.
5. Ellis, 1863, p. 8. Ellis's memoir and that of Isaac Ray are the sources of most of the biographical data on Bell.
6. Ellis, 1863, p. 44.
7. Ray, 1863, pp. 16–17.
8. *Proceedings of the Association,* July 1855, pp. 68, 70, 72–73.
9. Bell, Luther, letter to Dorothea Dix, 17 January 1854, by permission of the Houghton Library, Harvard University.
10. Ray, 1863, p. 17–18.
11. Rosenkrantz and Vinovskis, 1978, p. 116.
12. Bell, Luther, Annual Report, 1844.
13. Bell, Luther, Annual Report, 1840.
14. Bowditch, 1872, p. 172.
15. Bell, Luther, Annual Report, 1856.
16. Finch, 1853, pp. 185–186.
17. Bell, Luther, Annual Report, 1840.
18. Bell, Luther, Annual Report, 1843.
19. Bell, Luther, undated notes.
20. Bell, Luther, letter to Dorothea Dix, 4 February 1843, by permission of the Houghton Library, Harvard University.
21. Ibid.
22. Bell, Luther, "McLean Asylum for the Insane," 1838.
23. Dain, 1964, p. 13.
24. Sanborn, 1898, p. xi.
25. Deutsch, 1938, p. 190.
26. Bell, Luther, letter to Dorothea Dix, 5 June 1848, by permission of the Houghton Library, Harvard University.
27. Bell, Luther, letter to G. Peters, 18 August 1849, by permission of the Houghton Library, Harvard University.
28. Kaplan, 1980, p. 22.
29. Ellis, 1863, p. 56.
30. Sanborn, 1898, p. 273.

Chapter 4

1. Holmes, 1861.
2. Eliot, 1869–70, p. 18.
3. Holmes, 1872.
4. Holmes, 1869.
5. Haslam, 1809, p. 61.
6. Isaac Ray was a notable exception. He wrote a book called *Mental Hygiene* for laymen, pulished in 1863.
7. The relationship of the trustees to the railroad companies was probably more complicated than meets the eye in published reports. The trustees were men of substance and some of them, or their families, had financial interests in the offending railroad companies.
8. *Beyond the Neck*, 1982, pp. 90, 87.
9. "Dinner to Dr. Edward Cowles on his retirement from the McLean Hospital," 1904–05, p. 113.
10. Bowditch, 1872, p. 560.
11. Ibid. p. 683.
12. *American Journal of Insanity*, 1863–64, p. 359.
13. Beecher and Altschule, 1977, p. 157.
14. Whittemore's health improved. He returned to McLean as first assistant physician in 1874. The trustees elected him resident physician of the general hospital in 1876. The man appointed to his old position at the asylum, Charles E. Woodbury, had been on the job only a short time when a patient inflicted a severe injury on him. Woodbury's recovery progressed so slowly that he had to resign from the staff.
15. Cowles, "Report upon the Occupation of Patients," 1894, pp. 28–29.
16. Myers [1929?], pp. 56.
17. Bowditch, 1872, pp. 663–664.
18. Jelly, Annual Report, 1878.
19. For an intelligent discussion of moral treatment and Earle's statistical analyses, see Bockoven, 1956.
20. Folsom, 1886, pp. 127–128.

Chapter 5

1. "Dinner to Dr. Edward Cowles on his retirement from the McLean Hospital," 1904–05, pp. 115–116.
2. Cowles, 1896, p. 54.
3. Vogel, 1980, p. 40.

4. Trustee records, Vol. 8, 1888, p. 279.
5. Cowles, Annual Report, 1882.
6. Ibid.
7. Cowles, Annual Report, 1889.
8. Bolton, 1943, pp. 1, 3.
9. Cowles, Annual Report, 1882.
10. Tucker, 1887, p. 321.
11. Trustee records, Vol. 8, 1888, pp. 321, 325.
12. Cowles, Annual Report, 1888.
13. Cowles, Annual Report, 1890.
14. Hall, J.K., et al., 1944, p. 295.
15. Ibid. p. 296.
16. Mitchell, 1894, p. 101.
17. Cowles, 1896, p. 47.
18. Cowles, Annual Report, 1882.
19. Cowles, Annual Report, 1890.
20. Cowles, Annual Report, 1882.
21. Lamar, 1975, appendix.
22. Trustees, Annual Report, 1882.
23. Roper, 1973, p. 474.

Chapter 6

1. Amory, 1947, p. 194.
2. *Boston Evening Transcript,* 3 September 1895.
3. *Boston Globe,* 4 September 1895.
4. *Boston Evening Transcript,* 3 September 1895.
5. Hurd, 1896, p. 478.
6. *Boston Evening Transcript,* 1 October 1895.
7. Myers, [1929?], pp. 143–144.
8. Cowles, Annual Report, 1896.
9. Cowles, Annual Report, 1897.
10. Cowles, Annual Report, 1902.
11. Cowles, 1899, pp. 111–112.
12. Winters, 1950–52, Vol. 3, p. 516.
13. The difficulties of distinguishing between manic-depression and schizophrenia persist in the present, when misdiagnosis has more serious implications since different conditions may respond to different medications. A 1978 study by Joseph Lipinski and Harrison Pope of McLean reported that about 40 percent of patients diagnosed as schizophrenic in U.S. mental hospitals were suffering from other disorders.

14. Hoch, 1900, pp. 285–286.
15. Cowles, Annual Report, 1902.
16. For a discussion, see Levin, 1977.
17. Hoch, 1900, p. 285.
18. Winters, 1950–52, Vol. 2, p. 6.
19. The Adolf Meyer Papers [I/775/4] in the Alan Mason Chesney Medical Archives of The Johns Hopkins Medical Institutions, Baltimore, Maryland.
20. Winters, 1950–52, Vol. 3, p. 517.
21. Cowles, Annual Report, 1903.
22. Reiser, 1978, pp. 136–137.
23. Drinker, 1947, pp. 12–13.
24. Cowles, Annual Report, 1903.
25. Murchison, 1932, Vol. 2, pp. 104–105.
26. Cowles, Annual Report, 1903.
27. Hall, G.S., letter to Franz, 6 October 1916, G. Stanley Hall Papers, Clark University Archives.
28. Washburn, 1939, p. 23.
29. "Dinner to Dr. Edward Cowles on his retirement from the McLean Hospital," 1904–05, p. 126.
30. Cowles, letter to G.S. Hall, 5 June 1914, G. Stanley Hall Papers, Clark University Archives.
31. Franz, letter to G.S. Hall, 28 October 1916, G. Stanley Hall Papers, Clark University Archives.
32. Deutsch, 1938, pp. 483, 484.
33. Hall, G.S., letter to Franz, 6 October 1916, G. Stanley Hall Papers, Clark University Archives.
34. Cowles, letter to G.S. Hall, 5 June 1914, G. Stanley Hall Papers, Clark University Archives.
35. Franz, letter to G.S. Hall, 28 October 1916, G. Stanley Hall Papers, Clark University Archives.

Chapter 7

1. Eugene Taylor, Jr., associate in psychiatry at the Harvard Medical School, has recently reappraised the complicated relationships among Freud, James, G.S. Hall, and Putnam, adding insight into the development of theories of the unconscious.
2. Ross, 1972, p. 390.
3. James, 1920, Vol. 2, pp. 327–328.
4. Freud, 1955, 24th lecture.
5. Meyer, 1910, p. 385.

6. Burr, 1914, pp. 303–324.
7. Meyer, 1908, p. 245.
8. Grob, 1983, p. 150.
9. *Annual Report of the Massachusetts State Board of Insanity,* 1910, p. 29.
10. Winters, 1950–52, Vol. 2, p. 9.
11. MGH had established the first Social Service Department in American medicine in 1905. The service was the brainchild of Richard Cabot, a friend of Southard, Putnam, and other psychiatrically inclined physicians. Cabot, a free-spirited doctor interested in what became of his patients after they left the hospital, arrived at the belief that social workers could help insure long-term effectiveness of medical treatment. Though the logic of Cabot's argument applied powerfully to psychiatric patients restored to anxious families or suspicious employers, McLean failed to imitate its sister institution for several decades. The self-supporting classes served by McLean thought social workers helped poor immigrants and other destitutes, not people of their station. Accordingly, there was no Social Work Department at McLean until the mid-1950s.
12. Grob, 1983, p. 141.
13. Freud, 1955, 16th lecture.
14. Washburn, 1939, p. 24.
15. Abbot, 1927, pp. 385, 388–389.
16. Tuttle, Annual Report, 1915.
17. Bond, Earl, unpublished reminiscences, courtesy of Dr. Thomas C. Bond. See also Thomas C. Bond's "Looking Back: The Early Years of Earl D. Bond," *McLean Hospital Journal,* Vol. 6, Winter 1981.
18. Santostefano, 1976, p. 185.
19. Murchison, 1932, Vol. 2, pp. 106–107.
20. Wells, 1913, p. 4.
21. Hall, J.K., et al., 1944, p. 389.

Chapter 8

1. Packard, letter to Abbot, 22 October 1920.
2. Packard, Annual Report, 1919.
3. Packard, letter to Meyer, 12 December 1921.
4. Packard, letter to Abbot, 22 October 1920.
5. Tillotson, 1932, p. 12.
6. Packard, letter to Miss Roscoe, 14 June 1923.

7. Gifford, 1978, pp. 388–389.
8. Ibid. p. 371.
9. Tillotson, Annual Report, 1937.
10. Howard, personal communication.
11. Ibid.
12. Whitehorn, 1959, p. 4.
13. White, 1984, p. 224.
14. Tillotson, Annual Report, 1938.
15. Ibid.
16. Tillotson, Annual Report, 1939.
17. Myerson, 1939, p. 1204.
18. Bell, Whitfield, Jr., 1975, pp., 126–127.
19. Tillotson, Annual Report, 1939.

Chapter 9

1. Hall, J.K., et al., 1944, p. 420. My remarks on psychiatry during World War II are based on Albert Deutsch's excellent chapter in this volume.
2. Faxon, 1959, p. 374.
3. Gregg, 1944, pp., 285–291.
4. Wood, letter to George F. Weld, 25 March 1948.
5. Newspaper articles concerning the Tillotson and Salot affair are pasted in a scrapbook in the McLean archives. Unfortunately, the individual who clipped the stories neglected to include the names of the newspapers in which they appeared.
6. Armour, Alexander, personal communication.
7. Makin, Mildred, personal communication.
8. Howard, Annual Report, 1949.
9. de Marneffe, transcript, 1985.
10. Howard, Annual Report, 1955.
11. de Marneffe, transcript, 1985.

Chapter 10

1. Joint Commission on Mental Illness and Health, 1961, p. 193.
2. Ibid. p. 39.
3. Gifford, 1978, p. xxi. No one who has followed recent trends in psychiatry will be surprised to learn that the Boston Psychoanalytic Institute's rate of growth has slowed down considerably.
4. Joint Commission on Mental Illness and Health, 1961, p. 167.
5. "Future of the Psychiatric Services of the MGH and McLean," [undated].

6. Sullivan, 1973, p. xi.
7. Stanton's remarks were contained in a 14-page draft entitled "Some considerations regarding the psychiatric program at the Massachusetts General Hospital and the [McLean] Hospital." Stanton's corrections are pencilled in. The draft may have undergone additional changes.
8. Stanton, draft of memorandum to Lindemann, 21 September 1954.
9. Solomon, letter to Lowell, 17 May 1955.
10. Castleman et al., 1983, p. 175.
11. de Marneffe, transcript, 1985.
12. Kahne, Merton, personal communication.
13. Stanton, 1956, pp. 145, 146, 148.
14. Ibid. p. 147.
15. de Marneffe, transcript, 1985.
16. Stanton, 1965, p. 182.
17. Joint Commission on Mental Illness and Health, 1961, pp. 29–30.
18. Bockoven, 1956, p. 314.
19. Faxon, 1959, p. 314.
20. Stanton, 1965, p. 180.
21. Castleman et al., 1983, p. 172.
22. Joint Commission on Mental Illness and Health, 1961, pp. 266, 267.
23. Stanton, "The McLean Hospital: 1955–1962," 1962.
24. Ibid.
25. Frank Norton of McLean helped me understand Massachusetts Blue Cross/Blue Shield coverage. The oldest "nervous and mental" certificate went into effect February 1, 1950; the benefits covered 10 full days of hospitalization during the subscriber's lifetime. In July 1954, the Blues started offering a prolonged illness rider providing an additional $300 worth of benefits after the 11th day of hospitalization. The $12 per day/60-day program in force in 1960 permitted an individual to be discharged after the benefits ran out, stay out of the hospital for 90 days, and be eligible for another 60-day period if admitted on the 91st day after discharge. There was, however, a lifetime cap of $15,000 on payments for mental disorders. Since McLean had no contract with the Blues in 1960, the insurance company paid benefits directly to the subscriber, leaving the hospital to collect from former patients.

    Group Master Medical policies, which became available in the late 1960s, allowed full benefits to mental patients in general hospitals, and many of them had prolonged illness coverage that paid the full semiprivate rate at participating psychiatric hospitals for 60 days.

26. de Marneffe, transcript, 1985.
27. Stanton, letter to Lindemann, 23 April 1961.
28. Knowles, "The McLean Hospital," 1961.

Chapter 11

1. Frank, 1968, p. 1.
2. Foucault's argument apparently applies in some societies. But for a witty, realistic rejoinder see Gerald Weissmann's Chapter, "Foucault and the Bag Lady," in *The Woods Hole Cantata,* New York, Dodd Mead, 1985.
3. Castleman et al., 1983, p. 176.
4. Folsom, 1886, pp. 116–117.
5. de Marneffe, 1976, p. 334.
6. Though insurance companies have shown some signs of extending coverage since 1975, very few plans offer benefits for partial hospitalization.
7. Makin, "Implications and Recommendations for the Future of the McLean Hospital School of Nursing," 1964.
8. Annual Report, 1970.
9. Hirschowitz, 1971, Part I, pp. 47–48.
10. Ibid. summary, p. 5.
11. Ibid. Part I, p. 2.

Chapter 12

1. Altschule, Annual Report, 1954.
2. Grob and Singer, 1974, pp. 3, 32.
3. Kennedy, 1963.
4. Nicholi, 1978, p. 403.
5. Rothman, 1970, p. 260.
6. Nicholi, 1978, p. 297.
7. "McLean Review," Winter 1977–78.
8. Ibid.
9. "Outcome Evaluation Findings," 1982, pp. 1–2.
10. Ibid. pp. 3–4.
11. Levendusky, 1978, pp. 50–57.

Bibliography

Bibliographic Note

The bibliography, notes, and references are intended to aid the reader who may wish to consult sources and to provide occasional information supplementary to the text. For the purposes of simplicity I have divided the bibliography into two sections: 1) materials in the McLean archives which are either unpublished sources or printed hospital documents of limited circulation; 2) published sources, including books, papers, proceedings, and lectures. The bibliography lists all sources cited in the text, though by no means all sources consulted in the course of research.

I. Primary Sources

Letters, other unpublished materials, and McLean internal reports listed in the references are located in the McLean Archives unless otherwise noted. The following bibliography is limited to those records I consulted. Readers interested in a complete description of the rich archival materials are referred to the "Guide to the Archives of The McLean Hospital Corporation" compiled by Terry A. Bragg, archivist, in 1984.

A. Original Documents

1. Patient and Trustee Records

Patients Registers, 6 October 1818 to 16 December 1905, list patient number, name, date of admission, rate of board, and other information obtained at time of admission, as well as discharge data.

Patient Case Records, in bound volumes up to 1893, according to patient number; thereafter in file folders.

Incidents [Death and Disappearance] *Book,* 1 volume, 5 April 1856 to 23 September 1884.

Patient Restraint Records, 5 volumes, 1872–1910.

Records of the Visiting Committee, 5 volumes, 21 September 1818 to 17 May 1897.

Trustee Records [minutes of the meetings of the Board of Trustees]. Incomplete set of nineteenth-century bound volumes located at the Massachusetts General Hospital.

2. Correspondence

The McLean Archivist has organized letters in the "Office of the Superintendent" records. Until recent decades, these files contain correspondence received by superintendents. The farther back one goes in time, the less voluminous the files, and it is clear that nineteenth-century superintendents did not hold future historians in mind when they disposed of incoming mail. Dr. Cowles is believed to have destroyed his files before leaving McLean.

Letters originating from McLean during the nineteenth-century have been located in other archives. Drs. Tuttle, Packard, and Wood kept some carbon copies of outgoing mail. Dr. Stanton's papers, donated to McLean by his wife, are maintained as a separate collection and contain both correspondence he received and drafts or carbons of some of the letters he sent as psychiatrist-in-chief.

3. Miscellaneous

Bell, Luther. "McLean Asylum for the Insane." An unpublished manuscript dated 23 March 1838, containing autobiographi-

cal information and condensed histories of patients. Unpaginated.
de Marneffe, Francis. "Background information on the history of McLean." Transcript of tape recorded recollections made by Dr. de Marneffe in response to specific questions asked by this author, 1985. Used with his consent and available to scholars only with his written permission.
"General Rules, without minute details." Undated, handwritten document, probably written by Rufus Wyman as a draft for printed rules.

B. Printed or Photocopied Documents

"Address of the Board of Trustees of the Massachusetts General Hospital to the Public." 1814. Printed.
Annual Reports of the McLean Asylum/McLean Hospital," 1822–1985. The first annual report was published as part of the "Address of the Trustees of the Massachusetts General Hospital to the Subscribers and to the Public," March 1822, and after 1827 the publication of the annual report became a ritual. Until 1972 the annual reports, which usually included statistical data, were a rich mine of information. Beginning in 1972 the length of the reports was drastically reduced. However, McLean maintains unpublished reports of various departments and clinical services for those years. Annual reports are cited in the references as "Annual Report" with date and author, if authorship is a significant piece of information.
Armour, Alexander. "Some historic details of the McLean Asylum, Somerville, Massachusetts, 1811 to 1895." Unpublished manuscript, circa 1982.
Bolton, Annie R. "Glimpses of a pioneer nurse." Unpublished manuscript, 1943.
Cowles, Edward A. "Report upon the occupation of patients." 18 January 1894 [addendum to annual report].
"Future of the psychiatric services of the Massachusetts General Hospital and McLean, The Mental Health Services of the MGH." Undated report. Stanton Papers. Photocopy.
Hirschowitz, Ralph G. "McLean Hospital, 1971: Problems and

Prospects." Laboratory of Community Psychiatry, Harvard Medical School, 1971. Photocopy.

Knowles, John H. "The McLean Hospital." Report with covering letter to Ralph Lowell, dated 1 November 1961. Photocopy.

Makin, Mildred. "Implications and Recommendations for the Future of the McLean Hospital School of Nursing." 1964. Photocopy.

"Massachusetts General Hospital Asylum for the Insane, 'Rules of Admission.'" 1 September 1818. Printed.

"A program of development for McLean Hospital." June 1967. Photocopy.

"Reflections on social work practice at McLean, 1956–1981." 25th Anniversary of the McLean Department of Social Work, 24 April 1981. Photocopy.

"Services at the Laying of the Corner Stone of the Massachusetts General Hospital in Boston, July 4, 1818." 10 July 1818. Printed.

Stanton, Alfred H. "The McLean Hospital: 1955–1962." A report presented to the General Executive Committee, 21 February 1962. Photocopy.

II. SECONDARY SOURCES: BOOKS, PAPERS, LECTURES, AND PROCEEDINGS

Abbot, E. Stanley. "George Thomas Tuttle, M.D." *American Journal of Psychiatry,* Vol. 7, September 1927, pp. 384–389.

Amory, Cleveland. *The Proper Bostonians.* New York: E.P. Dutton & Co., Inc., 1947.

Arieti, Silvano, ed. *American Handbook of Psychiatry.* New York: Basic Books, 1959.

Beecher, Henry K., and Mark D. Altschule. *Medicine at Harvard.* Hanover, N.H.: The University Press of New England, 1977.

Bell, Luther. "On a form of disease resembling some advanced states of mania and fever, but so contradistinguished from an ordinarily observed or described combination of symptoms, as to render it probable that it may be an overlooked and hitherto unrecorded malady." *American Journal of Insanity,* October 1849, pp. 97–127.

Bell, Whitfield J., Jr. *The Colonial Physician and Other Essays.* New York: Science History Publications, 1975.

Beyond the Neck: The Architecture and Development of Somerville, Massachusetts. Cambridge, Mass., 1982.

Bockoven, J. Sanbourne. "Moral treatment in American psychiatry." *Journal of Nervous and Mental Diseases,* Vol. 124, August-September 1956, pp. 292–321.

Bond, Thomas C. "Looking Back: The Early Years of Earl D. Bond," *McLean Hospital Journal,* Vol. 6, Winter 1981, pp. 35–45.

Boorstin, Daniel J. *The Discoverers.* New York: Random House, 1983.

Bowditch, Nathaniel I. *A History of the Massachusetts General Hospital,* 2nd edition [with a continuation by Rev. George E. Ellis]. Boston, 1872.

Bromberg, Walter. *Psychiatry Between the Wars, 1918–1945.* Westport, Conn.: Greenwood Press, 1982.

Burr, Charles W. "A criticism of psychanalysis." *Proceedings of the American Medico-Psychological Association, 1914,* pp. 303–324.

Caplan, Ruth B. *Psychiatry and the Community in 19th Century America.* New York: Basic Books, 1969.

Castleman, Benjamin, David C. Crockett, and S.B. Sutton, eds. *The Massachusetts General Hospital, 1955–1980.* Boston: Little, Brown and Co., 1983.

Chittick, Rupert A. "Occupational therapy in its relation to a program of mental treatment." *Occupational Therapy and Rehabilitation,* Vol. 18, August 1939, pp. 231–234.

Cowles, Edward A. "The advancement of psychiatry in America." *Proceedings of the American Medico-Psychological Association, 1896,* pp. 47–70.

——. "Progress in the clinical study of psychiatry." *American Journal of Insanity,* July 1899, pp. 109–122.

Dain, Norman. *Concepts of Insanity in the United States, 1789–1865.* New Brunswick, N.J.: Rutgers University Press, 1964.

Dain, Norman, and Eric T. Carlson. "Milieu therapy in the nineteenth century: patient care at the Friends' Asylum, Frankford, Pennsylvania, 1817–1861." *Journal of Nervous and Mental Diseases,* Vol. 131, October 1960, pp. 277–290.

de Marneffe, Francis. "The psychiatrist-executive in the changing funding and political environment," *in* Hirschowitz, Ralph R., and Bernard Levy, eds., *The Changing Mental Health Scene.* New York: Spectrum Publications, Inc., 1976.

Deutsch, Albert. *The Mentally Ill in America.* Garden City, N.Y.: Doubleday, Doran and Co., Inc., 1938.

"Dinner to Dr. Edward Cowles on his retirement from the McLean Hospital." *American Journal of Insanity,* Vol. 61, 1904–05, pp. 113–128.

Drinker, Cecil K., et al. *Psychiatric Research.* Papers read at the dedication of the Laboratory for Biochemical Research, McLean Hospital, Waverley, Massachusetts, 17 May 1946. Cambridge, Mass., 1947.

Eaton, Leonard K. "Charles Bulfinch and the Massachusetts General Hospital." *Isis,* Vol. 41, 1950, pp. 8–11.

———. *New England Hospitals, 1790–1833.* Ann Arbor: University of Michigan Press, 1959.

Eliot, Charles W. "Annual report of the President of Harvard College." 1869–70.

Ellis, George E. "Memoir of Luther V. Bell, M.D., LL.D." Boston, 1863. [Reprinted from the *Proceedings of the Massachusetts Historical Society, 1863.*]

Faxon, Nathaniel W. *The Massachusetts General Hospital, 1935–1955.* Cambridge, Mass.: Harvard University Press, 1959.

Finch, Marianne. *An Englishwoman's Experience in America.* Richard Bentley, 1853. [Reprinted by Negro Universities Press, New York.]

Folsom, Charles F. *Mental Diseases.* Boston, 1886. [Reprinted from *American System of Medicine,* Vol. 5.]

Frank, Leo. "Crossroads in psychoanalysis." *New York Times Book Review,* 4 August 1968.

Freud, Sigmund. *A General Introduction to Psychoanalysis.* New York: Perma Books (paper), 1955. (Since so many editions of this book are in print, I refer to Freud's statements by lecture number rather than by page number.)

Gifford, George E., ed. *Psychoanalysis, Psychotherapy, and the New England Medical Scene, 1894–1944.* New York: Science History Publication/USA, 1978.

Gregg, Alan. "A critique of psychiatry." *American Journal of Psychiatry,* June 1944, pp. 285–291.

Grob, Gerald N. *Edward Jarvis and the Medical World of 19th Century America.* Knoxville: The University of Tennessee Press, 1978.

——. *Mental Illness and American Society, 1875–1940.* Princeton: Princeton University Press, 1983.

——. *Mental Institutions in America: Social Policy to 1875.* New York, Free Press, 1973.

Grob, Mollie C., and Judith E. Singer. *Adolescent Patients in Transition.* New York: Behavioral Publications, 1974.

Hall, J.K., et al., eds. *One Hundred Years of American Psychiatry.* New York: Columbia University Press, 1944.

Haslam, John. *Observations on Madness and Melancholy.* London, 1809.

Hendrick, Ives, ed. *The Birth of an Institute.* Twenty-fifth Anniversary, the Boston Psychoanalytic Institute, 30 November 1958. Freeport, Maine: The Bond Wheelwright Co., 1961.

Hoch, August. "On the clinical study of psychiatry." *American Journal of Insanity,* October 1900, pp. 281–295.

Holmes, Oliver W. "Borderlines of knowledge in some provinces of medical science." An introductory lecture delivered before the medical class of Harvard College, 6 November 1861.

——. "The medical profession in Massachusetts." A lecture of a course by the members of the Massachusetts Historical Society, delivered before the Lowell Institute, 29 January 1869.

——. *The Poet at the Breakfast Table.* Boston, 1872.

Hurd, Henry. "The new McLean Hospital." *American Journal of Insanity,* Vol. 52, April 1896, pp. 477–502.

——. *The Institutional Care of the Insane in the United States and Canada.* Baltimore: Johns Hopkins Press, 1916.

James, Henry, ed. *The Letters of William James.* Boston: Atlantic Monthly Press, 1920.

Joint Commission on Mental Illness and Health. *Action for Mental Health.* Final report of the Joint Commission on Mental Illness and Health. New York: Basic Books, 1961.

Kaplan, Justin. *Walt Whitman: A Life.* New York: Simon and Schuster, 1980.

Kennedy, John F. "Special message to the Congress on mental

illness and mental retardation, February 5, 1963." *Public Papers of the President, John F. Kennedy.* 1963.

Lamar, Margie. "A study of the history of landscape architecture; McLean Hospital, Belmont, Massachusetts." Masters Thesis. Harvard University, Cambridge, Mass., 1975.

Levendusky, Philip G. "Cognitive behavior therapy in cluster headache." *McLean Hospital Journal,* Vol. 3, Winter 1978, pp. 50–57.

Levin, Kenneth. "Edward Cowles on neurasthenia." *McLean Hospital Journal,* Vol. 2, Summer 1977, pp. 167–176.

Little, Nina F. *Early Years of the McLean Hospital.* Boston: The Francis A. Countway Library of Medicine, 1972.

Massachusetts State Board of Insanity. Annual Report, 1910.

Meyer, Adolf. "The dynamic interpretation of dementia praecox." *American Journal of Psychology,* Vol. 21, 1910, pp. 385–403.

——. "The problems of mental reaction-types, mental causes and diseases." *Psychological Bulletin,* Vol. 5, 1908, pp. 245–261.

Mitchell, S. Weir. "Address before the Fiftieth Annual Meeting." *Proceedings of the American Medico-Psychological Association, 1894,* pp. 101–121.

Murchison, Carl, ed. *A History of Psychology in Autobiography.* Worcester, Mass.: Clark University Press, 1932.

Myers, Grace W. *History of the Massachusetts General Hospital, June 1872 to December 1900.* Boston: Griffith-Stillings Press, [1929?].

Myerson, Abraham. "Theory and principles of the 'total push' method in the treatment of chronic schizophrenia." *American Journal of Psychiatry,* Vol. 95, March 1939, pp. 1197–1204.

Nicholi, Armand M., Jr., ed. *The Harvard Guide to Modern Psychiatry.* Cambridge, Mass.: The Belknap Press of Harvard University Press, 1978.

"Outcome evaluation findings: a decade of experience." [Presented at the McLean Hospital on the occasion of the 10th anniversary of the evaluative service unit], Report No. 50, December 1982.

Parkman, George. *Management of Lunatics with Illustrations of Insanity.* Boston, 1817.

Pinel, Philippe. *A Treatise on Insanity.* New York: Hafner Publishing Co., 1962. [Facsimile of the London 1806 edition.]

"Proceedings of the Association." *American Journal of Insanity,* July 1855, pp. 68–79.

"Psychiatry on the couch." *Time,* 2 April 1979.

Ray, Isaac. "Discourse on the life and character of Dr. Luther V. Bell." Paper read to the Association of Superintendents of North American Institutions for the Insane, 10 June 1862. Boston, 1863.

Reiser, Stanley J. *Medicine and the Reign of Technology.* Cambridge: Cambridge University Press, 1978.

Roper, Laura W. *FLO: A Biography of Frederick Law Olmsted.* Baltimore: The Johns Hopkins University Press, 1973.

Rosenkrantz, Barbara G., and Maris A. Vinovskis. "The invisible lunatics: old age and insanity in mid-nineteenth century Massachusetts," in Spicker, Stuart A., et al., eds., *Aging and the Elderly.* New Jersey: Humanities Press, 1978.

Ross, Dorothy. *G. Stanley Hall: The Psychologist as Prophet.* Chicago: University of Chicago Press, 1972.

Rothman, Theodore, ed. *Changing Patterns in Psychiatric Care.* New York: Crown Publishers, Inc., 1970.

Rush, Benjamin. *Medical Inquiries and Observations upon the Diseases of the Mind.* Philadelphia, 1812.

Sanborn, Frank B., ed. *The Memoirs of Pliny Earle.* Boston, 1898.

Santostefano, Sebastiano. "McLean then and now." *McLean Hospital Journal,* Vol. 1, Summer 1976, pp. 174–189.

———. "Shepard Ivory Franz, the father of research for clinical practice." *McLean Hospital Journal,* Vol. 1, Winter 1976, pp. 49–63.

Segal, Julius, ed. *Research in the Service of Mental Health.* Report of the Research Task Force of the National Institute of Mental Health. Publication No. 75-236. Washington, D.C.: Department of Health, Education and Welfare, 1975.

Stanton, Alfred H. "Some therapeutic mechanisms arising from psychiatric hospital structure." *Psychotherapy and Psychosomatics,* Vol. 13, 1965, pp. 165–185.

———. "The study of the psychiatric hospital as a therapeutic society." Centennial Papers, Saint Elizabeth's Hospital, 1956, pp. 143–152.

Stanton, Alfred H., and Morris Schwartz. *The Mental Hospital.* New York: Basic Books, 1954.

Starr, Paul. *The Social Transformation of American Medicine.* New York: Basic Books, 1982.

Sullivan, Harry S. *Clinical Studies in Psychiatry.* New York: W.W. Norton & Co., 1973.

Tillotson, Kenneth J. "Some newer trends in psychiatry." *New England Journal of Medicine,* Vol. 207, 7 July 1932, pp. 8–12, 45.

Tucker, G.A. *Lunacy in Many Lands.* Sydney, Australia: Charles Potter, Government Printer, 1887.

Tuke, Samuel. *Description of the Retreat, an Institution near York for Insane Persons of the Society of Friends.* Philadelphia, 1813.

Vogel, Morris J. *The Invention of the Modern Hospital.* Chicago: University of Chicago Press, 1980.

Washburn, Frederick A. *The Massachusetts General Hospital, Its Development, 1900–1935.* Boston, Houghton Mifflin Co., 1939.

Wells, Frederick Lyman. "On formulation in psychoanalysis." *Journal of Abnormal Psychology,* October-November 1913, pp. 3–13.

Werkman, Sidney L. *The Role of Psychiatry in Medical Education.* Cambridge, Mass.: Harvard University Press, 1966.

White, Benjamin V. *Stanley Cobb.* Boston: The Francis A. Countway Library of Medicine, 1984.

Whitehorn, John C. "Studies of the doctor as a crucial factor for the prognosis of schizophrenic patients." Henry Phipps Psychiatry Clinic, Johns Hopkins Hospital, 1959. [Mimeographed.]

Winters, Eunice, ed. *The Collected Papers of Adolf Meyer.* Baltimore: The Johns Hopkins University Press, 1950–1952.

Wyman, Morrill. "The early history of the McLean Asylum for the Insane, A criticism of the report of the State Board of Health for 1877." Cambridge, Mass., 1877.

Wyman, Morrill, Jr. *A Brief Record of the Lives and Writings of Dr. Rufus Wyman (1778–1842) and His Son, Dr. Morrill Wyman (1812–1903).* Cambridge, Mass., 1913.

Wyman, Rufus. "Mental philosophy as connected with mental disease." Paper delivered before the Massachusetts Medical Society, 2 June 1830.

Index